AF539497

EMERGING AREAS IN HOSPITAL SERVICES

EMERGING AREAS IN HOSPITAL SERVICES

(Encyclopaedia of Hospital Management—6)

DR. S.L. GOEL
Professor of Public Administration (Retd.),
Panjab University, Chandigarh
Editor, Indian Journal of Public Administration, IIPA, New Delhi
Former Member, UGC, Former Member Distance Education Council
Former Member All India Board of Management, AICTE
Member, Executive Council, IIPA, New Delhi.
Former Vice-President, IIPA, New Delhi.
Emeritus Fellow, University Grants Commission
Former Director, State Bank of India (Local Board) Chandigarh
Former Director, National Horticulture Board, Ministry of Agriculture,
Government of India, New Delhi.

and

DR. R. KUMAR
MBBS, MS, Ex. PGI
President, Chandigarh Ophthalmological Society, 2000-01,
Columnist on Health Education and Management,
Advisor on Health Care and Medical Tourism,
Member Tourism Advisory Forum,
Chandigarh Administration, Chandigarh

DEEP & DEEP PUBLICATIONS PVT. LTD.
F-159, Rajouri Garden, New Delhi-110027

EMERGING AREAS IN HOSPITAL SERVICES
(Encyclopaedia of Hospital Management—6)

ISBN 978-81-8450-221-3

Typeset by S.S. COMPOSERS
3190, Mohindra Park, Shakur Basti, Delhi-110034.

Printed in India at MAYUR ENTERPRISES
WZ Plot No. 3, Gujjar Market, Tihar Village, New Delhi-110018.

Published by DEEP & DEEP PUBLICATIONS PVT. LTD.
F-159, Rajouri Garden, New Delhi-110027.
Phones: 25435369, 25440916
E-mail: ddpbooks@yahoo.co.in • ddpubs@gmail.com
Showroom:
2/13, Ansari Road, Daryaganj, New Delhi-110002 • Telefax: 23245122

Contents

Preface

Premier institutes running courses for hospital administration across the country vouch that it was never so good for their students, with various health organizations now making a beeline at campus interviews. "It is mainly the corporate and trust hospitals which are recruiting professionals to manage their administrative operations," says Dr. C.A.K Yesudian, Head, Dept. of Health Services Studies, Tata Institute of Social Sciences (TISS), Mumbai.

According to Dr. S.V.N. Reddy, Principal Apollo Institute of Hospital Administration (AIHA), Hyderabad, it is not only hospitals which require management professionals. "A whole lot of specialized avenues such as lifestyle clinics, emergency medicine units, pharmaceutical firms, and hospital information systems, e-health ventures, credit rating firms, NGOs and health insurance now require trained manpower specialized in hospital administration." The remuneration packages offered to fresh graduates are attractive. Rating agencies like Crisil and Icra have absorbed many freshers in the recent past as health care consultants. "Moreover, an administrator or a manager gets to do those assignments in this segment that are not typical of their conventional role," he added.

New areas of health care management

1. It entails to deliberate in the emerging trends in planning and designing of health care facilities and to highlight the changing role of future hospitals in the evolving health care environment.
2. Establish dynamic networks between the diverse disciplines of medicine, architecture, financing and management and integrate them for evolving patient-focused and environment-friendly trends in hospital planning and design.
3. Assess the future projections for the health care sector and financing of health care facilities.
4. Explore the avenues for integration of Information Technology in health care delivery as a virtual outreach arm of multi-specialty care.

Deliberate on the issues concerned with strengthening of health care facilities in urban and rural setting at primary, secondary and tertiary levels.

Some of the thrust areas that require further study are the following:

- Planning principles and design considerations in health care facilities
- Emerging issues and strategic options in Medical Architecture
- Designing for Accreditation
- Healing Architecture
- Energy Efficient Hospitals
- Financing of Health Care Institutions
- Role of Public Private Partnership and Outsourcing in Health Care
- Intelligent Buildings
- Telemedicine and beyond
- Facility Management
- Patient focused Architecture
- Evidence-based Designs
- Environment-friendly hospitals and Green buildings
- Value-added Services
- Ambulatory Care Systems and Day Care Facilities
- Mobile Hospitals and Disaster units

While some of these areas are discussed elsewhere, the Authors have described some of the emerging areas in the following chapters:

1. Introduction
2. Prevention and Redressal of Patients Grievances: Key to Prevent Litigation
3. Health Insurance: Key Input in Health Care Management
4. Patient's Right to Health Care and Doctor's Right to Personal Safety
5. Promoting Health through Hospitals
6. Complementary and Alternative Medicines (CAM): India's Strengths
7. Injuries are a Major Challenge to Health Care: Trauma Hospitals
8. Palliative Medicine: An Emerging Concept for the Terminally Ill
9. Chronically Ill Patients with Bedsores: Challenge to Hospital's Management

Chandigarh

S.L. GOEL
R. KUMAR

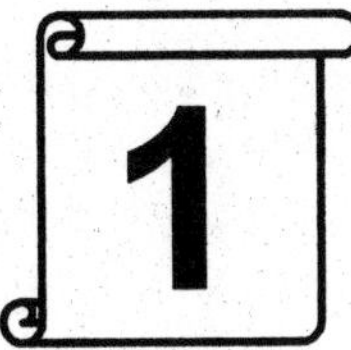

Introduction

There have been metamorphic changes in the recent past in the sphere of health care delivery. The planning, design and final architectural expression in health care is reflective of the gradual shift in outlook of health care institutions from merely treating the sick to a concerted approach to harness healthy living. This has been triggered by globalization, increased expectations of seekers and providers of health care and the participation of private players in the health sector. In the Indian situation lack of infrastructure and meager investment in the health care and hospitals is significant. Even in USA where huge sums are being spent on health care, the system has been described as a broken health care system. India has a long way to go to catch up with the rest of the world. With the change in perspectives of hospital management and expectations of the patients, certain new areas have emerged that require attention. **Obama's proposed Health Plan** Barack Obama has proposed sweeping changes in the health care system designed to provide health coverage to millions of uninsured Americans.

His plan would extend health coverage by expanding existing private and public programs with the help of federal subsidies and mandates. He has repeatedly claimed the reforms will lower the average family's health insurance premiums by about $2,500 a year. These reforms include:

- Requiring employers, except small businesses, to provide health insurance to their employees or contribute to the cost.
- Requiring that all children have health insurance.
- Expanding Medicaid and the State Children's Health Insurance Program (SCHIP).
- Creating a National Health Insurance Exchange to pool risk and give people the choice of competing private or public health plans.

According to an analysis group, the plan, if fully implemented, would reduce the number of uninsured Americans from a projected 67 million to 33 million over the next decade at a cost of $1.6 trillion. He has not provided a timetable for seeking his proposed reforms and has not said if he would present a comprehensive health care reform package or try for incremental change. Expansion Likely for State Children's Health Insurance (SCHIP) Program Experts agreed that expansion of the children's insurance program SCHIP is likely to be the first of the proposed reforms to be considered. The program will be up for congressional review next March, and experts say it will probably be the Obama administration's first chance to make good on a health care promise.

Medicare Reform More Problematic

Many of Obama's other proposals—from the expansion of Medicare to his National Health Insurance Exchange—will be much harder to win support for, even with a largely friendly Congress behind him. He says a key reason for the failure of President Clinton's 1993 health care reform effort is that his administration did not reach across the aisle. **Health Spending 'Not Sustainable'** Experts agreed that the nation's broken health care system must be addressed and that this must happen sooner rather than later.

- 45 million Americans have no health insurance.
- 25 million more have health plans but are considered underinsured because their policies offer only minimal coverage, according to the Commonwealth Fund.
- 42% of U.S. adults under age 65 are uninsured or underinsured, up from 33% in 2003.
- Total spending on health care represented around 16% of the gross domestic product in 2007, and the Congressional Budget Office says spending will rise to a quarter of gross domestic product by 2025.

The Rising Demand of Modern Hospital Administrators

Hospital administrators are in great demand. In fact, they are the most sought-after professionals in the health care sector today after doctors. Thanks to rapid corporatisation, a lot of medical graduates are taking up further specialization in hospital administration. Even non-medical professionals are increasingly taking the mantle of hospital administration. According to consulting and recruiting firm Hosmac, roughly 300 students are imparted training in hospital administration every year through 16 recognized institutes across the country. Around 90 per cent of them are readily absorbed by hospitals. The trend of recruiting business managers and not essentially a practicing medical professional was initiated by corporate hospitals. Now, even trust-based hospitals are following suit and experts point out that it is a matter of time before government hospitals too

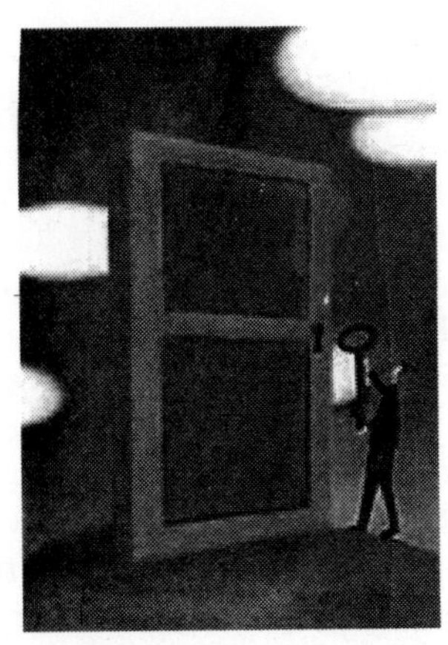

adopt the practice. Premier institutes running courses for hospital administration across the country vouch that it was never so good for their students what with various health organizations now making a beeline at campus interviews. "It is mainly the corporate and trust hospitals which are recruiting professionals to manage their administrative operations," says Dr. C.A.K. Yesudian, Head Dept. of Health Services Studies, Tata Institute of Social Sciences (TISS), Mumbai. A top favourite among health care recruiters, TISS had nearly 90 per cent of its students taken up within three days of its week-long placement programme held in January 2002.

According to Dr. S.V.N. Reddy, principal Apollo Institute of Hospital Administration (AIHA), Hyderabad, it is not only hospitals which require management pros. A whole lot of specialized avenues such as lifestyle clinics, emergency medicine units, pharmaceutical firms, hospital information systems, e-health ventures, credit rating firms, NGOs and health insurance now require trained manpower specialized in hospital administration." The remuneration packages offered to fresh graduates is attractive. "A management level cadre earns anywhere between Rs. 2.5-3 lakh per annum, while middle and lower level cadre earn between Rs. 2-2.5 lakh," says Dr. Yesudian. That's certainly good money for greenhorns when compared with remuneration offered in other industries. Freshers should focus more on gaining practical knowledge at the workplace than dreaming big salary packages, feels Dr. Satish Ratnaparkhi, Director, Garware Institute of Career Education and Development. The institute is one of the recent entrants into health care management education arena with its first batch of students to pass out in June 2002.

A majority of students at the Indian Institute of Health Management and Research (IIHMR), Jaipur belong to non-medical category, sources point out. Managers with a medical background command higher price in the market, confirms Dr. Reddy. Even though the industry has a preference for such people, non-medicos are putting a brave face on it. "Having a medical background definitely helps in better understanding of the hospital environment initially, but even non-medico can excel as what matters ultimately is how good are your managerial skills," says an MBA aspiring to be a hospital administrator.

Institutes conducting these courses are particular about one aspect making necessary modifications in the syllabus as per the requirements of the health care industry. "Therefore now we are emphasising more on topics like IT, quality and finance management in our syllabi," Dr. Yesudian says. He further explained that besides theory and internship at hospitals, a special five-week course has now been added at TISS wherein students visit emerging areas like health care consultancy firms and TPAs.

Apollo Institute has revised its syllabus for the third time recently. Says Dr. Reddy, "Since our institute is affiliated to Osmania University, we are awaiting their approval. The revised syllabus contains many new thrust areas like health insurance, entrepreneurship development, waste management, disaster management, supply chain management, customer relationship management, HIS to name a few." According to Dr. Ratnaparkhi, bringing in certain upgradation in the syllabus at least once in three years is essential.

The industry too seems to be upbeat with the availability of efficient manpower to handle managerial tasks in health care services. Says Anil V. Kamath, VP-business development, Wockhardt Hospitals Ltd., "There is a growing demand for managers in the health care sector due to increasing professionalisation of services. And the huge demand-supply gap in this segment is opening better avenues for freshers." He further noted that as a majority of professionals today are first level managers, 4-5 years down the line, the industry would benefit from strong force of well-experienced managers. "Grading of health care institutions is an area with lot of excitement and challenges for health care managers and they can learn newer concepts here," says Arun Panicker, director - Corporate Ratings, Crisil. Rating agencies like Crisil and Icra have absorbed many freshers in the recent past as health care consultants. Panicker admitted that interns as well as freshers were of great help during the company's grading process. "Moreover an administrator or a manager gets to do those assignments in this segment that are not typical of their conventional role," he added. According to George Mathew Molakal, MD ICAN Medicare Pvt. Ltd., a Pune-based TPA, doctors and administrators/managers form a crucial link in TPA operations. They can be assigned tasks like gate keeping functions, claim audit—technical evaluations, claim investigations, etc. "ICAN has employed several hospital administration staff in its processing centers across India. They are highly necessary for each and every TPA," Molakal says. To bridge the huge demand-supply gap in the professional management segment, experts feel that more teaching facilities should be set-up. And that explains the reason behind dubious hospital administration and health care management courses being floated by some institutes in the recent past. Dr. Yesudian says that hospitals are very choosy about the kind of people they want to recruit and the quality will separate wheat from chaff.

"The market is wise enough to recognize the right candidates. Therefore dubious programmes will die a natural death in due course of time," Dr. Ratnaparkhi opined.

According to a survey by the Association of British Health Care Industries (ABHI) in early 2000, there are over 15,000 hospitals in India. And more numbers are frequently being added up indicating that there is a tremendous opportunity for administrators in hospital sector alone for years to come not to mention related areas. Therefore, it is the right time to take a plunge into the health care administration and management arena.

NEW AREAS OF HEALTH CARE MANAGEMENT

1. It entails to deliberate in the emerging trends in planning and designing of health care facilities and to highlight the changing role of future hospitals in the evolving health care environment. 2. Establish dynamic networks between the diverse disciplines of medicine, architecture, financing and management and integrate them for evolving patient-focused and environment-friendly trends in hospital planning and design. 3. Assess the future projections for the health care sector and financing of health care facilities. 4. Explore the avenues for integration of Information Technology in health care delivery as a virtual outreach arm of multi-specialty care. Deliberate on the issues concerned with strengthening of health care facilities in urban and rural setting at primary, secondary and tertiary levels.

Some of the thrust areas are:

- Planning principles and design considerations in health care facilities
- Emerging issues and strategic options in Medical Architecture
- Designing for Accreditation
- Healing Architecture
- Energy Efficient Hospitals
- Financing of Health Care Institutions
- Role of Public-Private Partnership and Outsourcing in Health Care
- Intelligent Buildings
- Telemedicine and beyond
- Facility Management
- Patient focused Architecture
- Evidence-based Designs
- Environment-friendly hospitals and Green buildings
- Value-added Services
- Ambulatory Care Systems and Day Care Facilities
- Mobile Hospitals and Disaster units

The WHO has given the theme to Hospital Promoters, Health Care/ Hospital Policy-makers, representation from Financial Institutions, Facility Managers including Banking and Insurance Services, Health and Hospital Administrators, Hospital Planners and Project Consultants, Engineers, Architects, Equipment Manufacturers and Distributors and experts from the construction industry.

2

Prevention and Redressal of Patients Grievances: Key to Prevent Litigation

Grievance cell is assuming importance in India, as patients have become more conscious of their rights. Moreover, the accrediting and rating agencies insist on documentation of patient's feedback. The setting up of grievance cell enhances doctor-patient relationship. The patients and doctors are vulnerable to lawyers called as ambulance chasers, who incite the patient to file mischievous or frivolous litigation against the doctors. This has affected the doctor-patient relationship to a great extent.

WHAT IS A GRIEVANCE CELL?

According to Dr. Suganthi Iyer, assistant director, medical services, Hinduja Hospital, and a medico-legal expert, Grievance cell can be compared to a quasi-judicial body and is an internal inquiry cell within the hospital set-up in order to investigate as to what actually has transpired between the hospital and the patient.

In such a set-up, the aggrieved patient puts up his complaint or petition before the grievance cell. The cell should just not be defensive on behalf of the hospital and is supposed to give a fair hearing to both the parties concerned on the principles of natural justice in an unbiased manner, adds Dr. Iyer. The grievance cell has the power to investigate and make decisions. However, some experts believe that the role of the grievance cells is to explain the adequacy and rationale of the medical care delivered. Says Joe Curian, chief spokesperson, Association of Hospitals (AoH). The patient needs detailed explanation, when the cost of the treatment exceeds the indicated cost or there is a death due to a complication that has occurred during the course of the treatment.

IMPORTANCE OF GRIEVANCE CELL

The grievance cell helps to reduce frivolous litigation in consumer courts. Opines Dr. Lalit Kapoor, chairman, medico-legal cell, Association of Medical Consultants (AMC). The grievance committee ensures that any case of patient dissatisfaction is resolved at the earliest to avoid any medico-legal implication. According to Dr. R.K. Anand, medical director, Jaslok Hospital, the number of medico-legal cases in Consumer Courts can be reduced if patient's complaint is heard by the grievance cell in hospitals. During my tenure with the Association for Consumers Action on Safety and Health (ACASH), I observed most of the cases related to patient grievances were not due to medical negligence but were attributed to the lack of communication between the doctor and the patient. Twenty five per cent of the cases taken up by the grievance cells are sorted out by explaining to the patient, the nature of shortfall on the part of the hospital or hospital authority, say experts. The remaining 75 per cent of cases go to consumer courts (CCs).

Experts say that the patient should avoid approaching CCs as the judgment is delivered only after four to five years. The patient approach the CCs or the so-called patient friendly courts primarily because they do not have to hire a lawyer and pay any fees, informs Dr. Kapoor.

WHERE GRIEVANCE CELL COULD HAVE HELPED?

Amit went to see his younger brother Siddharth, who was operated for an ailment in a well-known Mumbai-based private hospital. Amit was denied entry into the ward, where his brother was staying, post-operatively and was asked to produce a consent letter duly authorized by the medical director to enter the ward. It was near to impossible for Amit to access the medical director at 7 in the evening, as the director was available only in the morning. After rounds of requests and an hour of waiting, the supervisor permitted Amit to see his brother. The case of Amit reveals the plight of many patients and their relatives, who are denied immediate redressal of their grievances. The case would not have been so time-consuming and frustrating, if a speedy and efficient grievance cell would have been in place to help him.

For Dr. Usha Sharma, a senior consultant, gynaecology, Royal Hospital, Muscat, getting a knee replacement surgery in the country turned into a harrowing experience, when she developed an infection after surgery. Narrating her experience, Dr. Sharma told Express Health Care Management (EHM) that just a few days after her total knee transplant surgery at one of the premier hospitals in Mumbai, she developed the wound swab. When the surgeon didn't act, Dr. Sharma went asking for in Delhi, where she had to undergo a repeat surgery. I went through unnecessary hassle, pain and agony and the doctor/hospital didn't take any responsibility, says an aggrieved Dr. Sharma. There are many patients like Dr. Sharma who suffer due to lack of virtually no redressal system in place in most of the hospitals across the country. According to Dr. P.M. Bhujang, medical director, Sir H.N. Hospital, no hospital can function effectively, unless it is sensitive to patients' grievances. According to Dr. Bidhan Das, vice-president, corporate affairs, Rockland hospital, it is important that patient is informed about his/her rights to seek justice, which is why it is imperative that all hospitals have Citizen's Charter, highlighting the rights of patients *vis-a-vis* the hospitals. However, the situation is bleak in government hospitals, private hospitals and nursing homes, more so in the former as the concept—consumer is the king—does not exist in government hospitals. According to Alok Mukhopadhaya, chief executive, Voluntary Health Association of India (VHAI), the private hospitals are overcharging and there is no check on them. In both the situations, the loser is the gullible patient and his relatives. There is no system of consumer redressal in primary and secondary health care institutions, he adds.

In big private hospitals in metros, the consumer redressal committees are on paper only, laments Mukhopadhaya and adds that there's need to initiate a consumer movement so that patients instead of being at doctors' mercy are informed of their rights. Though the concept of a patient grievance cell is gradually assuming significance in large private hospitals across the country, the hospital management have a long way to go in putting such a system in place as compared to the west, where the system has evolved manifold.

GRIEVANCE CELL IN VARIOUS HOSPITALS

Bombay Hospital

It has a team of administrators or a core team to look after the patient grievances. Says medical director Dr. D.P. Vyas. We are always accessible on any eventuality of patient grievance and our core team comprises of medical director, deputy medical director, medical superintendent, deputy medical superintendent, deputy officer on special duty and all the respective heads of the department.

Jaslok Hospital

According to medical superintendent Dr. J.P. Sharma, besides feedback form given to patients, there is a suggestion box, where the patients can post their complaints in written format. The box is opened by the medical superintendent under the strict supervision of a hospital staffer, deputed by the medical superintendent for ensuring confidentiality and security of the complaints.

Hinduja Hospital

The Hospital has a patient relationship department handled by a dedicated team of customer service executives (CSEs) for the redressal of patient grievances on a daily basis. According to Anupam Verma, director, administration, Hinduja Hospital, the cases are first taken up by the CSEs and then forwarded to the management team or the respective head of the departments. CSEs are empowered by the core committee of the hospital to solve cases of patient grievances on an urgent or priority basis. The core committee of the hospital comprises of the Administrator, Director (Professional Services), Director (Medical Quality and Ethics), CEO and the HR team. The patient relationship department resolves the grievances on a case-to-case basis within seven days. Generally, three to four cases of critical nature are resolved in a month.

Sir H.N. Hospital

The hospital has a floor supervisor and a public relation officer, who visits every patient daily and receives complaints and grievances. An officer looks after the administration of the hospital even in the night. Hospital administrators and trustees are always accessible to patients and relatives. When a patient is discharged from the hospital, he/she is given a feed back form. These grievances are studied and remedial actions are initiated.

Rockland Hospital, New Delhi

The hospital has a five-member redressal committee for attending to the complaints of patients. The hospital's complaint box is opened on a weekly basis to address the issues.

Post-graduate Institute of Medical Education and Research (PGIMER), Chandigarh

The hospital has a six member redressal committee under the chairmanship of a senior professor. Other members are from the medical fraternity, except the convener. Besides suggestion/complaint boxes, people can voice their grievances directly to the medical superintendent or even the director. The committee holds its meeting every month, the feasible suggestions are implemented and issues are taken up. The Citizen's Charter of PGIMER, Chandigarh is currently awaiting approval.

Dharamshilla Cancer Hospital

According to director Dr. S. Khanna, we have a very strong redressal system. There's a central complaint register at the front desk and satellite complaint registers at all counters. Complaint register is sent to the director on a daily basis. The hospital has a Preventive Action Group (PAG) comprising of five members, which include medical superintendent, deputy medical superintendent. The meetings take place every day with all the concerned departments. Patients are given customer feedback forms at the time of admission, which they are asked to fill up upon discharge. To enable government hospitals to constitute a grievance cell, experts suggest decentralization of medical services, whereby cases of patient grievance can be referred to secondary/tertiary care hospitals.

The Hospital CEO should Possess the following Qualities/Responsibilities

1. Overall operations of the acute-care facility.
2. Working with system management to develop and implement policies and procedures, short- and long-range goals, objectives and plans.
3. Providing leadership to hospital managers, directors and officers that will enroll support, create ownership of goals, and encourage active participate in decisions that impact the hospital.
4. Ensuring the hospital meets necessary regulatory and compliance approvals and quality accreditations in conjunction with the hospital's Chief Nursing Officer.
5. Partnering with physicians who use, or will use, the hospital; taking a leadership role in the recruiting and retention of physicians.
6. Assisting in planning new services that generate additional sources of profitable revenue.
7. Creating an environment that will encourage the recruiting and retention of qualified hospital employees.
8. Managing costs by continually seeking data that will identify opportunities and take action to eliminate non-value costs in conjunction with the hospital's Chief Financial Officer and Chief Nursing Officer.
9. Developing and maintaining positive relations with community that the hospital is located as well as the community leaders.
10. Analyzing areas in planning, promoting and conducting organization-wide performance improvement activities.
11. Representing the hospital at meetings including medical staff, hospital board of director meetings as well as relevant community meetings; participates with leaders in designing and providing patient care and services. At each monthly meeting the committee of visitors he shall state the number of patients received and discharged, the number of deaths, the manner of employment, the number remaining in the hospital, distinguishing sexes, the weekly cost of maintenance with such matters as may appear as desirable.
12. Participating in the hospital's monthly operation reviews as well as participating in corporate office meetings as deemed necessary.
13. He shall have full control over all attendants and servants and shall regulate their duties and have authority to suspend them whenever he shall deem it expedient reporting the same of the first meeting of the Committee of Visitors.
14. He shall be responsible for the management and condition of the establishment and of the patients therein and shall have the

direction of the medical, surgical and moral treatment of the patients and of all general arrangements within the hospital, and in case of emergency shall have the power of calling on the assistance of any physician or surgeon. He shall also in all cases of fatal or dangerous accident or other emergency immediately communicate the fact in writing to one of the committee or to their clerk.

15. He shall ensure examination of every patient on admission and make proper entries thereof and take care that such medicines as he may think proper for their certain and speedy cure be duly administered. He shall see every patient once a day and oftener, if requested. He shall order and be responsible for the drugs, surgical instruments and books belonging to the asylum and he shall report the case of every patient fit for discharge to one or more of the Committee of Visitors.
16. He shall classify the patient of both sexes and shall regulate and determine at all times the diet of the sick and infirm patients. He shall also have the power from time to time to examine and report on the quality of all provisions furnished for the use of the patients.
17. He shall never be absent himself for one night or for any longer period without the previous written consent of the Committee.
18. He shall sign all orders for the delivery of store or other articles for the use of the hospital such orders to be limited by the contract to be from time to time entered into by the Committee or if on an emergency he shall be given an extra order, it shall be reported to the next meeting of the Committee.
19. He shail be authorized to give directions for any requisite to buildings or works and shall report that same and other repairs needed to the Committee at their next meeting.

Setting up of a Public Relations Office (PRO) (A case study of Lucknow Deemed University Hospital)

A public relation office will help to make the patient aware and try to help him wherever possible. The hospital has a Public Relations Office situated in the main building. It functions round the clock throughout the year to provide information and assistance to patients and their attendants. This was started in 1964. At present it is manned by 3 Public Relations Officers, 1 Enquiry Assistant and 2 other staff members of the hospital. The PRO has a unique functioning and is an important link between the hospital administration and the patient. Besides helping the patients, the office manages all the administrative matters of the hospital after working hours and on holidays. It has a close link with the police and press. A good number of security and other staff are attached to this office to maintain law and order and help in keeping the campus clean with regular supply of water and electricity. The ambulances are also under the control of this office. The present PRO's are: Smt. Homa Jafar, Mr. Rahul Singh and Mr. Manoj Srivastava.

Human Resource Development is a Key to Prevent Grievances

Human resource is a critical asset and an important differentiator between a good and a great hospital. Therefore, it is essential not only to recruit the right people for the right job, but also to keep them engaged and delighted, provide them an environment to excel and ensure that they stay motivated. Needless to say, employees who bring direct revenue for the hospital are most valued employees. But apart from them, employees who perform their duty with ease and aplomb, demonstrate traits like initiative, creativity, incisive mind, quick decision-making, ability to guide others, high-level of commitment and sense of responsibility are described as Star Performers (SP). According to Dr. N.C. Borah, Chairman, Guwahati Neurological Research Centre, Guwahati, SPs add value to the brand image of the hospital and are very crucial, especially during the initial growth period of any new project. They also display keenness to contribute towards the goal and growth of the organization. What would ultimately differentiate them is the style of working. Super performers should be judged not just by mere outcome. The differentiating factor should be the method of working, which should be systematic.

As per Pareto's Law, 20 per cent employees in any organization drive the other 80 per cent. But these 20 per cent employees need not be in leadership positions. Any employee in any position can usher in positive changes in the way a particular process is executed or help device methodologies to enhance throughput and increase efficiency of the department, says Ankush Gupta, Manager, HR, PD Hinduja Hospital, Mumbai. In a hospital set-up where teamwork is crucial, interdepartmental productivity becomes an even more decisive factor for a SP. Scientific methods of recruitment, performance management system, feedback from colleagues and department heads are some tools that help identify SPs. Moving a step ahead from conventional tools, CMRI and B.M. Birla Heart Research Centre, Kolkata recently introduced the concept of 'balance score card' to evaluate an individual's performance. This concept, used for measuring a company's activities in terms of its vision and strategies, forces managers to focus on the important performance metrics that drive success. It balances a financial perspective with the customer, internal process and learning and growth perspectives.

Through balance score card, parameters are set prior to a person joining any department. Targets are maintained on a daily basis and performance is measured, explains Rupak Barua, Director, Growth and Development, B.M. Birla Heart Research Centre. The Hospital has also introduced a 'Talent Search' programme whereby management trainees are put on particular projects and monitored for six months to analyze their performance. (see box on how hospitals identify SPs).

How Hospitals Identify Star Performers' Hinduja Hospital

Relies on the concept of 'best employee of the month' to identify SPs. Based on parameters like discipline, sense of responsibility, decision-making ability and others, the Hospital assesses the social behaviour and performance of an individual. Every month, the HR department sends out a best employee nomination form to the heads of various departments, who rate their employees and send it back. A committee consisting of senior professionals screens the nominations to determine the best employee of the month.

Apollo Hospitals Group

Employs a scientific outlook to the idea of identifying and defining the targets for their employees. Their performance management system takes into cognisance two Ps—Performance and Potential of their employees. To analyse the performance of an employee, the hospital works on their key result areas (KRAs). At the beginning of the financial year, based on the annual operating plan of the unit, the heads of the units prepare KRAs which are cascaded down to the department heads and then the executives. The exercise is to align the organisational KRAs to individual KRAs. The job performance is evaluated in four major components like financial, customer perspective (as it is a service industry), employee perspective (because it is team effort) and process-related issues.

The test examines capabilities like whether an employee possesses the potential to get into higher responsibilities and has acquired the personality traits required to deal with his/her own work area. At the end of every year, the hospital tracks the individual's performance by incorporating results through performance management system.

Wockhardt Hospitals Group

It relies on performance appraisal system, the kind of business result that employees bring in and customer feedback to spot SPs.

Indian Spinal Injuries Centre (ISIC)

The SP is rewarded as the 'best employee of the year' award and honoured by placing his name on the department 'honour board'. He also gets the privilege to have a meal with the top management apart from a token of appreciation. Detecting talent also aids in examining whether the employee is apt for the work assigned to him. If a person from one department has a personality trait which can be best leveraged in another area, he or she can be shifted to that domain. This is done with an eye to enhancing the productivity of the employee. Once the super performer is identified, a detailed growth pattern should be chalked out for him/her. We give them higher responsibilities based on three factors—targets achieved on time, the potential to assume higher responsibilities and level of excellence with the customers, explains T. Karunakar, GM-HR, Apollo Hospitals, Hyderabad.

Roping in Stars

Any new induction obviously is based on the job specifications and the job description for the specific vacancy. It also depends on the level of hierarchy at which the person is to be inducted. If the position is that of a decision-maker and the person will impact the way a particular function is run, analysing the traits of a SP in him becomes *sine qua non*. In Apollo Hospitals Group, psychometric tools like Thomas Profiling are used for candidates during selection, to identify their behavioural traits. The test maps the behaviour of the applicant to his promised work profile, helping the company identify the right profile for the job. This in the long-term helps in choosing more SPs in the organisation. Though the test is not completely foolproof, it gives some insight into the person's ability to match the job profile. Since some jobs need less creativity while some require more creativity and problem-solving skill, one should be able to match skill set requirements with competencies and competencies with personalities, states Sangita Reddy, Executive Director-Operations, Apollo Hospitals Group. Initial right selection can obviously lead to harvesting potential star performers in the organisation.

Directing Star Power

The problems with managing creative employees are myriad. Often they leave the organization if they feel they are stagnating or their efforts have not been acknowledged. The biggest hurdle with managing SPs is meeting their expectations in terms of rewards, better salaries, better flexibilities, more authority and faster climb in the organisation, states Kumar S. Krishnaswamy, Group Head, HRD, Wockhardt Hospitals Group, Bangalore. And, there can be ego issues. Tensions can also occur in work environment when senior people have to work under a young and dynamic performer. When the SP gets restless and more lucrative job offers come in his way, he threatens to leave. This leads to organisations grappling with retention of their best talent. Organisations have realised that it is easy to lose a SP, but difficult to retain one and still more arduous to replace one. However, organisations are not always in a position to fulfil the demands and expectations of SPs in the process of retaining them. There are other employees in the organisation who are vital, and always heeding the demands of the SP might crush the growth of other employees. Thus, the approach for retaining should not be a last-minute one, when the person is calling it quits. Instead, the organisation should take a proactive approach. The three-tier strategy that most hospitals adopt is: appreciate them, train them and chalk a clear career path. Good appreciation of their efforts, involvement in challenging assignments, slightly non-routine job responsibilities, and clear growth in the organisation are the time-tested ways to manage and retain high performers, opines Gupta.

Nurturing the Star

Motivating and training star employees to deliver continuously is another issue. Talent needs to be nurtured and the right skill set has to be imbibed.

According to Dr. Ravindra Karanjekar, GM, Wockhardt Hospitals, Mumbai, the best method to hone the super performer is to continuously give him challenging situations and empower him to take decisions. Recently, in Wockhardt Hospital, Mumbai, a group from the administrative department was given a Herculean task of creating a liver transplant unit in just seven days. There was a time constraint as well as sterile conditions to be. Besides challenging tasks, it is mandatory that continuous training on behavioral as well as technical skills be imparted. Continuous training would ensure consistency of performance, explains Dr. Karanjekar. Confidence building is a constant process and SPs need to be taken into confidence through constant monitoring. Experts underscore the procedure of sensitisation, through which SPs are given the realisation that they are not indispensable and can make mistakes.

The Star in Spotlight

More than monetary benefits, it is essential to acknowledge them publicly. Thus, in the Star Programme at Apollo Hospitals, the employees are rewarded in front of everybody. Similarly, 'compliment a colleague' concept tracks the appreciation of one colleague's better performance by another. These strategies have helped Apollo Hospitals build the concept of oneness among all. Give them importance, recognise their contribution and at the same time tactfully make them understand that the contribution of other members of the team is equally important for his/her success, states Dr. Borah.

Motivation is the key for better performance and more enthusiastic employees, opines Dr. R.K. Anand, Medical Director, Jaslok Hospital, Mumbai. He cites a recent example to prove his point. The charity commissioner visited our hospital recently and the medical social worker (MSW) who was taking the commissioner around did exceptionally well in the task assigned to her. She not just knew every patient, but could also cite the medical diagnosis of that patient. After this incident, in the presence of the charity commissioner, we acknowledged her work, explains Dr. Anand. The result is a motivated employee, who is now working on many more projects. Money is not always a motivator. If someone is skilful, he will never really feel the dearth of money. Highlighting them in public gatherings as potential leaders and trainers will motivate them like nothing else, says Dr. Bidhan Das, Former Director, Operations, Rockland Hospital, New Delhi and now a consultant, Quality Council of India at Bhopal. They say that equipment and technology do not make a hospital. The employees do. And being able to make super performers of their employees will differentiate a good organisation from a great one. As one expert puts it, not having SPs is the failure of organization and not of employees.

Teaching Managerial Skills to Medical Students

The weakest link in the health care delivery system in most developing countries is the poor planning and management at different levels of health care services. This is mainly due to the lack of manpower trained in hospital and health management and also due to outdated policies and procedures. Hospital services are becoming more and more complex and sophisticated on the one hand, and health programmes on the other hand need to be more community and result-oriented. A well-trained workforce in health and hospital management is required for optimum utilization of scarce health care resources in the country, for improving public health. When the young medical graduates take up responsible positions in government hospitals, private hospitals, health centres and in national health programmes, they are given a lot of managerial responsibilities in addition to their technical role. Due to lack of training and exposure in health management they feel incompetent and insecure in their jobs, leading to frustration and low productivity. Management skills become more crucial at the peripheral health care institutions where a doctor is the team leader and has to implement a number of health programmes with the help of other health staff. So, skills like planning, leadership, supervision, monitoring and communication are a must for any doctor in order to make an impact on the health scenario of the country. Recognize the importance of following managerial skills in health care delivery services at different levels:

- Observe all activities of the Zonal Hospital and the district public health system;
- Familiarize oneself with activities at all levels of the health care system;
- Familiarize oneself with the mechanism of monitoring and supervision;
- Describe the Health Management Information System (HMIS); and
- Develop the skill to work as a group leader.

References

Abdel Rahim, I.M., Abdeen, A.Z., Faki, B.A., Mustfa, A.E., Nalder, S. Introducing training in Primary Health Care program management into the curriculum. *Med. Educ.* 1987; 21(4):288-92.

Agrawal, C.S. and Karki, P. Evolution of the second medical school in Nepal: A case study. *Medical Teacher.* 1999; 21(2):204-206.

Akpala Co. Medical education and primary health care in Nigeria: The Sokoto University experience. *Cent Afr J Med* 1991; 37(11):347-7.

Boelen C. Medical education reforms: the need for global action. *Academic Medicine* 1992; 67(11):745-749.

BPKIHS, Dharan, Nepal. The first version of MBBS curriculum 1996.

Flahault, D. and Roemer, M.I. Leadership for Primary Health Care. Public Health Paper No. 82. World Health Organization, Geneva, 1986.

Job, A.C., Coale, M.M., Kolasa, K., Willis, L., Irons, T.G. Leadership development for medical students beyond the prescription pad. *Fam Med.* 1993; 25(3):179-81.

McMohan, R., Barton, E. and Piot, M. *et al.* On being in change. World Health Organization, Geneva, 1992.

Naga Rani, M.A., Koirala, S., Das, B.P. and Rauniyar, G.P. A brief review of the pre-clinical curriculum of the B.P. Koirala Institute of Health Sciences, Dharan, Nepal. *Medical Education* 2002; 36:393-394.

3

Health Insurance: Key Input in Health Care Management

The need for insurance is not only for medical emergencies but also for elective surgical conditions like cataract, joint replacement and prostrate enlargement besides chronic conditions like diabetes, hypertension, and nervous system disorders requiring life long medical treatment. Leading a happy life, involves good planning for your health. Accidents happen and you need to be prepared for such situations. In times of high health cost, you need to get covered for health risks. The role of insurance in health care management is paramount.

COST OF TREATMENT TAKES ITS TOLL

Health treatment nowadays is very costly. More than the disease it is the cost of treatment that takes its toll. To get rid of health worries health/medical insurance is the answer. Health insurance policy not only covers expenses incurred during hospitalization but also during the pre as well as post-hospitalization stages like money spent for conducting medical tests and buying medicines. The cover will be to the extent of the sum insured. An added attraction of Medi-claim policies is the tax benefits which they attract under Section 80D. The maximum amount of deduction available under this section is Rs. 10,000. In case of senior citizens, the maximum limit is Rs. 15,000. Individuals also have the option of covering themselves for medical expenses by opting for the 'Critical Illness' (CI) rider available with life insurance policies. Life insurance companies have their own list of critical illnesses as defined by them. In case of a CI rider, on the occurrence of a 'critical illness' during the policy tenure, an amount as proposed in the policy will be paid out to the individual. This is irrespective of the expenses incurred by the individual on hospitalization, medicines and other such costs. In mid-80's most of the hospitals in India were government- owned and treatment was free of cost. With the advent of Private Medical Care the need for Health Insurance was felt and various Insurance Companies (New India Assurance, National Insurance Company, Oriental Insurance and United Insurance Company) introduced Mediclaim Insurance as a product. According to recent news report Health insurance continues to be the fastest growing segment with annual growth rate of 55%. Health Premium has risen to Rs. 3300 crores in 2006-07. As per the recent reports from various agencies the Health sector has the potential to become a Rs. 25000-crore industry by 2010. On August 15, 2007 Prime Minister announced Rs. 2000 Crores for Health Insurance for poor citizens. We foresee that this amount will be partly in the form of subsidy therefore during calendar year 2008 we can expect Health Insurance premium to touch figure in the range of Rs. 10,000 Crores.

In 2001 with entry of various private Insurance companies, the customers have choice of buying this insurance from 14 Insurance companies. The Companies, which offer Health or Mediclaim Insurance, are:

1. Apollo DKV Insurance Company Limited
2. Bajaj Allianz General Insurance Company Limited
3. Cholamandalam MS General Insurance Company Limited
4. HDFC Chubb General Insurance Company Ltd.
5. ICICI Lombard General Insurance Limited
6. IFFCO Tokio General Insurance Company Limited
7. National Insurance Company Limited
8. New India Assurance Company Limited
9. Oriental Insurance Company Limited
10. Reliance General Insurance Company Limited
11. Royal Sundram Alliance Insurance Company Limited
12. Star Health and Allied Insurance Company Limited
13. TATA AIG General Insurance Company Limited (Overseas Health Insurance only)
14. United India Insurance Company Limited.

India is the only country where hospitalization insurance policy was being sold as Mediclaim Insurance Policies. The very name gives a feeling to the insured that claim has to be lodged. If motor insurance policy is not sold as motor insurance claim policy and household insurance policy is not sold as household claim policy then why this is named as Mediclaim? In the recent years the trend has emerged that some Insurance companies have started calling this product as Health Insurance. Health Insurance and Mediclaim are two different names for the same product. The change has started coming and now we have started calling it Health Insurance. ICICI Lombard has even named it as Health Insurance Policy. Calling it as Health Insurance is a positive way of looking at this Insurance. It also gives us a feeling that we as a society have started moving from curative medical care to preventive medical care. According to sources in Oriental insurance it is being felt that mindset has started changing over the last couple of years. The new middle-class of India aspires for quality health caré service and doesn't mind going to expensive hospitals like Apollo or Escorts. There is no reason why health care insurance should not be successful with this class. Health insurance companies are offering innovative products to their customers these days. The latest product in this line is 'cashless hospitalization'. Here individuals do not have to pay for their hospital bills in case of hospitalization; the insurance company settles the bill directly. But certain conditions like the hospital needs to have a tie-up with the insurance company, the documents need to be in order have to be met.

HISTORY AND THE CONCEPT

The concept of health insurance was proposed in 1694 by Hugh the Elder Chamberlen from the Peter Chamberlen family. In the late 19th century, early health insurance was actually disability insurance, in the sense that it covered only the cost of emergency care for injuries that could lead to a disability. This payment model continued until the start of the 20th century in some jurisdictions (like California), where all laws regulating health insurance actually referred to disability insurance. Patients were expected to pay all other health care costs out of their own pockets, under what is known as the fee-for-service business model. During the middle to late 20th century, traditional disability insurance evolved into modern health insurance programs. Today, most comprehensive private health insurance programs cover the cost of routine, preventive, and emergency health care procedures, and also most prescription drugs, but this was not always the case.

A Health insurance policy is an annually or monthly renewable contract between an insurance company and an individual. With health insurance claims, the individual policy-holder pays a deductible plus co-payment (for instance, a hospital stay might require the first $1000 of fees to be paid by the policy-holder plus $100 per night stayed in hospital). Usually there is a maximum out-of-pocket payment for any single year, and there can be a lifetime maximum, or the upper limit of what the insurance company will pay over the covered individual's lifetime. Prescription drug plans are a form of insurance offered through many employer benefit plans in the U.S., where the patient pays a co-payment and the prescription drug insurance pays the rest. Some health care providers will agree to bill the insurance company if patients are willing to sign an agreement that they will be responsible for the amount that the insurance company doesn't pay, as the insurance company pays according to "reasonable" or "customary" charges, which may be less than the provider's usual fee. The "reasonable" and "customary" charges can.

Health insurance companies also often have a network of providers who agree to accept the reasonable and customary fee and waive the remainder. It will generally cost the patient less to use an in-network provider. Health Insurance companies are now offering Health Incentive accounts (HIA), to reward users for living healthy and making healthy choices, like stop smoking and/or losing weight, may get you funds added into your Health Incentive Account, which may lower your out of pocket costs. The health incentive accounts also carry over from year to year but once you leave the program you lose those benefits in the HIA. Inherent problems with private insurance. Any private insurance system will face two inherent challenges: adverse selection and ex-post moral hazard.

Adverse Selection

Insurance companies use the term "adverse selection" to describe the tendency for only those who will benefit from insurance to buy it. Specifically when talking about health insurance, unhealthy people are more likely to purchase health insurance because they anticipate large medical bills. On the other side, people who consider themselves to be reasonably healthy may decide that medical insurance is an unnecessary expense; if they see the doctor once a year and it costs $250, that's much better than making monthly insurance payments of $400 (example figures).

The fundamental concept of insurance is that it balances costs across a large, random sample of individuals. For instance, an insurance company has a pool of 1000 randomly selected subscribers, each paying $100 per month. One person becomes very ill while the others stay healthy, allowing the insurance company to use the money paid by the healthy people to pay for the treatment costs of the sick person. Adverse selection upsets this balance between healthy and sick subscribers by leaving an insurance company with primarily sick subscribers and no way to balance out the cost of their medical expenses with a large number of healthy subscribers.

Because of adverse selection, insurance companies use a patient's medical history to screen out persons with pre-existing medical conditions. Before buying health insurance, a person typically fills out a comprehensive medical history form that asks whether the person smokes, how much the person weighs, whether the person has been treated for any of a long list of diseases and so on. In general, those who look like they will be large financial burdens are denied coverage or charged high premiums to compensate. On the other side, applicants can actually get discounts if they do not smoke and are healthy. On the other hand, some companies insist on detailed medical examination and laboratory tests before giving an insurance policy.

Starting in 1976, some states started providing guaranteed-issuance risk pools, which allow individuals who are medically-uninsurable through private health insurance to be able to purchase a state-sponsored health insurance plan, usually at higher cost. Minnesota was the first to offer such a plan, and there are now 34 states which do. Plans vary greatly from state to state, both in their costs and benefits to consumers and to their methods of funding and operating. They serve a very small portion of the uninsurable market—about 183,000 people in the USA, but in best cases do allow people with pre-existing conditions such as cancer, diabetes, heart disease or other chronic illnesses to be able to switch jobs or seek self-employment without fear of being without health care benefits [5]. Efforts to pass a national pool have as yet been unsuccessful, but some federal tax money has been awarded to states to innovate and improve their plans.

Moral Hazard

Moral hazard describes the state of mind and change in behavior that results from a person's knowledge that if something bad were to happen, the out-of-pocket expenses would be mitigated by an insurance policy—in this case, one which provides reduced prices for medical care. In most cases the carriers have a 2 year window to go back and consider a condition pre-existing.

Other Factors Affecting Insurance Price

Because of advances in medicine and medical technology, medical treatment is expensive, and people in developed countries are living longer. The population of those countries is ageing, and a larger group of senior citizens requires more medical care than a young healthier population. (A similar rise in costs is evident in Social Security in the United States.) These factors cause an increase in the price of health insurance. Some other factors that cause an increase in health insurance prices are health-related: insufficient exercise; unhealthy food choices; a shortage of doctors in impoverished or rural areas; excessive alcohol use, smoking, street drugs, obesity, among some parts of the population; and the modern sedentary lifestyle of the middle classes.

In theory, people could lower health insurance prices by doing the opposite of the above; that is, by exercising, eating healthy food, avoiding addictive substances, etc. Healthier lifestyles protect the body from some, although not all, diseases, and with fewer diseases, the expenses borne by insurance companies would likely drop. A program for addressing increasing premiums, dubbed "consumer driven health care," encourages Americans to buy high-deductible, lower-premium insurance plans in exchange for tax benefits and utilization of Health Incentive accounts.

Some common complaints about private health insurance include:

1. Insurance companies do not announce their health insurance premiums more than a year in advance. This means that, if one becomes ill, he or she may find that their premiums have greatly increased (however, in many states these types of rate increases are prohibited).
2. If insurance companies try to charge different people different amounts based on their own personal health, people may feel they are unfairly treated.

3. When a claim is made, particularly for a sizable amount, insureds may feel as though the insurance company is using paperwork and bureaucracy to attempt to avoid payment of the claim or, at a minimum, greatly delay it.
4. Health insurance is often only widely available at a reasonable cost through an employer-sponsored group plan and online for individuals.
5. In the United States, there are tax advantages to Employer—provided health insurance, whereas individuals must pay tax on income used to fund their own health insurance, although a small number of pre-tax health plans exist.
6. Experimental treatments are generally not covered. This practice is especially criticized by those who have already tried, and not benefited from, all "standard" medical treatments for their condition.
7. The Health Maintenance Organization (HMO) type of health insurance plan has been criticized for excessive cost-cutting policies in its attempt to offer lower premiums to consumers.
8. As the health care recipient is not directly involved in payment of health care services and products, they are less likely to scrutinize or negotiate the costs of the health care received. The health care company has popular and unpopular ways of controlling this market force.
9. Some health care providers end up with different sets of rates for the same procedure. One for people with insurance and another for those without.
10. Unlike most publicly funded health insurance, many private insurance plans do not provide coverage of dental health care, or only offer such coverage with additional premiums and very low dollar-amount coverage.
11. Insurance Companies can influence the type or amount of treatment that the insured receives by setting limits on the number of visits, types of treatment, etc., it will cover.

National Insurance's Senior Citizen Health Scheme: India

This policy has been designed to cater to the needs of our Senior Citizens. It covers Hospitalization and Domiciliary Hospitalization Expenses under Section I as well as expenses for treatment of Critical Illnesses, if opted for, under Section II. Diseases covered under Critical Illnesses are as under:

- Coronary Artery Surgery
- Cancer
- Renal Failure, i.e. Failure for both kidneys
- Stroke
- Multiple Sclerosis

- Major Organ Transplants like kidney, Lung, Pancreas or Bone marrow
- Paralysis and blindness at extra premium

Critical Illness cover is an optional cover under the policy. Persons who will not opt for critical illness cover are entitled to Hospitalization and Domiciliary hospitalization expenses cover for those diseases categorized above as critical illness but up to the limit of Sum Insured under Section I, i.e. under Hospitalization and Domiciliary Hospitalization Expenses and the claim for those diseases will be paid on reimbursement basis or as cashless hospitalization. Person opting for Critical Illness cover may opt for claim either under Section I or Section II (if not hospitalized) or under both sections for those diseases categorized above as Critical Illnesses but claim under Section I will be paid either on reimbursement basis or as cashless hospitalization if it is otherwise admissible. If in any policy year a critical illness is diagnosed and claim paid thereafter, in subsequent renewals the person may avail cover both under Section I and II but with the exclusion, both under Sections I and II, of that particular critical illness which has been diagnosed and claim paid in the preceding policy year.

Sum Insured

Sum Insured is fixed per person. Under Hospitalization and Domiciliary Hospitalization Cover sum Insured is Rs. 1,00,000 and under Critical Illness cover Sum Insured is Rs. 2,00,000.

Age Group

For fresh entry in to the scheme—60 years to 80 years. However, for renewal, age limit will be extended up to 90 years in which case the premium of 76-80 age band will be loaded by 10% up to 85 years and 20% up to 90 years of age.

Pre-acceptance Medical Check-up

No Medical Check up is required if the insured was covered under any Health Insurance Policy of National Insurance Company or other Insurance companies uninterruptedly for preceding three years. Other persons have to undergo medical check up at their own cost for Blood/ Urine Sugar, Blood Pressure, Echo-cardiography and eye check up including retinoscopy.

I. Scope of Cover

In the event of any claim/s becoming admissible under this section, the Company will pay to the Insured person the amount of such expenses as would fall under different heads mentioned below and as are reasonably and necessarily incurred hereof by or on behalf of such Insured Person but not exceeding the Sum Insured in aggregate mentioned in the Schedule hereto.

Hospitalization Benefits	*Limits*
A (i) Room, Boarding expenses a provided by the Hospital/ Nursing Home (ii) If admitted in IC Unit	(i) Upto 1% of Sum Insured per day (ii) Upto 2% of Sum Insured per day Overall limit: 25% of the S.I. per illness/injury
B Surgeon, Anesthetist, Medical Practitioner, Consultants, Specialists Fees, Nursing Expenses	Upto 25% of Sum Insured per illness/ Injury
C Anesthesia, Blood, Oxygen, OT charges, Surgical appliances (any disposable surgical consumables subject to upper limit of 7% of Sum Insured), Medicines, drugs, Diagnostic material and X-Ray, Dialysis, Chemotherapy, Radiotherapy, cost of pacemaker, artificial limbs, Cost of stent and implants	Upto 50% of Sum Insured per illness/ Injury

(1) Company's overall liability in respect of claims arising due to Cataract is Rs. 10,000 and that of Benign Prostatic Hyperplasia is Rs. 20,000 only.

(2) Company's liability in respect of all claims admitted during the period of Insurance shall not exceed the Sum Insured for the person as mentioned in the Schedule.

(3) Liability of the company under Domiciliary Hospitalization clause is limited to 20% of the Sum Insured under Section I and within the overall limit of sum Insured under section I.

(4) Hospitalization expenses of person donating an organ during the course of organ transplant will also be payable subject to the sub-limits under 'C' above applicable to the insured person within the overall sum insured of the insured person.

(5) Ambulance charges up to a maximum limit of Rs. 1000 in a policy year will be reimbursed.

Section I—Hospitalization and Domiciliary Hospitalization Expenses Cover

In the event of any claim/s becoming admissible under this section, the Company will pay to the Insured person the amount of such expenses as would fall under different heads mentioned below and as are reasonably and necessarily incurred hereof by or on behalf of such Insured Person but not exceeding the Sum Insured in aggregate mentioned in the Schedule.

2. Definitions

2.1. Hospital/Nursing Home, means any institution in India established for indoor care and treatment of sickness and injuries and which either

(a) has been registered either as a Hospital or Nursing Home with the local authorities and is under the supervision of the registered and qualified medical practitioner; OR

(b) should comply with minimum criteria as under:
   (i) It should have at least 15 inpatient beds. In Class "C". towns condition of number of beds may be reduced to 10.
   (ii) Fully equipped Operation Theatre of its own wherever surgical operations are carried out.
   (iii) Fully qualified nursing staff under its employment round the clock.
   (iv) Fully qualified Doctor(s) should be in charge round the clock.

2.1.1 The term, 'Hospital/Nursing Home', shall not include an establishment which is a place of rest, a place for the aged, a place for drug addicts or place of alcoholics, a hotel or a similar place.

2.2 Surgical Operation means manual and/or operative procedures for correction of deformities and defects, repair of injuries, diagnosis and cure of diseases, relief of suffering and prolongation of life

2.3 Expenses of Hospitalization for minimum period of 24 hours are admissible. However, this time limit is not applied to specific treatments, i.e. day care treatment for stitching of wound/s, close reduction/s and application of POP casts, Dialysis, Chemotherapy, Radiotherapy, Arthroscopy, Eye surgery, ENT surgery, Laparoscopic surgery, Angiographies, Endoscopies, Lithotripsy (Kidney stone removal), D and C, Tonsillectomy taken in the Hospital/Nursing Home and the Insured is discharged on the same day. The treatment will be considered to be taken under Hospitalization benefit. This condition will also not apply in case of stay in Hospital of less than 24 hours provided—

(a) the treatment is such that it necessitates hospitalization and the procedure involves specialized infrastructural facilities available in Hospitals; and

(b) due to technological advances hospitalization is required for less then 24 hours only.

2.4 Domiciliary Hospitalization benefit means medical treatment for a period exceeding three days for such illness/disease/injury which in the normal course would require care and treatment at a Hospital/Nursing Home but actually taken whilst confined at home in India under any of the following circumstances, namely:

(i) The condition of the patient is such that he/she cannot be removed to the Hospital/Nursing Home, or

(ii) The patient cannot be removed to Hospital/Nursing Home for lack of accommodation therein. Subject to however that domiciliary hospitalisation benefits shall not cover:

(i) Expenses incurred for pre and post-hospital treatment, and

(ii) Expenses incurred for any of the following diseases:

1. Asthma
2. Bronchitis
3. Chronic Nephritis and Nephritic Syndrome
4. Diarrhea and all type of dysenteries including Gastroenteritis
5. Diabetes Mellitus and Insipidus
6. Epilepsy
7. Hypertension
8. Influenza, Cough and Cold
9. All Psychiatric or Psychosomatic Disorders
10. Pyrexia of unknown Origin for less than 10 days
11. Tonsillitis and Upper Respiratory Tract Infection including Laryngitis and Pharingitis
12. Arthritis, Gout and Rheumatism

Note: When treatment such as Dialysis, Chemotherapy, Radiotherapy is taken in the Hospital/Nursing Home and the Insured is discharged on the same day, the treatment will be considered to be taken under Hospitalization benefit section. Liability of the Company under this clause is restricted as stated in the Schedule attached hereto.

3.0 Any One Illness will be deemed to mean continuous period of illness and it includes relapse within 45 days from the date of last consultation with the Hospital/Nursing Home where treatment may have been taken. Occurrence of same illness after a lapse of 45 days as stated above will be considered as fresh illness for the purpose of this policy.

3.1 *Pre-Hospitalization*: Relevant Medical Expenses incurred during period up to 30 days prior to hospitalization/domiciliary hospitalization on disease/illness/injury sustained will be considered as part of claim mentioned under item 1.0 above

3.2 *Post-Hospitalization*: Relevant Medical Expenses incurred up to 60 days after hospitalization/domiciliary hospitalization on disease/illness/injury sustained will be considered as part of claim mentioned under item 1.0 above.

3.3 Medical Practitioner means a person who holds a degree/diploma from a recognised institution and is registered by Medical Council or respective State Council of India. The term Medical Practitioner would include Physician, Specialist and Surgeon.

3.4 Qualified Nurse means a person who holds a certificate of a recognized Nursing Council and who is employed on the recommendations of the attending Medical Practitioner.

3.5 TPA means a Third Party Administrator, who, for the time being, is licensed by the Insurance Regulatory and Development Authority, and is engaged, for a fee or remuneration, by whatever name called as may be specified in the agreement with the Company, for the provision of health services.

3.6 Preexisting Diseases means any ailment/disease/injury that the person is suffering from (known/not known, treated/untreated, declared or not declared in the proposal) whilst taking the policy. Any complications arising from pre-existing ailment/disease/injury will be considered as Preexisting Diseases.

4. Exclusions

The Company shall not be liable to make any payment under this Policy in respect of any expenses whatsoever incurred by any person in connection with or in respect of:

4.1 All diseases/injuries which are pre existing when the cover incepts for the first time. However, those diseases will be covered after one claim free year under this policy. Cost of treatment towards dialysis, chemotherapy and radiotherapy for diseases existing prior to the commencement of this policy is excluded from the scope of cover of this policy even after one claim free year.

Only two preexisting diseases (Diabetes and/or Hypertension) will be covered from the inception of the policy provided the company receives additional premium for covering these preexisting diseases and mentions the same in the schedule. However, any ailment already manifested or being treated and attributable to diabetes and/or hypertension or consequences thereof at the time of inception of insurance will not be covered even on payment of additional premium for covering diabetes and/or hypertension.

4.2 Any disease other than those stated in Clause 4.3, contracted by the Insured Person during the first 30 days from the commencement date of the policy. This condition 4.2 shall not however apply in case of the Insured Person having been covered under this Scheme or group insurance scheme with any one of the Indian Insurance Companies for a continuous period of preceding 12 months without any break.

4.3 During the first one year of the operation of the policy the expenses incurred on treatment of diseases such as Cataract, Benign Prostatic Hypertrophy, Hysterectomy for Menorrhagia or Fibromyoma, Hernia, Hydrocele, Congenital Internal Disease, Fistula in anus, Chronic fissure in anus, Piles, Pilonidal Sinus, Sinusitis, Stone disease of any site, Benign Lumps/growths in any part of the body, CSOM (Chronic Suppurative Otitis Media), joints replacements of any kind unless arising out of accident, surgical treatment of Tonsils, Adenoids and deviated nasal septums and related disorders are not payable. If these diseases (other than Congenital Internal Disease/Defects) are pre-existing at the time of proposal, they will be covered only after one claim free year as mentioned in column 4.1 above. If the Insured is aware of the existence of Congenital Internal Disease/Defect before inception of the policy, the same will be treated as pre-existing.

4.4 Injury or disease directly or indirectly caused by or arising from or attributable to War Invasion Act of Foreign Enemy Warlike operations (whether war be declared or not).

4.5 Vaccination or inoculation or change of life or cosmetic or aesthetic treatment of any description, plastic surgery other than as may be necessitated due to as accident or as part of any illness.

4.6 The cost of spectacles and contact lenses, hearing aids.

4.7 Any Dental treatment or surgery which is a corrective, cosmetic or aesthetic procedure, including wear and tear, unless arising from accidental injury and which requires hospitalization for treatment.

4.8 Convalescence, general debility, 'Run Down' condition or rest cure, congenital external disease or defects or anomalies, sterility, venereal disease, intentional self-injury and use of intoxicating drugs/alcohol, rehabilitation therapy in any form.

4.9 All expenses arising out of any condition directly or indirectly caused to or associated with Human T-Cell Lymphotrophic Virus Type III (HTLB-III) or Lymphadinopathy Associated Virus (LAV) or the Mutants Derivative or variations Deficiency Syndrome or any Syndrome or condition of a similar kind commonly referred to as AIDS.

4.10 Charges incurred at Hospital or Nursing Home primarily for diagnostic, X-Ray or laboratory examinations or other diagnostic studies not consistent with nor incidental to the diagnosis and treatment of positive existence or presence of any ailment, sickness or injury for which confinement is required at a Hospital/Nursing Home.

4.11 Expenses on vitamins and tonics unless forming part of treatment for injury or disease as certified by the attending physician.

4.12 Injury or disease directly or indirectly caused by or contributed to by nuclear weapons/materials.

4.13 Treatment arising from or traceable to pregnancy childbirth including caesarean section.

4.14 Naturopathy treatment.

5. Payment of Claim

All claims under this section shall be payable in Indian currency. All medical treatments for the purpose of this insurance will have to be taken in India only.

6. Cumulative Bonus

Sum insured under this section shall be progressively increased by 5% in respect of each claim free year of insurance subject to maximum accumulation of 10 claim free years of insurance. In case of claim under the policy in respect of insured person who has earned the cumulative bonus, the increased percentage will be reduced by 10% of sum insured at the next renewal. However, basic sum insured will be maintained and will not be reduced.

N.B.: (1) For existing policy holders (as on date of implementation) the accrued amount of benefit of cumulative bonus will be added to the sum insured, subject to maximum 10 claim free years.

(2) Cumulative Bonus will be lost if policy is not renewed on the date of expiry.

Waiver

In exceptional circumstances where policy is renewed within 7 days from expiry date, the renewal is permissible to be entitled for cumulative bonus although the policy is renewed only subject to Medical Examination and exclusion of diseases developed during the break period.

However, insured has the option either to avail Cumulative Bonus or claim 5% discount in renewal premium will be allowed in respect of each claim free year of insurance subject to maximum of 10 claim free years of insurance. This discount will not be applicable to the S.I. increased if any by the insured at renewal.

7. Cost of Health Check Up

In addition to the cumulative Bonus, the insured shall be entitled for reimbursement of the cost of medical check up once at the end of block of every three underwriting years provided there are no claims reported during the block. The cost so reimbursable shall not exceed the amount equal to 2% of the amount of average sum insured excluding cumulative bonus during block of three underwriting years.

What is Important?

For Cumulative Bonus and Health Check-up provision as aforesaid: Both Health check-up and Cumulative bonus provisions are applicable only in respect of continuous insurance without break except however, where in exceptional circumstances, the break in period for a maximum of seven days is approved as a special case subject to medical examination and exclusion of disease during the break period. Health check up benefit will be accrued after completion of three years continuous claim free insurance.

8. Co-payment

Insured has to bear 10% of all the admissible claims (Compulsory Excess). However, 20% co-payment will be considered if the insured opt for the same. In such cases 10% additional discount in premium will be allowed. Insured has to bear additional 10% of all admissible claims if the claim arises out of pre-existing diseases for which the insured opted cover and paid additional premium. This provision is in addition to the compulsory excess stated herein above and applicable only for claims arising out of Pre-existing Diseases

9. TPA Services

Services of TPA will be available under this policy.

10. Premium

	Sum Insured	Premium			
		60-65 years	*66-70 years*	*71-75 years*	*76-80 years*
Mediclaim	1,00,000	4180	5196	5568	6890
Critical Illness	2,00,000	2007	2130	2200	2288
	TOTAL	6187	7326	7768	9178

10.1 For fresh entrants to National Insurance above premium will be loaded by 10%.

10.2 Under Mediclaim Section (Section I), if the insured intends to cover pre-existing diseases of Hypertension and/or Diabetes from the inception of the policy he/she has to pay additional premium @10% for either hypertension or diabetes and 20% for hypertension and diabetes for first year of the policy. However, if a fresh entrant suffers from blood pressure/hypertension and/or diabetes and opts for Critical Illness cover, the same may be covered at additional premium @10% for either hypertension or diabetes and 20% for hypertension and diabetes provided no organ of the proposer is affected in consequence of blood pressure and/or diabetes. If the medical report indicates occurrence of any such consequential complication, those proposals will be declined.

Loading for preexisting Diabetes and/or Hypertension to be applied on Total Premium for first year and on Critical Illness Premium only from 2nd year onwards.

10.3 At the time of taking this policy, if a person suffers from any of the terminal diseases referred under Critical Illness cover mentioned below, that particular disease will never be covered under Section II of this policy even on payment of additional premium.

10.4 Cover for Paralysis and Blindness under Critical Illness.

Paralysis and Blindness may be covered under Critical Illness by loading the Critical Illness premium by 15% in each case or 25% in case of both covers together.

10.5 Under Group Policy, if the incurred claim ratio of the group exceeds 70% then the renewal premium will be loaded on 70% as if basis, i.e. if the incurred claim ratio of any policy year exceeds 70% renewal premium will be loaded in such a way that the incurred claim ratio of 136 expiring policy becomes 70%.

11. Claims Procedure

11.1 Section I:

Upon the happening of any event, which may give rise to a claim under this section notice with full particulars shall be sent to the Company within 7 days from the date of Injury/Hospitalization/Domiciliary Hospitalization.

Claim must be filed within 30 days from date of discharge from the Hospital and where post-hospitalization treatment is not completed, it shall be within 30 days from the date of completion of Post-hospitalization treatment.

Note: Waiver of this condition may be considered in extreme cases of hardship where it is proved to the satisfaction of the Company that under the circumstances in which the Insured was placed it was not possible for him or any other person to give such notice or file claim within the prescribed time limit.

Claims will be settled by the Third Party Administrators (TPA). They will send details of the claims procedure for emergency/planned hospitals.

Documents to be submitted

1. Claim form
2. First consultation document
3. Copy of admission advice
4. Discharge Summary
5. Prescription with bills and receipts
6. Test Reports
7. Any other document required by TPA pertaining to this insurance contract/policy.

Procedure for Availing Cashless Access Services in Network Hospital/ Nursing Home

Claims in respect of Cashless Access Services will be through the list of network Hospitals/Nursing Homes and is subject to pre-admission authorization. The TPA shall, upon getting the related medical information from the insured persons/network provider, verify that the person is eligible to claim under the policy and after satisfying itself will issue a pre-authorization letter/guarantee of payment letter to the Hospital/Nursing Home mentioning the sum guaranteed as payable, also the ailment for which the person is seeking to be admitted as a patient.

The TPA reserves the right to deny pre-authorization in case the insured person is unable to provide the relevant medical details as required by the TPA. The TPA will make it clear to the insured person that denial of Cashless Access is in no way construed to be denial of treatment. The insured person may obtain the treatment as per his/her treating doctor's advice and later on submit the full claim papers to the TPA for reimbursement subject to admissibility of claim under the terms and conditions of the policy.

The TPA may repudiate the claim, giving reasons, if not covered under the terms of the policy. The insured person shall have right of appeal to the insurance company if he/she feels that the claim is payable. The insurance company's decision in this regard will be final and binding on TPA.

11.2 Section II

Upon detection of any critical illness, which may give rise to a claim under this section, notice with full particulars shall be sent to the Company within 15 days from the date of diagnosis of the disease. Claim documents as mentioned hereunder must be submitted to the company after 30 days from the date of diagnosis of the disease.

(1) Doctor's certificate confirming diagnosis of the critical illness along with date of diagnosis.
(2) Pathological/other diagnostic test reports confirming the diagnosis of the critical illness.
(3) Any other documents required by the company.

Section II: Critical Illness Cover (Optional)

Under this section the Company shall pay to the Insured Person, the compensation as set against such Insured Person's name in the schedule, should an Insured Person be diagnosed, during the period of insurance set in the schedule, as suffering from a critical illness stated hereunder, symptoms (and/or the treatment) of which were not present in such Insured Person at any time prior to inception of this Policy.

1. Stroke

2. Cancer
3. Renal failure
4. Major Organ Transplant
5. Multiple sclerosis
6. Coronary artery surgery
7. Paralysis and Blindness at additional premium

Waiting Period

No claim will be paid, if a critical illness as specified in the policy incepts or manifests during the first 90 days of the inception of the policy.

Survival Period

The insured person needs to survive for 30 successive days after the diagnosis of the critical illness in order to make his claim.

Provisos

1. Each of the above illnesses mentioned in the Policy, must be confirmed by a registered medical practitioner appointed by the company and must be supported by clinical, radiological, histological and laboratory evidence acceptable to the company and to be reconfirmed by a Registered Medical Practitioner appointed by the company.
2. The Company shall compensate the Insured on behalf of the insured Person only once in respect of any particular Critical Illness.
3. The Cover under the Policy will cease upon payment of the compensation on the happening of a Critical Illness and no further payment will be made for any consequent disease or any dependent disease.

Exclusions

The Company shall not pay any benefit to any insured Person who suffers an event giving rise to a Critical Illness which arises or is caused by or associated with directly or indirectly by any one of the following:

1. The ingestion of drugs other than those prescribed by a practicing and duly qualified member of the medical profession.
2. The ingestion of medicines, prescribed or not, for treatment of drug addiction and any treatment relating to drug addiction.
3. Any attempt by the Insured Person at suicide or any injury, which is self inflicted or in any manner willfully caused by or on behalf of the Insured Person.
4. Where the Insured Person at any time suffered from the condition commonly known as AIDS or was infected by the commonly called HIV virus. The terms AIDS and HIV will be

interpreted as broadly as possible so as to include all or any mutants, derivatives or variations thereof. The onus will always be on the Insured Person to show that any event was not caused by or did not arise through AIDS or HIV.

5. The Company will not be liable for a Critical Illness and/or its symptoms (and/or the treatment) of which were present in the Insured Person at any time before inception of the Policy or the date on which cover was granted to such Insured Person, or which manifest themselves within a period of 90 days from such date, whether or not the Insured Person had knowledge that the symptoms or treatment were related to such Critical Illness. In the event of any interruption in cover, the terms of this exclusion will apply as new from recommencement of cover.
6. No claim will be payable if the Insured Person smokes 40 or more cigarettes/cigars or equivalent tobacco intake in a day.
7. No claim will be payable if a critical illness is caused directly or indirectly or contributed to by or arising from:
   (i) Ionising Radiations or contamination by radioactivity from any nuclear fuel or from any nuclear waste from the combustion of nuclear fuel or nuclear weapons materials.
   (ii) War, Invasion, Act of Foreign enemy, Hostilities, Civil War, Rebellion, Revolution, Insurrection, Mutiny, Military, or Usurped Power, Seizure, Capture, Arrest, Restraints and Detainment of all Kings, Princes and People of whatever nation condition or quality whatsoever.

Special Note: The company reserves the right to review the premium rate, terms and conditions of this policy at the time of renewal.

This policy has been designed to cater to the needs of our Senior Citizens. It covers Hospitalization and Domiciliary Hospitalization Expenses under Section I as well as expenses for treatment of Critical Illnesses, if opted for, under Section II. Diseases covered under Critical Illnesses are as under:

1. Coronary Artery Surgery
2. Cancer
3. Renal Failure, i.e. Failure for both kidneys
4. Stroke
5. Multiple Sclerosis
6. Major Organ Transplants like kidney, Lung, Pancreas or Bone marrow
7. Paralysis and blindness at extra premium

Critical Illness cover is an optional cover under the policy. Persons who will not opt for critical illness cover are entitled to Hospitalization and Domiciliary hospitalization expenses cover for those diseases categorized above as critical illness but up to the limit of Sum Insured under Section I, i.e. under Hospitalization and Domiciliary Hospitalization Expenses and the claim for those diseases will be paid on reimbursement basis or as cashless hospitalization. Person opting for Critical Illness cover may opt for claim either under Section I or Section II (if not hospitalized) or under both sections for those diseases categorized above as Critical Illnesses but claim under Section I will be paid either on reimbursement basis or as cashless hospitalization if it is otherwise admissible. If in any policy year a critical illness is diagnosed and claim paid thereafter, in subsequent renewals the person may avail cover both under Section I and II but with the exclusion, both under Sections I and II, of that particular critical illness which has been diagnosed and claim paid in the preceding policy year.

Sum Insured: Sum Insured is fixed per person

Under Hospitalization and Domiciliary Hospitalization Cover sum Insured is Rs. 1,00,000 and under Critical Illness cover Sum Insured is Rs. 2,00,000.

Age Group: For fresh entry in to the scheme-60 years to 80 years. However, for renewal, age limit will be extended up to 90 years in which case the premium of 76-80 age band will be loaded by 10% up to 85 years and 20% up to 90 years of age.

Pre-acceptance Medical Check-up

No Medical Check-up is required if the insured was covered under any Health Insurance Policy of National Insurance Company or other Insurance companies uninterruptedly for preceding three years. Other persons have to undergo medical check up at their own cost for Blood/ Urine Sugar, Blood Pressure, Echo-cardiography and eye check up including retinoscopy.

Health Insurance in the United States

According to the latest United States Census Bureau figures, approximately 85% of Americans have health insurance. Approximately 60% obtain health insurance through their place of employment or as individuals, and various government agencies provide health insurance to over 29% of Americans. In 2005, there were 41.2 million people in the U.S. (14.2 percent of the population) who were without health care insurance for at least part of that year. (*ibid*) For many people, however, this does not boil down to a simple question of affordability. Part of this population might include young and healthy individuals with low risk of serious illness who don't believe that health insurance would be cost-effective. In fact, approximately one-third of these 41.2 million live in households with an income over $50,000, with half of these having an income of over $75,000. Additionally, one-third of these 41.2 million are eligible for public health insurance programs but have not signed up for them. People living in the western and southern United States are more likely to be uninsured.

Medicare

In the United States, government-funded Medicare programs help to insure the elderly and end stage renal disease patients. Some health care economists (Uwe Reinhardt of Princeton and Stuart Butler among others) assert that (the third party payment feature) these programs have had the unintended consequence of distorting the price of medical procedures. As a result, the Health Care Financing Administration has set-up a list of procedures and corresponding prices under the Resource-Based Relative Value Scale. Starting in 2006, Medicare Part D provides a program for the elderly to buy insurance for the purchase of prescription drugs.

Medicare Advantage

Medicare Advantage plans expand the health care options for Medicare beneficiaries. The option for Medicare Advantage plans is a result of the Balanced Budget Act of 1997, with the intent to better control the rapid growth in Medicare spending, as well as to provide Medicare beneficiaries more choice.

Medicaid

While Medicaid was instituted for the very poor, beginning in 1972, the number of individuals in the United States who lacked any form of health insurance for any period during the year increased each year, every year with the exceptions of the years 1999 and 2000. It has been reported that the number of physicians accepting Medicaid has decreased in recent years due to relatively high administrative costs and low reimbursements.

Private: Employer-Sponsored Medical Expense Insurance

Health insurance paid for by business entities generally on behalf of their employees and other immediate stakeholders. Broadly classified as "Traditional/Indemnity" and "Managed/Preferred Provider." Most private health coverage in the U.S. is employment-based, and the employer typically makes a substantial contribution towards the cost of coverage.

Many small employers provide employee health insurance, but the percentage offering is not as high as it is for larger employers. The types of coverage available to small employers are similar, but they do not have the same options for financing their benefit plans. In particular, self-insuring the benefits is not a practical option for most small employers. [6]

Private: Individually Purchased Medical Expense Insurance

Policies of health insurance obtained by individuals not otherwise covered under policies or programs elsewhere classified. Generally major medical, short-term medical, and student policies. Fewer Americans are covered by individually purchased medical expense insurance than by employer-sponsored coverage. The range of products available is similar, however. Average premiums are generally somewhat lower than those for employer-sponsored coverage, but vary by age. Deductibles and other cost-sharing is also higher, on average, and the individual consumer pays the entire premium without benefit of an employer contribution.

Private: Long-term Care Insurance

Long-term care (LTC) insurance is growing in popularity in the U.S. Premiums have remained relatively stable in recent years. However, the coverage is quite expensive, especially when consumers wait until retirement age to purchase it. The average age of new purchasers was 61 in 2005, and has been dropping.

Managed care in the U.S.

Through the 1990s, managed care grew from about 25% of U.S. employees to the vast majority.

	Rise of managed care in the U.S.				
Year	*Conventional plans*	*HMOs*	*PPOs*	*POS plans*	*HDHPs*
1998	14%	27%	35%	24%	~
1999	10%	28%	39%	24%	~
2000	8%	29%	42%	21%	~
2001	7%	24%	46%	23%	~
2002	4%	27%	52%	18%	~
2003	5%	24%	54%	17%	~
2004	5%	25%	55%	15%	~
2005	3%	21%	61%	15%	~
2006	5%	20%	60%	13%	4%

According the Centers for Medicare and Medicaid Services, nearly 100% of large firms offer health insurance to their employees. Although much more likely to offer retiree health benefits than small firms, the percentage of large firms offering these benefits fell from 66% in 1988 to 34% in 2002.

New Types of Medical Plans in the United States

On December 8, 2003, President Bush signed The Medicare Prescription Drug, Improvement and Modernization Act of 2003 into law, creating tax-deductible Health Savings Accounts. This gives consumers a new alternative to pay for health care expenses. The HSA is a private bank account which is un-taxed and only penalized if spent on non-medical items or services. Because it must be part of a high deductible insurance plan, the HSA insurance generally has a reasonably priced monthly premium and allows mostly healthy people to bank money for their own health care expenses rather than give it to the insurance company. Limited Medical Benefit Plans pay for routine care and do not pay for catastrophic care. Most people would be well served by such a plan, but financial security is not guaranteed like a major medical plan. Annual Benefit Limits can be as low as $2000. Life time maximums can be very low as well.

Medicare Part D Prescription Drug Plan (PDP) is a prescription benefit available to Medicare eligible individuals.

Common Medical Insurance Terms

- *Annual Limit*—A benefit may be limited to a certain dollar or utilization limit (example: chiropractic care may be limited to 20 visits per calendar year).
- *Alternative Funding Arrangement*—A hybrid funding arrangement that features benefits of both self-funding and fully insured arrangements (ASO, Minimum Premium, *et. al.*).
- *Birthday rule*—Many insurance companies have adopted this rule to determine which parent is primary payer when both parents cover the same dependents. Who ever has the earlier date of birth, excluding the year, is designated primary insurance carrier. Exceptions to this rule usually arise when there is a court order for one of the parents to be the primary carrier.
- *Co-insurance*—Generally expressed as the percentage that you pay of any covered medical services after you have paid the deductible and co-pay.
- *Co-insurance limit*—The dollar amount you have to pay with Co-insurance before the insurance company begins paying your bills at 100% for the remainder of the plan year.
- *Co-ordination of benefits (COB)*—How your plan pays when it is coordinating with another plan. There are three principle methods in US health plans.
- *Co-pay*—A fixed fee you pay for services rendered. Most plans cover 100% after the co-pay for services rendered, however this can be adjusted to any amount depending on how the plan is set-up.
- *Deductible*—The fixed amount you have to pay before your insurance starts to pay.
- *Deductible carry-forward*—Amounts for benefits incurred in the previous year may be subject to the prior year's deductibles.
- *Employee Assistance Plan*—A health-related benefit for non-medical, work-place issues or employees that commonly develop into medical issues such as marital counseling, absenteeism, suicidal ideation, etc.
- *Experimental/Investigational*—Most insurance companies will deny coverage for any procedures or tests which have not been medically verified by clinical trials conducted by recognized bodies of physicians or scientists. Many medical providers use

tests which they believe in but have not been clinically validated.

- *Fully Insured*—The insurance company collects the premiums and pays claims from its own money.
- *Incurred But Not Paid (IBNP)*—Under insurance-based accrual accounting, a liability for claims that have not been paid, but may or may not be received. Incurred But Not Reported (IBNR) plus Reported But Not Paid (RBNP) equals IBNP. IBNP is a significant balance sheet item for insurers.
- *In-Network/Participating/Par Providers*—Medical providers who have an established relationship with an insurance company.
- *Life time maximum*—The total your policy will pay out over the life of the contract. Many plans have a yearly restoration amount which will replenish the total so that after the policy money is exhausted there will still be some money in the following plan year for new claims. Life time maximums are easily avoided by switching policies or re-enrolling.
- *Self-Insured*—Many major U.S. and world corporations hire insurance companies and Third Party Administrators as claims and eligibility administrators to manage a health plan or trust. Many state laws do not apply to these plans due to ERISA exemption.
- *Reciprocity*—Most insurance plans deal with networks of doctors. If for example you have an HMO plan that allows you to see any HMO provider anywhere in the country, it is called Full Reciprocity, but if it only allows you access to local area networks of providers it is called Limited Reciprocity and if you can only go to select networks that your company has purchased access to, it is called No Reciprocity.
- *No-fault*—This is generally for automobile insurances, however if your auto policy is no-fault and you are injured, the medical insurance will become a secondary payer and will not be able to process claims until explanation of benefits are received from the auto insurance carrier.
- *Out-of-Network/Non-Participating/Non-Par Providers*—Medical providers without an established relationship with an insurance company.
- *Out of Pocket Maximum*—The total dollar amount paid out by a subscriber (deductible plus co-insurance).
- *Subscriber*—The primary member on the insurance policy. Also, "enrollee", "contractee".
- *Reserve*—refers to the amount that must be set aside for statutorily required funds for dissolution (terminal liability).

Necessity for Health Insurance in India

DoctorNDTV.com conducted a survey on the necessity for health insurance in India. The results of the survey have indicated that health insurance has become a necessity in view of the escalating cost of medical treatment, which is making it beyond the reach of the common man. Access to quality health care in the private sector till now is limited by the high cost. 400 people participated in the survey, out of which 93% considered that health insurance should be compulsory for all employers. Eighty-six per cent people voted in favor of covering pregnancy under medical insurance, 89% wanted free medical aid for people above the age of 65 and 67% people wanted that it should be free for the poor. There was an inclination towards foreign participation but only 42% people voted in favor of private ownership. Seventy-three per cent people wanted it to be cashless. The results thus suggest that in case of a medical emergency, health insurance provides much needed financial relief.

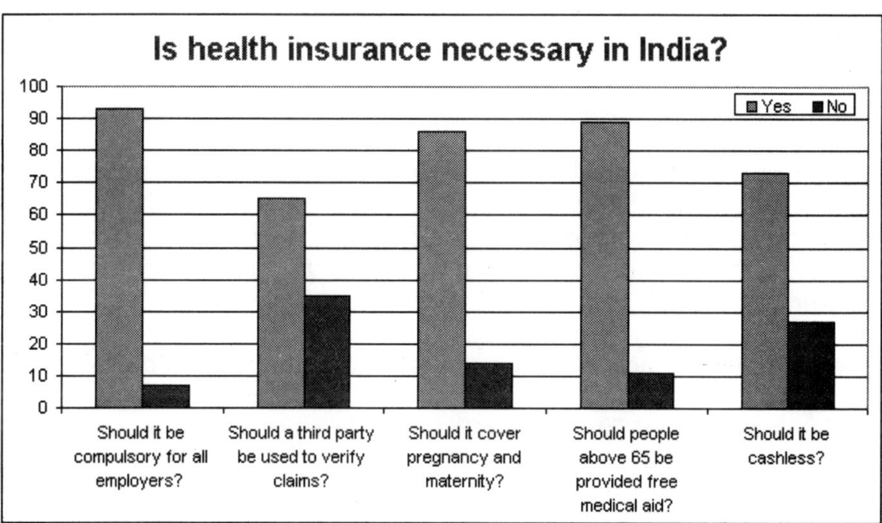

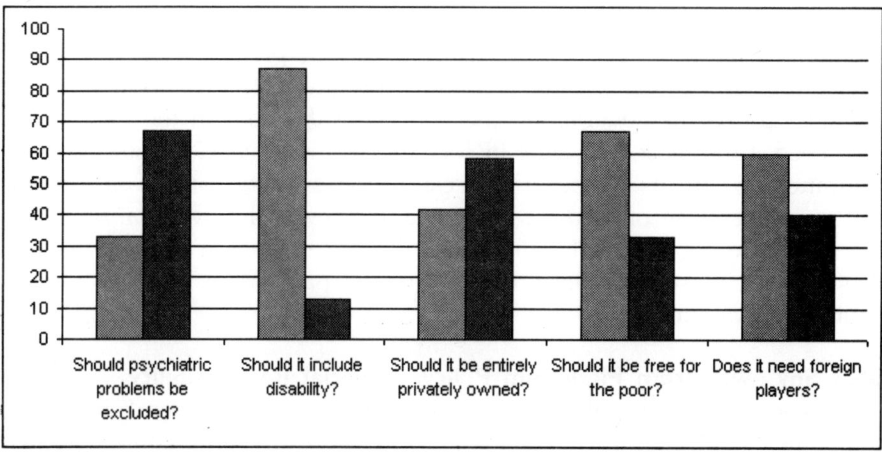

Health insurance is destined to grow exponentially in the coming years with large and diverse players having entered the fray and enticing consumers with an ever growing array of schemes. Less than 10% of India's population today has some sort of health insurance cover: either voluntary or as part of the Employees State Insurance, Central Government Health Scheme or Community Insurance. Private players in the voluntary health insurance sector saw spectacular growth in their collections last year. Health Care insurance premium collected in 2005-06 registered a growth of 35% over year 2004-05. The private players registered a growth of 77% over year 2004-05 and public players a growth of 25% over 2004-05. These figures are only likely to further increase. In addition, Community Health Insurance (CHI) schemes are also slowly penetrating the rural market. There are more than 25 schemes covering over 8 million lives all over India. With the Insurance Regulatory and Development Authority (IRDA) stipulating that 5% of the business for insurance companies be from the rural sector, a slew of innovative schemes and better coverage is being seen. The entry of pure Health Insurance companies into the marketplace in 2007 promises a plethora of innovative products. They estimate a potential of US$ 7,700 million in health insurance premium by 2015. Foreign Direct Investment (FDI) limit in health insurance may be raised from 26% to 49%, which would result in surge of international players and even more customized offerings targeting all sections of society. In the event of the minimum capital requirement of US$ 22 million being reduced to US$ 11 million, a number of standalone players would enter the fray as is the trend across the world for health insurance.

Dr. Devi Shetty of Narayan Hrudalaya, Banglore health city is in the process of offering health insurance coverage to the farmers of Karnataka. In the Phase-I they are going to cover 10 per cent of the State's population, that is roughly about 50 lakh farmers. Each farmer-member is expected to contribute Rs. 5 to Rs. 10 a month and he/she will be insured for all types of operations starting from appendices to heart surgery. These procedures will be totally free and other than this free service they will also get medical treatment at a concessional rate. The private sector has an estimated premium potential of over Rs. 4,500 crore. But the private sector will target only those who can afford its premiums. Private insurance companies are unlikely to provide coverage to the poorest of the poor in the rural areas, who need it the most. The state in collaboration with NGOs should provide insurance to all its citizens; especially those who cannot afford the treatment/premium of medical insurance. However, the overcharging from the insurance companies by the hospitals concerned is a serious malady. This if not checked can lead to the ruinous path of 'American system', letting the system go haywire.

GICs Shy away from Mediclaim Policy: A Social Responsibility

The other side of the story is that for most general insurance companies (GIC), health is a loss-making portfolio and companies are currently facing claim ratios of over 100%. A huge base still remains to be covered by different kinds of innovative products." The potential that health insurance holds can be seen from the fact that LIC of India has recently said that it wants to start a company exclusively offering health cover, though with a lower capital requirement. However, Insurance Regulatory and Development Authority (IRDA) chairman C.S. Rao's proposal of a higher minimum capital requirement of Rs. 100 crore as against expected Rs. 50 crore for standalone health companies could prove to be a hurdle in developing the health insurance sector. Till date, only one standalone health insurance company, Star Health and Allied Insurance Company Ltd. has come up. Promoted by a number of individuals, in association with Oman Insurance Company and few overseas partners, Star Health will have a capital base of Rs. 105 crore and will be headed by V. Jagannathan, former CMD of United India Insurance (UII). At present, most of the activity in health insurance is concentrated on the mediclaim policy, marketed by the public sector insurance companies. According to Gopal Verma, director, E-Meditech Solutions, a third-party administrator, "Between undercutting and stagnant pricing of policies, most of the market growth is lost. While actual cost of medical procedures and related issues like medicines, medical tests, room rates have gone up by 150%, the pricing structure has been revised upwards only by 5-6%. A regular re-pricing at least once in three years is absolutely necessary." A recent Parliamentary committee report pointed out that an additional burden had been thrust upon the insured by increasing the premium costs by 6% to meet the cost of service rendered by TPAs. It had also said that TPAs lacked the competence and necessary infrastructure to handle the huge number of claims successfully. Moreover, companies are cross-subsidizing health with more lucrative tariff products. Insurance companies also complain about the absence of any correlation between the premium paid and the type of room chosen. Further, many a time, there is a nexus between doctors, hospitals and the policy holders to cheat insurers by inflating the bills, doctoring the medical reports and other methods. In order to arrest the rampant abuse of health insurance facilities by medical-providers, standardization of services with appropriate acquisition cost should be done with immediate effect at all levels, say experts. Again, there is cross-subsidization in the health insurance segment—rural and semi-urban policy holders subsidize urban policy holders as the premium rates are uniform throughout the country. And between the individuals and the corporate houses, individual policy holders subsidize the latter. Agrees Verma, "The pressure to accept a lower premium rate is much more in the case of a corporate client as nobody wants to lose bulk business." However, the rural health insurance remains largely ignored. "Lack of awareness about various schemes has been one of the major challenges in spreading rural health insurance. The other challenges are selecting an appropriate distribution channel to meet the needs of the widely dispersed population and tying up financial support for premium funding in the economically weaker sections," says Jacob.

Presently, around 25 micro-health insurance schemes are being run across the country, mostly attached to micro-finance institutions, catering to local populations. Says Jacob, "Our Gramin Arogya Raksha benefits the rural sector. It covers critical illness, hospital expenditure and personal accident. It has been spread across the country with over 1,11,000 lives insured since its launch in April 2005." According to Pranav Prashad, head, rural and agri business, ICICI Lombard General Insurance Company, the two basic areas of concern are the availability of health infrastructure and distribution of health insurance policies. "In the absence of accessible health centres, where do villagers go to claim the health services? Also, specialised products are required to address the needs of rural patients." The company has an Arogya Raksha Yojana health insurance scheme run in Anekal Taluk and Kanakapura Taluk of Karnataka in collaboration with Biocon Foundation and Narayana Hrudayalaya IRDA needs to separate health from other insurances since claims incidence is extremely high and need health management expertise. Also, rural health schemes need to cover OPD and day surgeries as the rural poor find it expensive to stay in a hospital for more than a day as they lose wages. A premium financing mechanism is also important, as these people find it difficult to pay even the specially structured low rates of premiums. Till then, the health insurance sector in India will continue to have a lot of potential, without it being actually realized.

ICICI Lombard Health Plan

The policy covers the following medical expenses:

- Incurred as an inpatient during hospitalization for more than 24 hours, including room charges, doctor/surgeon's fee, medicines, etc.
- 30 days prior to hospitalization.
- 60 days post-hospitalization.
- Day Care expenses incurred on advanced technological surgeries and procedures like Dialysis, Radiotherapy, and Chemotherapy requiring less than 24 hours of hospitalization.

Key Benefits

- One Policy-One Premium for the entire family.
- Income Tax benefits under Section 80D.
- No health check up required up to the age of 45 years (as on last birthday).
- 5% discount on premium for every claim-free year.
- Digitally signed policy available 24x7 online. You can take prints instantly.
- Hassle free claims procedure.
- Cashless claim facility at over 3,500 network hospitals in more than 175 cities across India.

Additional Benefits

- FREE Health Checkup coupon—A FREE Health Checkup coupon for the senior most member of the family being insured.
- Up to 2-year Cover—We offer a continuous 2-year protection with no increase in premium in the second year. This one time payment of premium for 2 years takes care of your renewal hassles next year. Option for 1 year cover also available.

Policy Exclusions

All health policies have following set of temporary and permanent exclusions:

30 Days Exclusion

Medical charges incurred, except those arising out of accidental injuries, within the first 30 days from the start date of the policy are not covered. This clause does not apply for subsequent renewal (without a break) of this policy.

2 Years' Exclusions

Expenses incurred on treatment of following diseases within the first two years from the start date of the policy are not covered:

- Cataract
- Benign Prostatic Hypertrophy
- Myomectomy, Hysterectomy unless because of malignancy
- Hernia, Hydrocele
- Fistula in Anus, Piles
- Arthritis, Gout, Rheumatism
- Joint replacement, unless due to accident
- Sinusitis and related disorders
- Stone in the urinary and biliary systems
- Dilatation and Curettage
- Skin and all internal tumors/cysts/nodules/polyps of any kind, including breast lumps, unless malignant/adenoids and hemorrhoids
- Dialysis required for chronic renal failure
- Surgery on tonsils and sinuses
- Gastric and duodenal ulcers

These above diseases are covered from third year, if the policy is renewed with us for two consecutive years (4 years, if these are pre-existing diseases at the time of inception of the policy).

Permanent

- Any internal congenital illness.
- Non-allopathic treatment, pregnancy and childbirth related diseases, cosmetic, aesthetic and obesity related treatment.
- Expenses arising from HIV or AIDS and related diseases, use or misuse of liquor, intoxicating substances or drugs as well as intentional self-injury.
- War, riots, strike, terrorism acts, nuclear weapon induced treatment.

Cashless Settlement

Cashless claims facility is available only at specified network hospitals. This list of network hospitals is enclosed with your policy. Under this facility you just sign the bills at the time of your discharge and they shall settle the amount directly with the hospital. Under cashless facility, claims can be of two types:

Planned: Where the insured or covered family member(s) is aware of the hospitalization 2-3 days in advance.

(a) Contact Third Party Administrator (TPA) TTK Health Services help-line at 1800 42 58885/1800 42 57878 (Toll Free and Accessible only in India). You can also fax them at the toll free number 1800 425 2626 and call at their landline number 080-40125678. The same is mentioned on the Health Identity Card.
(b) Fax/submit the pre-authorization form to TPA with doctor's comments. This form is available online and also at all our network hospitals.
(c) The TPA faxes pre-authorization form with approval within 2-3 hours.
(d) Avail the health treatment. On your discharge, the TPA settles bills with the hospital.

Emergency

Where the insured or covered family member(s) meets with a sudden accident or suffers from a bout of illness that requires immediate admission to the hospital. After showing their Insurance card or policy copies the Policyholder can be hospitalized in emergency and are supposed to fill an undertaking form at the emergency reception. They should complete pre-authorizations formality filled by the concerned doctor. TPA will issue an authorization letter for the coverage as per the policy to the concerned hospital. The answer will come from TPA in the form of authorization letter. Rush the patient to the hospital. Patient avails the treatment. Family contacts TPA help-line at 1800 42 58885/1800 42 57878 (Toll Free and Accessible only in India) as mentioned on the health card. You can also fax them at the toll free number 1800 425 2626 and call at their landline number at 080-40125678. Family submits the pre-authorization form to TPA with doctor's comments. This form is available online and with all network hospitals. The TPA faxes pre-authorization form with approval within 2-3 hours. On discharge, the TPA settles bills with the hospital.

Policy holder can directly approach the hospital Admission Counter for admission with the ID Card and one copy of the authorization letter will be given to the Admission/IP billing counter. Hospital will extend cashless treatment to the policyholder up to the authorized amount. In case the authorized limit get exhausted get in touch with Insurance helpdesk. At the time of discharge, policyholder has to inform the Insurance desk and is supposed to sign the claim form. Insurance help desk is only helping you to get your claim processed by TPA. In the event of the cashless authorization request being rejected by TPA, the patient has to pay the bill to the hospital and try to claim the expenses subsequently from the Insurance company or TPA.

Do's

1. Obtain pre-authorization form from Insurance Helpdesk 3-4 days prior to the admission for planned hospitalization.
2. Pre-authorization form is to be filled in by treating doctor.
3. Check about the pre-authorization approval at the Insurance helpdesk within next 24 hrs.
4. You can avail cashless treatment at the hospital after receipt of written authorization from TPA for the covered.
5. Leave back all the original documents and signed claim form with the hospital at the time of discharge.
6. Contact local TPA office in case of any query.
7. Make payment to the hospital for the expenditure over and above the TPA approved limit and for the treatment not covered under the package.

Don'ts

1. Don't insist upon admission at the hospital merely for investigation, evaluation or Health check-up, as these are not approved by TPAs.
2. Don't insist on admission on cashless basis at the Hospital without obtaining the pre-authorization approval from TPA.
3. Don't carry back any original documents at the time of discharge from the hospital, if your cashless hospitalization is approved by the TPA.
4. Don't forget to sign the claim form.

Health Insurance in Canada

Most health insurance in Canada is administered by each province, under the national law that requires all people to have free access to basic health services. Collectively, the public provincial health insurance systems in Canada are called Medicare. Private health insurance in Canada cannot cover the same services provided by the universal Medicare services paid by the government. Private health insurance in Canada is allowed only for services the public health plans do not cover; for example, semi-private or private rooms in hospitals and prescription drug plans. Canadians also must use private insurance for medical services such as Lasik surgery, plastic surgery such as liposuction, and other non-basic medical procedures. Private health care cannot cover physician fees which are covered by Medicare. Private sector services not paid for by the government accounted for nearly 30 percent of total health care spending [Canadian Institute for Health Information: National Health Expenditure Trends, 1975-2003 (2003)].

In 2005, the Supreme Court of Quebec ruled, in Chaoulli *v.* Quebec, that the prohibition on insurance for health care already insured by the state constitutes an infringement of the right to life and security. It is yet to be seen if this ruling will change the overall delivery of health insurance across Canada.

Insurance Waiting Lists and Comparisons to US Health Care

Waiting lists in Canada are essentially different for each hospital system. There is no true system-wide average wait time, as wait times change on a daily basis as patients come in to receive services, and waiting lists are different for each hospital. A Canadian patient has the choice to visit a different hospital system if the primary care they received at the original hospital is found to be unacceptable. For example: If hospital A has a waiting list of five weeks for a surgery, the patient can go to hospital B that may have no waiting list at all. It is important to note that only elective surgeries, such as hip replacement, have waits associated with them. Emergency procedures are performed as soon as medically necessary, based on doctor opinion. This triage system is essentially the same as used in American hospitals where PPO, POS, and HMO managed-care plans may schedule elective surgeries several weeks or months out, but emergency procedures are carried out as soon as medically necessary based on doctor opinion. The American and Canadian systems are more similar than many people realize, and in effect only different in how the majority of insurance claims are paid. Both the Canadian and American health systems are undergoing major debate for each respective system in order to get more access to health care for the people who need it, in order to lower mortality rates. Each system has unique problems that need attention, mostly dealing with funding and insurance issues. Canada has a slightly lower mortality rate on average, particularly when involving HIV mortality. The US rate for HIV mortality is approximately 4x higher; however, there are not 4x more HIV cases per capita in the United States.

Health Insurance in Australia

The public health system is called Medicare. It ensures free universal access to hospital treatment and subsidized out-of-hospital medical treatment. It is funded by a 1.5% tax levy. The private health system is funded by a number of private health insurance organizations, the largest being Medibank Private (which is government-owned, but operates at arms length from government; the John Howard government has announced it will be sold in 2008 assuming it is returned to office at the 2007 election). Some private health insurers are 'for profit' enterprises, and some are non-profit organizations. Most aspects of private health insurance in Australia are regulated by the Private Health Insurance Act 2007.

LIC of India to File its Health Insurance Plan

Life Insurance Corporation of India (LIC) will lodge its first long-term health insurance plan with the insurance regulator, IRDA, this month (6 Oct, 2007), said the insurance major's executive director-health insurance DD Singh. The product will have elements of a unit-linked insurance plan and a hospital cash policy.

References

California Insurance Code Section 106 (defining disability insurance). In 2001, the California Legislature added subdivision (b), which defines "health insurance" as "an individual or group disability insurance policy that provides coverage for hospital, medical, or surgical benefits."

Cunningham P, May J. "Medicaid patients increasingly concentrated among physicians." *Track Rep.* 2006 Aug;(16):1-5. PMID 16918046.

Dr. David Gratzer, senior fellow at the Manhattan Institute. Interviewed in the Sun, in the article Momentum Grows on Health Care.

Hannah Yoo, Karen Heath and Tom Wildsmith, "Small Group Health Insurance in 2006,"Americ-'s Health Insurance Plans, September 2006.

http://www.ahipresearch.org/pdfs/FINALSmallGroupPaper.pdf

http://209.217.72.34/HDAA/ReportFolders ReportFolders.aspx? CS_referer '&CS_ChosenLang'en

http://www.amsa.org/studytours/WaitingTimes_primer.pdf

http://www.cms.hhs.gov/TheChartSeries/downloads/private_ins_chap4_p.pdf

http://www40.statcan.ca/l01/cst01/health30a.htm

Income, Poverty, and Health Insurance Coverage in the United States: 2005." U.S. Census Bureau. Issued August 2006.

Navigating your health benefits for dummies. Charles M Cutler MD Tracey A Baker CFP ©2006 ISBN-13:978-0-470-08354-3

R. Adams, CSR Aetna Ins. Tampa fl.

Teresa Chovan, Hannah Yoo and Tom Wildsmith, "Individual Health Insurance: A Comprehensive Survey of Affordability, Access, and Benefits," America's Health Insurance Plans, August 2005 http://www.ahipresearch.org/pdfs/Individual_Insurance_Survey_Report8-26-2005.pdf

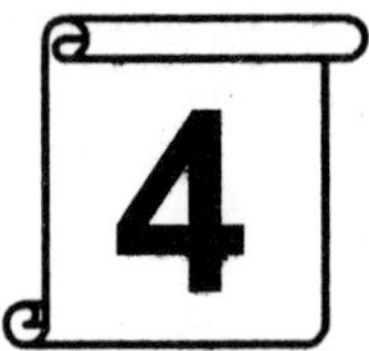

Patient's Right to Health Care and Doctor's Right to Personal Safety

Most people agree that everyone deserves the basic right to health care, but how far that right goes has been the center of debate all over the world. Within the existing social structure, inequities in access to health care are widespread. Because of numerous inequities in health care that often involve such factors as race, socio-economic status, and gender, politicians have tried for many years to change the health care system. While health care system and hospitals have been set-up to help patients, the doctors engaged in helping them have to work hard and with skill and dedication. There has been emphasis on the patient's rights and patient safety, but the doctors working round the clock to give relief/cure to them have not found mention in the matter of their respect, comfort, compensation and even their safety against the assaults on their person or their property. There is no dearth of cases where despite the best of efforts by doctors could not save the patients and subsequently the relatives or street mobs indulged in uncalled for violence. The doctors have been abducted when they agreed to go to attend emergency. The doctors also became victims of police apathy or deliberate criminal designs. The Draconian law 'consumer protection act' (COPRA) extended to doctors some years ago has the potential of taking away the life time wealth/ income of a doctor and damage of reputation in no time. The list is long. In this chapter we shall touch those issues as well, where the safety of the doctors is endangered. All citizens must now begin to wonder: "Will a surgeon be there" when I need one? "Will an obstetrician be there" when I need one? "Will an emergency room physician be there" when I need one? "Will a family physician be there" when I need one? If this patient access crisis is not resolved very soon with real reform, there is no limit to how far-reaching the implications could be.

INADEQUATE HEALTH CARE ALL OVER THE WORLD

There is no doubt that ideal health care system is yet to evolve even in the developed countries like USA. In developing countries like India the state of affairs is dismal in most parts of the country. Let us first talk of America, where the expectations are high and the present system has been described as 'broken health care system' by none other than the new President of USA. One the setbacks to universal health care in America was the failure of President Clinton's health care plan for national health care coverage to pass through Congress in 1994. America's health care system consists of a patchwork of health care programs and insurance that includes private health insurance, HMOs, Medicaid, and Medicare, among others. However, more than 40 million Americans (about 50 millions at present) are uninsured, and the government has been forced to pass various laws in order for America's health care system to provide more equal care. An example of such a law is the Consolidated Omnibus Budget Reconciliation Act (COBRA). The COBRA regulations are federal legislation that mandates an evaluation of patients who seek medical attention at emergency facilities. If an emergency care institution refuses to provide care, the institution and health care providers are held responsible and liable. These regulations prevent health care institutions from refusing needed care to people without money or health insurance. Together, the COBRA laws and the Emergency Medical Treatment and Active Labor Act (EMTALA) refer to federal laws related to patient screening and transfer. They require Medicare-participating hospitals to do the following:

- Perform an appropriate medical screening examination by a qualified provider to determine whether an emergency condition exists.
- Provide further examination and treatment to stabilize the patient, and if necessary and appropriate, to arrange a transfer.
- Consider patients in labor unstable for transfer.

EMTALA requires that Medicare-participating hospitals screen anyone who is in active labor or is seeking emergency care. If such a screening reveals the presence of an emergency medical condition—such as severe pain, serious threat to life or limb, or active labor—the hospital is required to perform stabilizing treatment to the best of its capabilities. In order to provide continuing health insurance for the recently unemployed, COBRA provisions also permit continuation of coverage through the workplace. Recently, many federal and civil lawsuits have been filed against HMOs for failing to provide needed care because of the drive to reduce health care costs. What the outcome of such lawsuits will be is unclear, but the quality of provided care is on the minds of all who obtain health care.

Doctors are Over-worked and Harried Lot even in US

India has a large population of about 125 crores of people and the corresponding facilities and manpower is not adequate. Most of the doctors are over-worked in public sector hospitals as well as private hospitals. However, even in USA the Primary care doctors feel overworked, and nearly half plan to either cut back on how many patients they see or quit medicine entirely, according to a survey released recently. More than half—60%—of 12,000 general practice physicians would not recommend medicine as a career.

> "The whole thing has spun out of control. I plan to retire early even though I still love seeing patients. The process has just become too burdensome," the Physicians' Foundation, which conducted the survey, quoted one of the doctors as saying.

The survey adds to building evidence that not enough internal medicine or family practice doctors are trained or practicing in the United States, although there are plenty of specialist physicians.

Health Care reform is near the top of the list of priorities in US and doctor's groups are lobbying for action to reduce their workload and hold the line on payments for treating Medicare, Medicaid and other patients with federal or state health insurance.

The Physicians' Foundation, founded in 2003 as part of a settlement in an anti-racketeering lawsuit among physicians, medical societies, and insurers, mailed surveys to 270,000 primary care doctors and 50,000 practicing specialists. The 12,000 answers are considered representative of doctors as a whole, the group said, with a margin of error of about 1%. It found that 78% of those who answered believe there is a shortage of primary care doctors. More than 90% said the time they devote to non-clinical paperwork has increased in the last 3 years and 63% said this has caused them to spend less time with each patient.

Eleven percent said they plan to retire soon and 13% said they plan to seek a job that removes them from active patient care. Twenty percent said they will cut back on the number of patients they see and 10% plan to move to part-time work. Seventy-six percent of physicians said they are working at "full capacity" or "overextended and overworked." Many of the health plans proposed by members of Congress, 'insurers and employers' groups, as well as Obama's, suggest that electronic medical records would go a long way to saving time and reducing costs.

Medical Residents' Fatigue and Patient Safety

A new report by the Institute of Medicine (IOM) recommends strategies to reduce medical resident fatigue-related errors and improve patient safety and medical training by reducing residents' duty hours, increasing their sleep hours, and increasing supervision of work hour limits. The report, titled "Resident Duty Hours: Enhancing Sleep,

Supervision and Safety," was funded by the US Department of Health and Human Services Agency for Health Care Research and Quality (AHRQ) and was published online December 2.

"The [IOM] study provides the clear evidence to prove what we have long-believed is true—fatigue increases the chance for human error," AHRQ Director Carolyn M. Clancy, MD, said in a news release. "Most importantly, this report provides solid recommendations that can improve patient safety, as well as increase the quality of the resident training experience."

An IOM committee performed a 15-month study examining the associations between residents' work schedules, their performance, and quality of care provided. Residents suffering acute and chronic fatigue are more likely to make errors, according to the study findings.

"The impact of resident fatigue caused by long work hours is still a major concern," Joanne Conroy, MD, chief health care officer, Association of American Medical Colleges, told Medscape Medical News when asked for independent review of the IOM report. "We believe that improved management of the resident work day may lead to a safer clinical environment, although the data has not yet demonstrated this statistically."

Dr. Conroy noted that studies published more than a decade ago first demonstrated the effect of fatigue on performance levels.

"When Dawson and Reid first published the effect of fatigue on performance and equated it with alcohol impairment, the medical community took notice," Dr. Conroy said. "Anecdotally, we also recognize the tremendous variation among physicians in terms of their ability to recognize and manage their own fatigue."

Current rules of the Accreditation Council for Graduate Medical Education (ACGME) permit a maximum 30-hour shift for residents, including direct patient care for 24 hours and training or transition activities for the remaining 6 hours. These rules also permit a maximum 80-hour work week.

On the basis of their study results, the IOM committee recommends several changes to these rules. Specific recommendations are as follows:

- Residents who complete a 30-hour shift may treat patients for only up to 16 hours, followed by a 5-hour protected sleep period between 10 PM and 8 AM, during which time patient care would be managed by other nonsleeping residents or additional staff members.
- Supervision of work hours should be increased because of frequent, often underreported lack of compliance with ACGME limits. The IOM committee recommends periodic independent reviews of hours worked by residents, as well as increased protections for those who report failure to comply with current work hour restrictions.
- Moonlighting restrictions should be increased so that both internal and external moonlighting count against the ACGME

80-hour weekly limit. Only internal moonlighting, defined as additional paid health care work at the same health care facility, is currently considered to be part of the 80-hour weekly limit. Because moonlighting outside residency training affects strategically designed periods for rest and sleep and may hinder residents' abilities to complete their primary duties, the IOM recommends that both internal and external moonlighting be counted toward the total work week hourly limit.

- To facilitate recovery after working long shifts, the IOM report recommends guaranteed 5 days off per month, with 24 hours off each week and one 48-hour period-off each month.
- Hospital on-call periods for residents should be limited to no more than every third night.
- Because the risk for motor vehicle accidents more than doubles when residents drive home after working extended shifts, hospitals should provide safe transportation to residents who are too fatigued to drive home.
- Residents should receive more training on better communication, using a structured team approach, during change-of-shift handovers. These handovers will increase as resident shift duration decreases, possibly increasing the risk for adverse events unless training and team communication improve.
- Residents should be more involved inpatient safety activities and in adverse event reporting not only to improve quality of care but also to enhance their educational experience.

"Patient safety is a top priority for educators, administrators, and clinicians," Dr. Conroy said. "The challenge will be how to develop a strategy to ensure that these changes don't impact the continuity of patient care and the quality of the educational experience."

When asked whether there are barriers to widespread implementation of recommendations in the IOM report, Dr. Conroy cited "trying to create an optimal work environment that also produces the best-trained physician."

If these recommendations are widely implemented, Dr. Conroy pointed out that data are currently insufficient to determine the effect on health care.

"There will always be unintended consequences," Dr. Conroy concluded. "We would expect, however, that there will be additional costs."

On December 3, the *New England Journal of Medicine* published online a perspective on the IOM's recommendations, noting tensions among 3 main objectives that are sometimes in conflict: patient safety, resident safety, and resident education.

The Committee of Interns and Residents (CIR) in New York City, an advocate for resident work hours reform, contributed to the debate on this issue. "The recommendations in this new report are an important corroboration of our advocacy over the course of many years about the dangers of long hours to patient care and to resident well-being."

What are Patient's Rights?

As one who knows your body, your aches and pains, your specific needs related to your injury, you have the right to two-way communication with your doctor about your long-term care concerns. You have the right to whatever information you need about your injury and possible complications arising from the injury. Kievman, in her book, For Better or For Worse, suggests that you also have other rights, such as:

- having adequate access to your doctor
- participating in major decisions related to your care
- changing doctors if your best interests are not being served
- knowing whom to contact if your doctor is unavailable
- having your records handled confidentially
- knowing what you will be charged for, and how much those charges will be
- being seen within a reasonable time of your scheduled appointment
- asking for a second opinion

Never be afraid to ask questions. There is no such thing as a dumb question as far as your health is concerned. You have a right to know and understand. You have a right to express your concerns, doubts and fears, and to be heard.

What are Your Responsibilities

In addition to your rights, you have responsibilities to your doctor. You need to tell him your medical history, what other doctors you may be seeing, what medications you use or have used, and what is your alcohol or drug history. If you have a right to the best treatment available, then you have the responsibility to share with your doctor information that will help him or her diagnose, medicate or treat your particular problems. If you keep things from your doctor, then the treatment you receive may be ineffective or dangerous.

It is also your responsibility to tell your doctor everything you know about your injury, its possible long-term effects, and complications.

Additional Responsibilities?

In addition, you are responsible for:

- telling your physician about your symptoms,
- understanding in detail what is wrong with you and what treatment is available and planned for you,

- following your doctor's directions, reporting symptoms or complications or making sure your doctor knows why you cannot do so, and
- keeping scheduled appointments, paying bills on time, and limiting other calls unless they are vital to your well being.

The principal rights fall in the following categories

1. Right to adequate health care.
2. Right to information.
3. Right to privacy and confidentiality.
4. Right to self-determination.

Your Doctor has Rights, too...

Among your doctor's rights are:

- to know about your life-style, particularly if it has an impact on your SCI or complications from the injury, or proposed treatment, and
- to withdraw from treating you if he or she feels that there is an ethical or personal conflict with you to privacy.

...and Responsibilities

While this seems obvious, physicians are accountable for:

- thoroughly discussing with you diagnoses, tests, and treatments in a non-technical way,
- recommending reasonable alternative treatments or medications,
- notifying you of non-office hour coverage, keeping good patient records, and informing you of services not covered by insurance,
- recognizing when his or her knowledge is limited and asking for a second opinion, and
- developing a partnership with you in your quest for wellness.

As you age with your spinal cord injury, you need people to work with you to keep you healthy and to improve your quality of life. Your doctor is the key to your health. As part of your team, your physician wants you to understand the rights and responsibilities you both have. How to keep the patients happy:

1. The patient is never an interruption to work: the patient is our work. Everything else can wait !
2. Greet every patient with a friendly smile, patients are people and they like friendly contact. They usually return it.
3. Call patients by name. Make a game of learning patients' names, and see how many you can remember.

4. Teach your staff members that for patients, all staff members are as important as the doctor !
5. Never argue with a patient, the patient is always right (in his or her own eyes). Be a good listener, agree with them where you can and do what you can to make them happy.
6. Never say, "I don't know". If you don't know the answer to a patient's question, say, "That is a good question. Let me see if I can find out the answer for you."
7. Remember that the patient pays your salary: treat him like your boss !
8. Choose positive words when speaking to a patient. This a valuable habit that will help you become an effective communicator.
9. Brighten every patient's day, and you'll soon discover that your own life is happier and brighter.

Always go that extra mile, do just a little more than the patient expects you to do. For example, make it a habit to phone the patient after discharge from the hospital, to ensure that he is doing well. Exceeding patient expectations is the best way to keep your patients happy—and keep them as your patients for life !.

Violence against Doctors a Worldwide Phenomenon; it Curtails Patient's Right too

Statistics suggest that a third of doctors will experience some form of violence in their workplace. As part of the 2002 NHS Plan the government sought to tackle violence in GP surgeries through involvement of the PCTs in their Zero Tolerance campaign. Despite statistics that suggest violent attacks have fallen by 1,690 in 2005/6, we cannot afford to be complacent about this very real threat. As part of the GMS contract, practices may offer to see violent patients on behalf of other surgeries as part of a direct enhanced service.

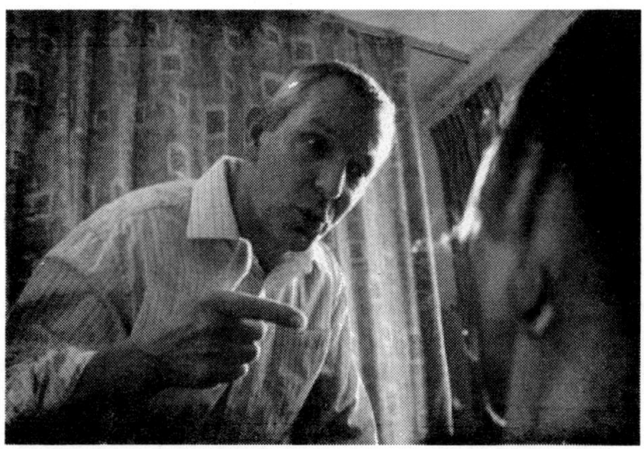

Staying Safe in the Surgery

Before you start seeing patients, look around your consulting room and make a risk assessment.

Examine the layout of the room. Seat yourself closer to the door than the patient so you can get out if you need to. Consider if there is anything in the room that could be used as a weapon. Move sharp items out of sight and don't place hot liquids between you and the patient.

It is important to ask where the panic alarms are in each room. These may be actual buttons or linked in with the computer system. Thankfully, in most surgeries these are not used very often. This may mean that the staff forgets to tell you of their existence unless you specifically ask.

Signs of possible violence

Patients, or their relatives, may become violent for a multitude of reasons. They may be angry at being kept waiting, annoyed by the attitude of staff or upset about a clinical error. Very often you will start to have a sense that the consultation is not going well before overt signs appear.

The patient may start to avoid your gaze, interrupt you, swear or raise their voice. They may start to use intimidating gestures, such as pointing or thumping their fist on the desk. They may stand too close to you, raise their fists, pace the room or start to throw objects around while making verbal threats.

Keeping in control

Violence is an escalating process, so the key is to spot the early signs of possible danger and deal with them.

With an angry patient or relative, give them time to vent their feelings. Acknowledge their anger but don't antagonize them by telling them that you understand how they feel. Speak in a calm reassuring tone and try not to be defensive or argue back.

Use open body language and look at the patient's face. Find out exactly why they are angry and how they would like the matter resolved.

Resist the urge to blame other members of staff if you realize that you are not in the wrong and don't make comments about third party conversations unless you know exactly what was said.

Once you have established the problem, discuss possible solutions with the patient and how these will be resolved. Strongly encourage them to put their complaint in writing.

If you feel that the patient may be physically violent, it is best to leave the room as quickly as possible. Try not to antagonize the patient by making sudden moves. If your way out of the room is blocked, activate the panic alarm, shout for help or try to talk calmly to the patient, attempting to defuse the situation.

Conflict resolution courses are excellent for providing advice on how to do this. Courses also teach techniques to deflect common assaults safely.

Check the practice policy for dealing with certain groups of patients where your personal safety could be at risk. Examples of such patients include drug abusers trying to obtain more supplies of a particular medication, or patients with a previous history of violence.

Safety on home visits

Home visits may present dangers, especially when visiting new patients. Let staff know where you are going and when you are likely to return.

Take a fully charged mobile phone with you and let the surgery have the number.

If you are unsure about visiting, don't go alone. You might want to have a pre-arranged phrase you could use when calling the surgery to indicate that you are in difficulty (for example, 'can I speak to Barbara Davies please?'). This will alert staff without arousing suspicion.

When entering a house always have the relative lead you up to the patient, especially when going upstairs. This makes it more difficult if someone is planning to ambush you.

Try to minimize your appearance as a target. Think very carefully if it is appropriate in some areas to carry your equipment in a typical doctor's bag and weigh up the pros and cons of carrying controlled drugs in your bag if you are not likely to need them. If you are a woman, dressing modestly may help deflect unwanted male attention. www.RCGP-curriculum.org.uk

Learning Points

1. Consider the layout of your room and keep any potentially dangerous items out of sight.
2. Know where the panic alarms are in each room.
3. Recognize aggressive behavior and learn how to defuse potentially violent situations.
4. When attending home visits take a mobile phone and ensure the practice staff knows where you are going.
5. Consider attending a conflict resolution course.

Dedicated Indian doctor languishing in a filthy jail

Doctor Binayak Sen is an unusual 58-year-old. He inspires people as a doctor, a kind, gentle human being and passionate human rights defender, a fighter for the rights of the poverty stricken tribal people to whom he has dedicated his life. Yet, after 30 years of committed work for the poor, he is currently languishing in a filthy jail in Chattisgarh, central India. The story is a long one.

Binayak graduated from the Christian Medical College (CMC), Vellore, one of India's premier institutions. Even as a student he was something of a legend—charismatic, caring, concerned about every last patient. Stories are being exchanged on the web about him. Dr. Sara

Bhattacharji, one of his contemporaries, writes: 'As a new intern, in CMC Vellore, at the end of a grueling day he realized he had written a prescription for Lasix (a diuretic) for a patient, without also including the required potassium supplement. The patient had of course left by this time. Binayak went to the medical records department and looked up the patient's address, then to the pharmacy where he bought the potassium, then sallied forth taking various bone-rattling village buses (remember this is a Bengali floundering without the local language, in rural Tamilnadu) to the patient's village, where he delivered the medicine to the patient.' That was early Binayak.

Mine workers

He became a pediatrician, then focused on community health, which was his passion. Binayak met, wooed and married Ilina. He was fortunate to have found a soul-mate as committed to eradicating poverty as himself. Ilina—warm, caring, compassionate—is one of those rare individuals adored by everyone who knows her.

The doctor's heart was always with the poor, so he joined an organization run by the Quakers in Hosangabad. Here, in addition to the general work, he was involved in the care of tuberculosis patients. He began to visit some of the mine areas in South Madhya Pradesh (now Chhattisgarh). Contact with the extreme poverty and the plight of the unorganized mine workers moved him. He was invited to join them by their leaders and was primarily responsible for developing a low-cost clinic in Dalli Rajahara.

The mine workers had employment—the hospital was run on their modest donations. The trade union was strong. Volunteers from the union helped to organize the people and work for education, and better social and environmental conditions. They also conducted anti-alcohol and anti-tobacco campaigns. This helped to keep costs down and left the doctors free to provide low-cost, good-quality clinical care. The hospital has now grown to a 90-bed facility.

New models

When he felt it could run without his help, Binayak moved on. He worked for some time in a mission hospital, nearby in Tilda. He treated patients and trained village health workers. Though he was happy doing this, he felt the necessity to do more than just treat the few who were able to access services.

So they moved to Raipur and started a trust called Rupantar to explore models of development that reflect the people's aspirations. The new place was totally different from Dalli Rajahara. The people lived in scattered villages. Most of them had a long history of being displaced by the damming of the Mahanadi river, especially the Hirakud Dam.

After a significant struggle, 12 of 18 villages were recognized and given amenities. The other six were destroyed, causing further displacement of people. Regular work was a problem. So getting people organized was hard. The issues needing attention were livelihood, education and health. As Binayak started to set-up clinics and train health workers he also realized that the main problems were malaria, TB, high mother and child mortality. He experienced the slowly dawning realization that the people were chronically undernourished. This underlying malnutrition became an important focus for them, leading them to look at food security. An agricultural programme grew out of this.

Another issue identified was violence against women. Ilina worked with the community to address this problem. As the health work grew, the problem of access to health care became evident. So it was logical to train local people in health. From the health centre they began satellite clinics for surrounding areas. Yet there were many people who still had to travel long distances to access care. Slowly malaria mortality began to decrease; antenatal care and immunization improved. Deaths from diarrhoea and dehydration came down and respiratory illnesses in children were treated.

TB and malaria were still huge problems, both in terms of diagnosis and treatment. Health workers learned to take blood and sputum smears, give antenatal care, health education, to diagnose and treat common illnesses. A trained lab-tech added greatly to the quality of the care.

Recognition

The state recognized their work. Both Binayak and Ilina were part of the planning and setting up of the government health resource centre in the new state of Chhattisgarh. They greatly influenced the health worker programme, called the Mitanin model. Binayak was also asked to be part of the process of the planning for the National Rural Health Mission (NRHM) and was responsible for the training of Accredited Social Health Activists (ASHAs).

In 2004 his alma mater, CMC, Vellore, gave him the prestigious Paul Harrison award for his work. The citation read: 'Dr. Binayak Sen has been true to the spirit and vision of his alma mater and has carried his dedication to truth and service to the very frontline of the battle. He has broken the mould, redefined the possible role of the doctor in a broken and unjust society, holding the cause much more precious than personal safety. CMC is proud to be associated with Binayak and Illina Sen.'

The Naxalites

Meanwhile, in Chattisgarh, a different kind of drama was unfolding. The state had a problem with the Naxalites (a Maoist-Leninist revolutionary army that believes in violence to achieve justice). The Naxalites had approached the very poor villagers and organized them to demand better wages. However, the Naxalites had their own agendas, and often used brutal violence. The state, in retaliation, started the Salwa Judum movement—supposedly a spontaneous response of the people to the violence. The government armed the tribal people—those who refused to fight were branded Naxalites. Many tribal people were trapped between the Salwa Judum and the Naxalites.

The government brought in a draconian special security act. Binayak, with his long experience of the oppression and injustice meted out to the simple people in the area, found himself in the middle of a state-*versus*-terrorist war. Innocent tribal people were being tortured and beaten up mercilessly, women were gang raped, families were massacred, men killed in fake 'encounter' deaths and villages razed to the ground. All this was documented and reported by several newspapers.

Human rights

Binayak began to investigate and make public the human rights violations, through the Peoples' Union for Civil Liberty. He called for the violence to stop.

'For the past several years,' he said, 'we are seeing all over India—and, as part of that, in the state of Chhattisgarh as well—a concerted programme to expropriate from the poorest people in the Indian nation their access to essentials, common property resources and to natural resources, including land and water. The campaign called the Salwa Judoom in Chhattisgarh is a part of this process, in which hundreds of villages have been denuded of the people living in them and hundreds of people—men and women—have been killed. Government-armed vigilantes have been deployed and the people who have been protesting against such moves and trying to bring before the world the reality of these campaigns—human rights workers like myself—have also been targetted through state action against them.

At the present moment the workers of the Chhattisgarh PUCL (People's Union for Civil Liberties), of which I am General Secretary, have particularly become the target of such state action; and I, along with several of my colleagues, am being targeted by the Chhattisgarh state in the form of punitive action, illegal imprisonment. And all these measures are being taken especially under the aegis of the Chhattisgarh 'Public Security Act.'

This infuriated the local police. They filed trumped up charges against him, branding him a Naxalite and accusing him of smuggling letters for a jailed prisoner he was treating medically. He was arrested and jailed on 14 May 2007.

The campaign

On 12th June, in an interview with ABC Radio National (Australia), the noted Indian commentator P. Sainath said: 'You have a number of studies, reports and investigations done by the People's Union for Civil Liberties, of which Binayak is a leading member, on "fake encounters". The word "encounter" has a very special meaning in India. It means the police kill someone, he may be unarmed, he may be tied to a chair. Then he posthumously becomes a Maoist. That's immediately conferred on you in death. [There have been] a number of studies on these .encounters., and on fake killings, and on a vigilante war that the government is waging on the Maoists... That's what got Binayak Sen into trouble. . . The charges brought against him - it's very interesting. The police now have sort of outsourced the smear campaign to the media. So the media bring incredible charges against him which the police then do not repeat in the court."

Noam Chomsky and several other prominent figures issued a Press Statement dated 16 June 2007 alleging that: 'The fake encounters, rapes, burning of villages and displacement of adivasis [indigenous tribals] in tens of thousands and consequent loss of livelihoods have been extensively chronicled by several independent investigations. Dr. Sen's arrest is clearly an attempt to intimidate PUCL and other democratic voices that have been speaking out against human rights violations in the state.'

'The word "encounter" has a very special meaning in India. It means the police kill someone, he may be unarmed, he may be tied to a chair. Then he posthumously becomes a Maoist. That's immediately conferred on you in death.'—P. Sainath. On 31 August the Supreme Court of India issued notice to the Chhattisgarh Government on a petition seeking Dr. Sen's release from alleged illegal detention. The bench of Justices sought response from the Chhattisgarh Government after senior counsel Soli Sorabjee claimed that Dr. Sen had been illegally detained since 14th May on fabricated charges of supporting Naxalites.

Other protests against Dr. Sen's arrest have come from Nobel Prize winner Amartya Sen, Magsaysay Prize winner Aruna Roy, Booker Prize winner Arundathi Roy, retired judge Rajinder Sachar of the Delhi High Court, film maker Shyam Benegal and many eminent medical professors and scientists in India, the US, Britain, Australia and beyond. Ilina Sen, friends and colleagues who have been inspired by Binayak, urge like-minded people from all over the world to join the protest to fight for justice both for Binayak Sen and the thousands of adivasi people suffering oppression in Chhatisgarh.

Communal virus attacks the doctors left and right

Doctors in the riot hit Indian city of Ahmedabad have not been working in its Muslim neighborhoods for several weeks, because of security concerns and a disruption in medical services. Consultants and general practitioners belonging to the majority Hindu community are avoiding visits to Muslim localities in Ahmedabad, where religious riots between Hindus and Muslims have claimed more than 400 lives in the past 10 weeks.

Security concerns for doctors surfaced after individuals posing as patients stabbed and injured a Hindu doctor last month in his clinic in a Muslim neighborhood. The incident prompted the Ahmedabad Doctors' Forum to urge Hindu doctors not to venture into Muslim localities unless their safety was guaranteed.

The forum has asserted that its call was not intended to deny medical services to Muslims but to ensure the safety of doctors. Religion is not an issue at all, Dr. Bharat Amin, president of the forum told the *BMJ*. All patients are equal to us, he said. But doctors concede that medical services in Muslim localities are in disarray. Less than 200 of the city's 4500 doctors are Muslims, and they simply cannot handle all the Muslim patients, said Dr. Vijay Bhatia, vice-president of the Indian Medical Association's Ahmedabad branch. Personal safety or professional duty—that's the dilemma that doctors in this city are facing, Dr. Bhatia said. Hindu doctors have stopped visiting hospitals in Muslim localities. At the Al Amin Hospital, for example, 70 out of 82 consultants are Hindus. All but two have stayed away from the hospital for several weeks, Dr. Sadiq Kazi, medical superintendent at Al Amin told the *BMJ*.

Its Muslim consultants have also stopped visiting because of safety concerns about traveling around the city.

Safety first, naukari later at Lucknow

The minister for medical and health Ramapati Shastri hints at suspension and even termination of government doctors who fail to report at the rural primary health centers and community health centers, the terse warning, for once has fallen on deaf ears. "Safety first, naukari later" is the latest slogan doing the rounds among the 11,391 strong provincial medical health service cadre, which has 7,000 physicians/surgeons specially earmarked for rural postings only. And they are a worried lot. With growing cases of assault and robbery against doctors, rural postings over the years have become extremely unsafe for the cadre. They list at least a dozen such crimes which have gone unheard during the last six months. What adds to their shock value is the fact that none of them has been worked out by the police so far. Topping the list has been the brutal assault on Dr. Kashyap, medical officer in Tiloi, Rai Bareli in February. The miscreants who broke into his official residence hurt him grievously, fracturing both his arms and legs. Kashyap has not yet fully recovered and the culprits are still at large. The medical officer Tamkuhi deoria was attacked and robbed in January and so were medical officers from Mehmoodabad and district hospital, Lakhimpur. The attacks on the two eminent doctors all within a month had sent a shock wave in the district and had led to a local strike in Lakhimpur. But till date the police has not been able to make any headway in the case. Similarly, Dr. Anil Rao posted at mandi Tateri PHC in Baghpat was roughed up and looted in his house in May, while Dr. O.B. Srivastava, deputy CMO and his physician son were killed by unknown miscreants in Meerut. Alarmed at the growing cult of violence, the association had submitted a proposal to the state government last year to provide for security, but has failed to evoke any response.

Superintendent of medical college hospital at Kolkata Attacked

Superintendents of various city hospitals were divided on how to react following the attack on the superintendent of medical college hospital, Sachidananda Sinha. Observers said on Monday that the CPM has managed to drive a wedge between them. Seven hospital superintendents met at medical college hospital during the day. While a few expressed their desire to begin a peaceful agitation from tuesday, the majority differed. a few supers said that they would go to work as usual but not sign the attendance register in protest. a majority of them, however, refused to do so, said a doctor at MCH. Superintendent of the SSKM Hospital was not present at the meeting. City doctors affiliated to various organizations, however, openly expressed their displeasure following the bail given to three persons on monday arrested on sunday for charges of assault. They also criticized the failure of the police to take any action against left front chief whip Lakshmi Dey. In the evening, rebel Trinamul Congress leader Ajit Panja visited mch though neither the superintendent nor the college principal was there to meet him. College secretary Mahendra Chakraborty claimed that they had been summoned to writers' buildings and said that he would not comment on the incident as he was not in office on sunday. Sources, however, said that Dr. Sinha had been forcibly admitted to sskm hospital to prevent him from speaking to Panja or the media. Sinha's wife Soma broke into tears in front of Panja . . . after beating up my husband and son, they are now calling us up and asking us not to speak to the media, she said . . . please do something for us. These illegal structures were criminal dens. My mother is sick and she had to watch us being beaten up by hooligans while Lakshmi Dey stood by the police arrived after the mob had left, Sinha's 19-year-old son Rupam told Panja. Incidentally, Dr. Sinha is already in trouble with the state government as he has resisted at least two attempts to transfer him and cases are still pending in court. I have never heard of such an incident in my 40 years of political life. We support the government in their move to evict squatters. It is a conspiracy and the government is standing behind Dey and the others. We will give them till friday to arrest Dey. If not done, we will start an agitation, said Panja. The state health services association has condemned the attack on Sinha and demanded action against the criminals. According to president of the association, Dr. Sanjib Mukherjee, we are distressed to note that the hooligans belonged to the ruling party. We feel that political interference in government hospitals is a hindrance to proper functioning. The Indian Medical Association, Kolkata branch, has demanded the arrest of those named in the fir, failing which they would begin an agitation in all the medical colleges. The IMA will also observe Tuesday as 'protest day' and doctors will wear black badges to work. Speaking about Sunday's incident, Lakshmi Dey said, .out of the 27 workers, six would be rehabilitated as they had worked regularly for the director of the school of tropical medicines. after I was assured of this I left the hospital . . . it is sad that I am being blamed for the incident. It is being wrongly said that I was present when the superintendent was attacked. I am deeply hurt at such accusations," he said.

Junior doctors strike in Surat

The strike called by nearly 150 junior doctors of the Junior Doctors' Association (JDA), New Civil Hospital (NCH), on Sunday, was called off on Monday evening as the hospital authorities assured the agitating doctors of meeting their demands. The strike was called after a junior doctor was allegedly beaten by a patient's relative on Sunday evening. Dr. Chintan Patel was allegedly slapped. by one Rashid Mirza, elder brother of patient Ayub Mirza, at the E-1 ward of New Civil Hospital (NCH), on Sunday evening.

According to hospital sources, Ayub (28) was admitted to the hospital on Wednesday afternoon with severe burn injuries. On Sunday afternoon, Dr. Chintan called Ayub for a dressing to be done. With the patient reporting late, the doctor apparently rebuked him, following which he succumbed to his injuries.

When Rashid arrived at the hospital and learnt from his relatives that Dr. Chintan Patel had allegedly kicked the patient, he went to Dr. Chintan and apparently slapped him before the patients and other hospital staff. The security guards and other doctors arrived at the scene and controlled the situation.

The members of the Junior Doctors' Association (JDA), irked by the incident, declared a strike from Sunday evening. Dr. Chintan later lodged a complaint against Rashid with the Umra police station.

New Civil hospital Superintendent M.K. Wadhel office met the agitating doctors today and assured them that security would be stepped up on the hospital premises. Following which, the doctors called off their strike.

JDA vice-president Dr. Devendra Choudhary said, "We had earlier demanded the higher authorities to increase the security of doctors as a similar incident had taken place earlier. We also apprised him of the other problems like lack of drinking water, no reading room and high rates charged by the canteen."

Dr. Choudhary added, "We called off the strike as our tutors and professors had already booked their tickets for Diwali vacations and if we continued with the strike, they would have to attend the patients."

Hospital superintendent Dr. M.K. Wadhel said, "The relatives of the patient had alleged that Dr. Chintan kicked the patient. After the incident, we have increased the security and there are 15 security persons deployed in the hospital area."

He added: "We had called extra staffers from all the community health care centres and they are on duty in the hospital. Work was not stopped as the tutors and professors were also asked to treat patients."

Ludhiana IMA gives strike call to protest the assault on doctors

On a call given by the Indian Medical Association (IMA), Ludhiana, doctors and medical students held a demonstration and took out a protest march from Batra Hotel to the Mini Secretariat today, in order to protest the assault on doctors and registration of cases against doctors under Section 304A of the Indian Penal Code. The doctors also presented a memorandum to the administration demanding action against those who indulge in violence against the doctors, and not to register case against the doctors under section 304A of the Indian Penal Code. The protest was organised following a recent incident of ransacking of a hospital at Jamalpur owned by Dr. Rakesh Aggarwal. Dr. Aggarwal was threatened with dire consequences and his staff beaten, following a case of alleged negligence in which a patient had died.

The association representatives stated that in the recent case, the police did not act against the unruly mob which attacked the doctor and hospital, and rather booked him under section 304A. They said that even now the doctor was getting constant threats. Such incidents have created a feeling of insecurity and panic among the doctors, they said.

"A doctor cannot be treated like a criminal since unless there is complete evidence to prove it", said Dr. Arun Mitra, president of IMA, Ludhiana. While citing the Supreme Court ruling on death in a hospital, Dr. Rajeev Gupta added that since no doctor would deliberately do something that results in the death of a patient, a doctor should not be treated like a criminal.

Members of Punjab Medical Representatives Association, doctors from DMC and other hospitals also participated in the protest.

A deputation comprising Dr. Arun Mitra, Dr. Rajeev Gupta, Dr. Narotam Dewan, Dr. Savita Nauhria, Dr. Manoj Sobti, Dr. Subhas Batta, Dr. Karamveer Goyal, Dr. Kulwant Singh and Dr. Gurpreet Singh Wander met the Deputy Commissioner in this regard. The members of the association also met Senior Superintendent Police R.K. Jaiswal.

According to the members of the delegation, the SSP assured the doctors of registering case against those who indulged in violence and withdraw case against Dr. Rakesh Aggarwal. Dr. Gupta said the SSP added that he would look into the security aspect of the doctors.

Himachal Pradesh assures to protect the doctors

Chief Minister Prem Kumar Dhumal today announced that the State Government would make an appropriate law to deal with instances of doctors being manhandled and their private infrastructure being damaged by relatives of patients. Speaking on the occasion of the third Annual Conference of the State Chapter of Indian Medical Association (IMA), the Chief Minister said cases of public are against doctors was on the rise and a law needed to be made to protect them. "If a patient suffers because of the negligence of the doctor, then the doctor would have to face the legal consequences, but if the patient dies despite the best efforts of the doctor, the government will ensure that the doctor gets due protection for his life and property," the Chief Minister said.

The Chief Minister said Medical Advisory Council would be formed to advise the government on bettering the health services and the State of health infrastructure in the State. He asked Health Minister Rajiv Bindal to ensure that the process of formation of the Council was expedited. On the occasion Mr. Dhumal also honoured some eminent doctors of Himachal Pradesh, who were providing super specialty services at the PGI, Chandigarh or other hospitals in the neighbouring states.

Punjab also passes a bill to protect doctors

Welcoming the decision to pass the Bill pertaining to the assault on doctors by the Punjab Assembly, the Indian Medical Association (IMA), Chandigarh Chapter today thanked the state Government for taking care of the interests of the medical fraternity. A Bill to provide for the protection of Medicare Service Persons and Medicare Service Institution and for the prevention of violence and damage to property was passed in the state assembly recently. Dr. Zora Singh, president of IMA, said: "The absence of the Act was causing problems to genuine patients who were being referred to other hospitals, because of the fear that some anti-social elements may ransack the hospital and assault the doctors if there is any complication in the case or in the view of the death of a patient."

Maharashtra doctors cry for safety

Doctors across the city of Mumbai observed a one day token strike to protest against the spate of incidents where medical practitioners have been assaulted, and the hospital property has been destroyed. The Indian Medical Association (IMA-Maharashtra) representing over 22,000 doctors, has asked for stringent laws so that attacks on doctors becomes a non-bailable offence, like it is in some southern states like Tamil Nadu, Kerala and Andhra Pradesh.

Chembur Ghatkopar Plus spoke to Dr. Vinod Kharkhare, owner of Shree Hospital, situated at Central Avenue Road, Chembur, to know more about the mob attack at his premises recently. Spelling out the details of the riot, Dr. Kharkhare, a senior doctor who has been practising since 1978 says, "This is the first time in 28 years that my hospital has been targeted. On September 28, a patient named Balasaheb Punde, aged 50 years, came to my clinic. He had been suffering from TB since 1983. His condition was serious, and I was told that two other hospitals had refused him admission. Moreover, he did not have the required cash to pay the deposit money. We admitted him on humanitarian grounds in the ICU. Following detailed investigations by our doctors, it was detected that he also suffered from heart problems. Next day he suffered a cardiac arrest; despite our intensive treatment, we could not save his life. Hearing this news, the patient's younger son made a hasty phone call and all of a sudden a mob of over 80 persons stormed into the hospital. Three staff members, including the young consultant present at that time was manhandled. Telephones, computers, furniture, glass panes, flower pots, etc. were all damaged by the mob. Almost 30 police personnel were needed to control the crowd.

Dr. Kharkhare adds, "While I insisted on conducting a postmortem, the senior police inspector Raut, from Chembur police station, who was at the site, took down a written statement from the relatives of the patients stating that they had no complaints against the doctors and the hospital. Even after chasing the police for two days, no FIR was lodged. As per law the police could have booked them under various sections of the IPC. In desperation, I approached a popular regional newspaper. It was only after the news was flashed that the DCP Dilip Sawant took action and lodged an FIR. Till date only one arrest has been made, although the police present at the site saw a mob of 80 attacking us. I have now written letters to all the top officials like the police commissioner, revenue minister Narayan Rane and home minister R.R. Patil, because more than my own safety, I feel responsible towards my staff."

Supporting the cause, Dr. Anil Brado, the president of IMA, Chembur unit, says, "Such disturbing incidents are taking place almost every fortnight, in some parts of the city. This kind of mob attack on doctors is unacceptable. Nobody likes mortality, but death is inevitable, which the public has to understand. Doctors as a group feel that such assaults are a direct attack on the medical fraternity. The culprits indulging in such acts know very well that they can get away easily because in Maharashtra this is a bailable offence

Dr. Swaroop Bhale Patil is hoping that the order passed by the Andhra Pradesh government on Monday to hold assault against doctors as a non-bailable offence, punishable with imprisonment up to three years, is implemented across India. Bhalepatil left Mumbai after he was assaulted earlier this year. Bhalepatil, who was part of the team of doctors at the Bhagwati Morgue, was beaten up by NCP workers for allegedly demanding money to release bodies of victims of the Laxmi Chhaya building collapse in Borivli this July. While those who had assaulted him and blackened his face were released on bail within three days, Bhalepatil said he was so humiliated that he moved out of Mumbai three-and-a-half months ago to avoid further harassment. Speaking to MID DAY from Nashik, Bhalepatil said, " Just like the residents of Laxmi Chhaya, my life changed forever after the incident. My family is still traumatized. My wife, who was a lecturer at an engineering college, had to leave her job at short notice. The AP rule should not only be implemented in Maharashtra, but all across India, so that doctors can practice without fear. Bhalepatil is now a forensic medicine professor at Maratha Vidya Prasarak Samaja's Medical College in Nashik. The Maharashtra Association of Resident Doctors (MARD), which had supported Bhalepatil's cause, now plans to push for the new rule here too. Dr. Mahadev Bansode, president, MARD, said such incidents take place at least twice a month and have left doctors feeling insecure. "The only way to make our voices heard is to go on strike. But we can't do that every second day and put our patients in jeopardy, said Bansode.

However, some believe this new law won't be too useful. Dr. Arun Bal of Association for Consumer Action in Safety and Health said assault is already a criminal offence that warrants arrest. "This, however, rarely happens. Any new law will also need to be implemented by the police. What's the point of getting a new law when the current one hasn't made any difference?" he said.

Meanwhile, on Saturday, Police Commissioner D.N. Jadhav issued a circular to all stations stating that if any person assaults a doctor, a case needs to be registered. The matter was recently raised in the Assembly as well.

Bangalore branch of IMA condemns assault on doctors

In a press release here on Friday, the IMA supported the protest staged by its Shimoga branch. The IMA has demanded, among other things, police protection for doctors on duty and an Ordinance to make assault on doctors and other hospital staff a non-bailable offence.

Tension prevailed at Rajnagar since last night after the death of a 14-year old boy in the Rajanagar Public Health Centre allegedly due to wrong diagnosis and negligence of the doctors.

Some irate relatives of the deceased boy along with some locals allegedly assaulted the doctors last night. They also staged road blockade by laying the dead body on the road at Gopalpur under Rajnagar police station, said Officer-in-Charge of Rajnagar Police station Subash Panda.

According to police Abhaya Kumar Roul of Badaolara village was suffering from fever. Dr. K.C. Mishra, a paediatric doctor of the PHC allegedly treated him for typhoid. But later a medicine specialist diagonised that he was suffering from cerebral malaria and advised his relatives to take him to SCB Medical College and Hospital, Cuttack after his condition deteriorated. The boy died while being taken to Cuttack. Later the relatives of the boy assaulted the doctors and blocked the road and demanded compensation to the family members of the deceased. The blockade was removed this afternoon after the intervention of the Chief District Medical Officers and other senior officials.

The CDMO assured to order a departmental inquiry and take action if the doctors were found guilty. Three cases were registered in connection with the incident while two cases were filed by both the parties and a case was filed for illegal road blockade.

Haryana to follow Punjab

Haryana is going to follow Punjab in passing a bill that extends protection to doctors, vulnerable to be assaulted by aggrieved attendants of patients. Modalities are being worked out to form a Haryana protection for medicare service persons and medicare service institutions (Prevention of violence and damage to property, Ordinance)', for which the Punjab model is being studied. Punjab's initiative to pass such an ordinance, becoming third state in the country to do so, has spurred private practitioners in Haryana to step up their efforts for a similar bill in the state to protect interests of doctors. The state branch of Indian Medical Association has submitted memorandums to the Haryana health minister and the chief minister, demanding such a legislative solution.

V.K. Bhatia, president of IMA, Panipat, who led the delegation of doctors to meet the chief minister on Wednesday informed *The Times of India*, "There have been at least 50 cases of assault on doctors across Haryana in the past six months. This is a very worrying condition for us since doctors stand to lose hardearned reputation besides being mentally harassed." Such a bill, added he, will also work in the interest of the patients as it will empower the doctor to take up serious cases without fear. "As of now, doctors prefer to play it safe and there is a certain restlessness in taking up very serious cases," he said.

"We are studying Punjab model of the bill passed to work out modalities as to how a similar bill can be worked out in the state," said Avinash Sharma, Director General, Health Services, Haryana.

Two weeks ago, a patient died in a private hospital in Jhajjar, after being rushed there in a critical condition. His relatives threatened the doctor, manhandled him besides shouting slogans against him.

In another case, a fortnight ago, a doctor's clinic in Bahadurgarh, was attacked by relatives of a patient, who died due to alleged negligence of the doctor.

The bill in Punjab, as in Andhra Pradesh and Tamil Nadu, has prohibited violence against medicare service persons or damage to property. Any offender found guilty of this is liable to face an imprisonment of three years along with a fine of up to Rs. 50,000, besides being liable to pay a penalty of twice the amount of purchase price of medical equipment damaged. (*The Times of India,* September 18th, 2008).

Doctors rapid burnout: need for counseling

The overwork and poor working conditions expose the doctors to early and rapid burnout. This has to be prevented by various ways including improvement of the working conditions of the doctors and their counseling. A study carried out on Norwegian doctors seemed to indicate the need and the benefits of such counseling to the doctors.

"A short-term counseling intervention was effective in reducing burnout and stress in a cohort of Norwegian clinicians, according to the results of a study published online November 12 in the *British Medical Journal.*

"Research on the mental health of doctors has led to a call for preventive interventions to lower the risk of burnout and mental distress," write Karin E. Isaksson Rø, MDr, from the Research Institute, Modum Bad, in Vikersund, Norway, and colleagues. "Early intervention programmes could ensure that practising doctors in trouble get help in time, before their problems interfere with care of patients and give rise to medical errors, but such programmes have been poorly investigated."

At a Norwegian resource center, 227 physicians participated in a counseling intervention during 2003 to 2005 and completed a self-reported assessment at 1 year. The intervention consisted of individual counseling lasting 1 day or group-based counseling lasting 1 week, aimed at motivating reflection on and acknowledgement of the physicians' situation and personal needs. Primary endpoints were levels of burnout, measured with the Maslach burnout inventory, and predictors of reduced emotional exhaustion, based on linear regression.

Of 185 physicians (81%) who completed 1-year follow-up, 88 were men and 97 were women. On a scale of 1 to 5, the mean level of emotional exhaustion significantly decreased from 3.00 ± 0.94 to 2.53 ± 210 (0.76 to 6.76; P< 001), which was similar to the level found in a representative sample of 390 Norwegian physicians. In addition, participants had decreased their working hours by 1.6 ± 11.4 hours/week.

The proportion of physicians on full-time sick leave decreased from 35% (63 of 182 physicians) at baseline to 6% (10 of 182 physicians) at follow-up, and the proportion that had undergone psychotherapy increased from 20% (36 of 182 physicians) to 53% (97 of 182 physicians). After adjustment for sex, age, and personality dimensions, reduction in emotional exhaustion in the overall cohort was independently associated with reduced number of work hours per week (ß = 0.17; P = .03). Among men, "satisfaction with the intervention" was an independent predictor of reduced emotional exhaustion (ß = 0.25; P = .04).

"A short-term counseling intervention could contribute to reduction in emotional exhaustion in doctors," the study authors write. "This was associated with reduced working hours for the whole cohort and, in men, was predicted by satisfaction with the intervention."

Study limitations include an inability to determine causality, lack of further analyses of subgroups possibly causing a false negative finding (type 2 error), regression analyses for each sex also subject to possible type 2 errors, and possible recall bias.

"Considering doctors' reluctance to seek help, despite high levels of distress, it is important to offer interventions that facilitate access and that can enhance motivation to reconsider personal and professional priorities when necessary," the study authors write. "The indications of factors possibly contributing to reduction in emotional exhaustion need to be further investigated with a more controlled design."

The Norwegian Women's Public Health Association and Modum Bad psychiatric hospital supported this study. Dr. Rø has been employed at the resource center, Villa Sana, and was reimbursed for a presentation of preliminary results at an internal meeting of the Norwegian Medical Association. (*BMJ*, Published online November 12, 2008.)

Doctor's liability is a big issue

Five reforms are essential to solve the medical liability crisis. The following proposals have come from USA:

A. First, a new medical tort and liability insurance system modeled after the one enacted in California, which has stabilized that state's system and maintained open access to courts for all patients.

1. Liability rates up 168 percent in California compared to national average of 420 percent.
2. Cost of settlements in California 53% lower than national average.
3. California cases settled in average of three years *vs.* national average of four.
4. Injured patients compensated more quickly in California than in any other state but Minnesota.
5. California reforms have lowered health care costs by estimated six percent—saving patients $6 BILLION every year on health care.
6. California now has a system working for benefit of patients—not trial lawyers.

B. The second major reform is; It is Not fair for a doctor not in same specialty to be an expert witness in a malpractice case—just as it does not make sense for a plumber to evaluate the work of an electrician. Expert witnesses should be:
   - Practicing same specialty in Maryland;
   - Board certified;
   - Specially licensed by State;
   - Subject to peer review and subject to sanctions in the event of false testimony.
   - Court brings witnesses to eliminate bias or incentives to give certain testimonies.

C. Third, stronger "Good Samaritan" protections are called for. Don't punish doctors for donating care to critically ill, often uninsured patients. Make volunteer care economically feasible to keep retiring doctors practicing. Establish immunity for ER/ trauma care officials who cannot get patient consent.

D. Fourth, a Health Care Court can block frivolous lawsuits from making it to court and further cut down on legal costs.
   1. This reform is already working in Indiana.
   2. System evaluates merits of malpractice claims before they go into the legal system.
   3. One attorney and three health care professionals define standard of care and decide whether it has been violated.

E. Fifth, medical liability insurance reform that includes accountability, transparency and a healthy respect for competition among providers of malpractice coverage to Maryland doctors.
   1. Accountability means requiring Med Mutual to disclose its rate setting practices to doctors—because it's "doctor-owned."
   2. Transparency means letting doctors know about Med Mutual's practices, full investigatory authority for the Maryland Insurance Commissioner and full disclosure to

any legislative body that seeks oversight without throwing up protections that information is proprietary, etc.

3. Competition means looking into the potential or actual conflict of interest of MedChi and Med Mutual in allowing commissions to be paid to Med Mutual. Competition also means possible changes in the criteria at the Maryland Insurance Administration to allow more companies full access.

"Why should I care if doctors get a pay cut or loses his job or is hauled up in a court of law?" a patient recently asked me. Therein lies the delicate dilemma physicians face today. While the common perception is that the medical profession is well-compensated, there are serious implications in targeting physician pay to control medical spending. Congress recently passed a bill protecting doctors from a 10.6% cut in Medicare payments, overriding President Bush's veto in the process. The U.S. boasts the world's most expensive health care system. The Costs exceed $2 trillion annually and outpaces inflation and growth in national income. In an attempt to cut costs, Medicare has instituted a formula that calls for regular decreases in physician payment of more than 20% by 2010.

The number of physicians who do not accept new Medicare patients is dramatic; in states like Texas, this number can exceed 40%. No wonder, as Medicare pays less than half of doctors' fees. This scenario comes as a record number of Boomers approach Medicare age. Those without Medicare are not spared the consequences. Seniors sometimes delay their care, leading to expensive treatment in the emergency department. Doctors who lose money seeing Medicare patients could pass on the costs to the privately insured.

According to the Kaiser Family Foundation, there are more significant drivers of health costs, including new prescription drugs, technology and administrative needs. Princeton economist Uwe Reinhardt estimates that physicians' take-home pay represents roughly 10% of national health care spending. Cutting physician pay by 20% would only reduce spending by 2%.

A more effective option would be for the government to enhance the nation's primary care by paying physicians to coordinate care between specialists, install electronic medical records and encourage patient communication via e-mail or telephone. *The New York Times* recently reported that a pilot program increasing primary care spending in North Carolina saved Medicaid upwards of $160 million in 2006.

Furthermore, improving access to providers such as internal medicine and family physicians would provide timely care and keep patients out of the hospital and emergency room. With medical spending estimated to rise nearly 10% annually, costs need to be curbed. But by focusing on physician payments, government alienates the profession for little in return. Dutch doctors have welcomed a Supreme Court ruling that a patient can be ordered to give blood for an HIV test in order to limit injury to a doctor during treatment. After an appeal process lasting more than two years, the court concluded that the need to limit the damage to a doctor outweighed the relatively minor infringement of the patient's rights. The judgment goes beyond previous similar cases, which involved a rape or biting by someone suspected of being HIV positive. In such cases, a patient not accused of deliberately or irresponsibly spreading an infection was still required to cooperate.

In 2001 a doctor in a dental surgery at the Alkmaar Medical Centre, north of Amsterdam, removed a molar from a remand prisoner. In doing so, he cut his finger on an instrument used in the treatment, resulting in blood contact with his patient. The patient was considered to have an increased risk of HIV infection because of a history of drug misuse. However, the doctor's request for a blood sample was rejected for fear it could influence the patient's forthcoming trial. The doctor successfully took legal action to order the patient to give blood, with the results being made known only to the doctor and the patient's legal representative. Meanwhile, he had begun prophylactic treatment despite possible .serious and damaging side effects.

The case was appealed finally to the Supreme Court on the grounds that it violated rights to privacy and physical integrity enshrined in the Dutch constitution. The Supreme Court concluded that the violation of the patient's right was .relatively minor as the blood test involved no danger to the patient's health and the results could be restricted to only those who needed to know. This was outweighed by the doctor's interest in knowing if he was infected with HIV especially if he was considering beginning treatment with serious side effects.

The court argued the medical treatment agreement could involve reasonable and fair. limits to rights, including a degree of care towards each other. The patient can be required, even after the end of the agreement, to act within reasonable limits, to restrict damage caused to the doctor during treatment.

Johan Legemaate, coordinator of legal policy for the Royal Dutch Medical Association (KNMG), said the case had a big psychological impact on doctors, who have felt that discussions aboutpatients' rights were often one sided. It does not change the overall situation of patients' rights and doctors' duties but it is very important for doctors to feel that, in specific situations, they have rights too, he said.

Doctor's Rights; USA takes a lead

In July, Deborah Kotz wrote about a possible new federal rule designed to protect health care providers from being denied employment or fired if they, say, refused to administer emergency contraception or certain forms of birth control because of their religious or moral beliefs. Dozens of health organizations, including the American College of Obstetricians and Gynecologists and the American Medical Association, voiced their fierce opposition, saying that such a rule would deny women access to full reproductive care. In a poll, 92 percent said they were against the regulation, while 8 percent favored it. As it turns out, this draft rule was formally proposed at the end of last month and could become a reality on September 25 after the period ends for submitting comments.

The proposed rule states: "Any entity, including a state or local government, that carries out any part of any health service program funded in whole or in part under a program administered by the Department of Health and Human Services . . . shall not require any individual to perform or assist in the performance of any part of a health service program or research activity funded by the Department if such service or activity would be contrary to his religious beliefs or moral convictions."

Women's health activists are continuing to voice their collective dissent; as, for example, in this op-ed by Sen. Hillary Clinton of New York and Cecile Richards, president of Planned Parenthood, which was recently published in the *New York Times*.

I asked attorney Judy Waxman, vice-president for health and reproductive rights at the National Women's Law Center, to discuss how this new regulation could affect our medical care. I was surprised to hear her say that "the rule is not just about abortion and birth control."

Could a woman be denied an abortion at, say, a Planned Parenthood clinic that accepts federal funds for family planning services? It's possible, but I'm more concerned about what's going to happen in doctor's offices. The rule is so broad that it includes not only physicians but nurses, lab technicians, receptionists, and anyone else who works there. For instance, a receptionist could theoretically refuse to schedule an appointment for a woman wishing to have an IUD inserted because the device may cause the expulsion of a fertilized egg, which the receptionist considers to be abortion. A maintenance worker may refuse to clean rooms used for abortions.

Does the rule still define pregnancy as fertilization of an egg, as the previous draft rule did?

No, that part was taken out, but the latest version basically leaves the question open, leaving it up to individual health care workers to decide whatever it is that they morally object to. A nurse, for example, could refuse to provide counseling to cancer patients about freezing eggs or sperm before chemotherapy if he or she morally objects to artificial fertility treatments. And, in an effort to discourage promiscuity, a pediatrician may decline to provide the vaccine that protects against the sexually transmitted HPV virus to teenagers.

What about the rights of patients in all of this?

We're certainly most concerned about this. Women are the ones who will lose out here, and this proposed rule contradicts other laws on the books that protect employers' rights—which in this case would be the health care facility trying to provide these services to patients. Title VII of the Civil Rights Act has a provision that says that an employer is obligated to accommodate an employee's religious beliefs *unless it presents a burden for the employer*. So a large pharmacy chain with several pharmacists on duty can afford to have one pharmacist who won't dispense birth control if others behind the counter will. A small family-owned shop may not be able to do that.

Will you take legal action to combat this rule?

We're hoping that the Department of Health and Human Services comes to its senses, after reading all the public comments, and doesn't issue a final regulation. But we'd consider bringing a lawsuit if this goes forward.

Reforming Health Care and Parents' Rights

In pursuing health care reform, federal and state policymakers alike need to respect and protect parental rights and responsibilities. Currently, they are not doing so, said Daniel P. Moloney.

A 14-year-old grade-school girl in Kentucky arrives at the local health clinic seeking birth control. Who should decide whether she receives it? The doctor? The girl? Or her parents? The state legislature says that the girl is not even old enough to consent to sexual activity. Yet public officials, under authorization from Congress, have written rules that allow the girl to enroll in one of a number of federal programs, and this federal law would overrule state law and prohibit the clinic from informing her parents.

A Common Problem

Thousands of similar situations occur each year— not surreptitiously, but legally, under the authority of policies and laws, some of which have been in place for decades. In exercising this authority, government intrudes into some of our most intimate living arrangements, separating parents from children, and putting the family doctor at odds with the wishes of the parents.

As a result, the moral values of ordinary people are often replaced by those of a health care establishment composed of government bureaucrats, liberal professional organizations, industry lobbyists, and major hospital systems. Because they control the funding and set the health care policies, they can, and often do, pre-empt many Americans from making health care decisions that reflect their own values.

In the continuing debate over major reforms in federal health care policy, these moral concerns are often overshadowed by other challenges— such as controlling health care costs and providing accessible health insurance to low-income Americans. But in addressing these problems, policymakers at the state and federal level must not choose solutions that would override individuals' deeply held convictions. This is especially important in our religiously and morally pluralistic society.

The debate over health care solutions is focused on two broad and very different approaches to comprehensive reform. One is a government-controlled insurance program, either centrally managed and regulated or based almost exclusively on government payment. The other is based on personal choice and market competition, where individuals and families make the key financial decisions, particularly when it comes to insurance coverage, benefits, medical procedures, and treatments. On the question of whose moral values are controlling the sensitive matter of health care decision-making, these two approaches are worlds apart.

A national health insurance program, government-run or government-controlled, would centralize control over health care financing and delivery, and would centralize the power of approved third-party payers to impose their values on a morally pluralistic society. Political decisions would, in effect, supplant moral ones. A reform based on personal choice and competition in a pluralistic market would ensure that patients—or in the case of minors, their parents—exercise the primary control over how their health care dollars are spent, allowing them to make health care decisions that are consistent with their values. A market-based reform, in other words, is inherently compatible with parental authority.

The Bureaucratic Suppression of Moral Decisions

Current federal health insurance programs routinely govern the health care of minors in ever larger numbers, and in so doing, government officials pre-empt or interfere with important decisions that should be made by parents. In contrast, new policies that would inject principles of consumer choice and competition into the financing and delivery of health care can restore respect for the primary relationships between parents and children, leaving families free to live according to their moral convictions.

To better understand how government currently intrudes on these relationships, consider again the 14-year-old girl in Kentucky requesting birth control at a health clinic. Examine further the details from this real-life case.

The girl told the doctor that she was not yet sexually active, but that the mother of her boyfriend, who had driven her to the clinic, wanted her on birth control so that her son would not father a child out of wedlock if they were to have sex. The girl wants her boyfriend to like her, she told the doctor, and she wanted to remain on good terms with his mother. That's why she was asking to be put on prescription birth control. However, she does not want her parents to find out. Because the girl requested confidentiality, the doctor had her enroll in a federal program to pay for the contraception, so that the charges would not show up on her parents' insurance bill.

Unless they pay close attention to the health care debates in state legislatures, typical Americans are unaware of the intrusiveness of current government policy. Representatives of professional health care organizations often argue that minors should be allowed to receive reproductive health care without their parents' knowledge or consent. The American Association of Pediatrics states bluntly, "Comprehensive health care of adolescents should include a sexual history that should be obtained in a safe, non-threatening environment through open, honest, and nonjudgmental communication, with assurances of confidentiality. . . . The primary reason adolescents hesitate or delay obtaining family planning or contraceptive services is concern about confidentiality." Specifically for this reason, Congress enacted a federal law, popularly known as Title X, which provides that whenever a sexually active minor seeks confidential birth control, she is to be treated independently from her parents. Therefore, she can accept birth control without consulting her parents, and if she requests confidentiality without parental knowledge, the government will foot the bill for her contraception and related medical costs, regardless of her parents' income.

Under current law, Congress makes confidential access to birth control for school-age girls such a priority that it picks up the tab even for services that the girl's family insurance would cover. Since federal law trumps state law, it does not matter that the laws of her state deem her too young to consent to sex.

Limiting Medical Judgment

Doctors make delicate decisions about teen health care every day, but current federal confidentiality rules can render it nearly impossible for a doctor to perform the medical action that his professional judgment demands. Consider, for example, the case of the 16-year-old boy in North Carolina who went to his pediatrician complaining of severe daily headaches. The doctor questioned the boy after his mother stepped out of the room, and discovered that the boy regularly used marijuana and cocaine, and occasionally LSD, hallucinogenic mushrooms, and Ecstasy. The doctor informed the boy that his headaches might be related to his drug use, and recommended that he undergo treatment for substance abuse. The doctor asked for permission to tell his mother, and the boy said no. He said he was not afraid of his parents' reaction; he simply thought he had his drug use under control, it was no big deal, and his parents would not care. Under North Carolina law, if the child is on private insurance and the doctor judges the matter "essential to the life or health of a minor," he can ignore the boy's request for confidentiality and tell the mother about his addiction. In this case, the doctor did tell the mother, and the boy was enrolled in a drug treatment program a few weeks later.

The Medicaid Angle

If the child's family had been on Medicaid instead of private insurance, the story would have been different. Under federal law, Medicaid prohibits any doctor from breaching the confidentiality of any patient, even to the parents of children. Had the boy's family been enrolled in Medicaid, the law would have enforced his right to confidential medical care, deferring to the short-term self-interest of a drug-addicted minor and overruling the doctor's expert judgment regarding his objective medical needs.

In both of these real cases, federal laws and the reigning ethos of the professional health care associations intrude on intimate health care choices of parents and families. In both cases, they exclude parents from key decisions regarding the welfare of their own children. In both cases, they impose one set of values on the entire country, trampling on local and state laws reflecting their communities' deliberate moral judgments.

Government Health Programs Separate Parents and Children

Problems of parental choice and control are typical in federal health care programs, especially in Medicaid, SCHIP, and Title X.

Medicaid, for instance, prohibits parental notification for any medical procedure it covers. This means that children are not required to notify their parents if, while on Medicaid, they receive any of the following medical services (this list is not exhaustive):

- abortions (in the cases of rape, incest, and the life of the mother),
- birth control,
- pregnancy tests,
- the morning-after pill,
- tests for sexually transmitted diseases,
- gynecological exams,
- prescription drugs,
- treatment for drug abuse,
- treatment for psychiatric disorders (including depression, suicide, and attention deficit disorder),
- sexual-orientation counseling, and
- personalized sexual education.

As in the example of the drug-using teenager above, the doctor is prohibited from informing the parent of a child on Medicaid about the case, even if the doctor believes it is in the best interests of the child, unless he can obtain the consent of the minor.

SCHIP. Medicaid is a welfare program. While children from working and middle-class families are not eligible for Medicaid, they are often eligible for another federal program called the State Children's Health Insurance Program (SCHIP). In a number of states, however, this program is an extension of Medicaid and offers many of the same services—including abortion, birth control, psychiatric treatment, substance-abuse treatment, prescription drugs, and sex education—but specifically for children.

Under SCHIP each state can elect to apply Medicaid's rules, or to design an entirely different program from scratch. Despite this flexibility, however, all 50 states continue to offer Medicaid-style family planning services for children, and most states have also continued Medicaid's policies regarding confidential care for minors. As a result, children from middle-class families are frequently able to receive these services without their parents' knowledge.

Title X. In addition to Medicaid and SCHIP, which pay for a full range of medical care, the federal government also has a special program that funds only reproductive health care and activities related to population control, the above-mentioned Title X. Under Title X, a clinic charges its clients based on their ability to pay for its services, from wealthy clients who pay full price to lower-income patients who pay a nominal fee or nothing at all.

While Medicaid and SCHIP only pay for children who qualify for their programs, the Title X program will completely cover confidential birth control for any child who is not independently wealthy. Once a girl asks that her parents not be notified, as in the case of the 14-year-old Kentucky girl, the government pays for her services, which include birth control, the morning-after pill, gynecological examinations, and abortion. The Alan Guttmacher Institute, the research arm of Planned Parenthood, says that Title X is the "gold standard" of teen confidentiality rules, and it lobbies federal and state lawmakers to incorporate these rules into every expansion of government control over health insurance.

Because Title X confidentiality rules are so strong and apply to children, clinics supported by the program can even facilitate statutory rape, whereby adult men molest minor girls. In January of 1996, a 13-year-old girl went to the McHenry County Health Clinic in Illinois to request Depo-Provera, a long-term contraceptive injection. She told the doctor that she was sexually active and that she did not want her parents to know, so she received confidential services just like the 14-year-old Kentucky girl. After she received a prescription for the injection, her sex partner—her 37-year-old former teacher at Crystal Lake Middle School--drove her home from the clinic. They returned for follow-up shots on multiple occasions before she finally told her parents in February 1997. More than two years later, when the parents tried to sue the clinic for facilitating statutory rape, a county judge ruled that the doctor's actions were legal under Title X.

Finally, parents should be aware that health clinics based in public schools receive funds from all three of these federal programs, and therefore are often governed by their rules prohibiting parental access to their children's health records. Nearly three-quarters of school-based clinics receive funds from Medicaid, and over half also receive funds from SCHIP. Many of these clinics receive Title X funds themselves or have contracts with Title X clinics to provide reproductive services and sex education programs. In a school-based clinic that receives Title X funds, for example, a wealthy minor on private insurance can, at the discretion of the doctor, enroll in a government program that permits confidential access to birth control, STD testing, abortion, and more. Indeed, the movement toward including more elaborate clinics in public schools was in part to ensure that teenagers had access to confidential birth control.

Sound Health Care Reform can Return Power to Parents

Parents have the primary responsibility for their children, and thus ought to play a paramount role in any decisions affecting their children's lives. Doctors and government officials should certainly be allowed to contribute their professional advice or financial support, but the parents must have the ultimate right, in all but extraordinary circumstances, to raise their children the way they deem best. Medicaid, SCHIP, Title X, and other government health insurance programs routinely violate this most basic of principles. Members of Congress and state legislators alike should, therefore, take decisive steps to reform all three programs.

Obstacles to Change

Reform-minded legislators must be prepared, however, to overcome certain obstacles. Poorer parents often have no choice but to enroll in a government program such as Medicaid or SCHIP, and so are at the mercy of the health care establishment that sets the rules for the program. Because the government provides their health care, it determines the requirements to remain eligible—and the result is that it removes the right of the parent to make many of the key moral decisions that are only the parents' responsibility. Parents' only practical alternative is to accept those rules or not have any health insurance at all. If parents had the ability to choose from a variety of health care options, they could walk away from a situation in which they were not happy and seek better treatment elsewhere.

Most people receive their health insurance through the government or their employer, and do not have the personal power to change insurance companies except at a very high cost. As a result, insurance companies, hospitals, and doctors are not required to be as responsive to the demands of the patients as are suppliers of other goods and services in a normally functioning competitive economy. If more Americans controlled their own health insurance, and could easily switch insurance companies whenever a better health plan became available, the entire health care sector of the economy would become much friendlier to consumers and patients. Greater personal control over health care dollars, including where to purchase health insurance and from whom, would lead to a health care system far more responsive to people's needs than it is today— including their wish to have their deeply held moral views respected in the financing and delivery of care.

Key Principles of Sound Reform

Any reform that gives parents control over the health care decisions for their families should be based on four principles:

1. Individual patients, not employers or government bureaucrats, should be able to choose their health insurance coverage for themselves and their families.
2. Each person must be able to change insurance companies easily, without requiring an employment change or suffering major tax or regulatory penalties as in effect today.

3. Each person should have a variety of insurance plans from which to choose, including health plans that reflect different life situations and respect individual values.
4. Americans should be given ownership of their health insurance coverage so that an unaccountable third party does not have control over its contents and quality—and the values it embodies.

Parental Values

Parents have the right to pass on their moral values to their children. That right is often disregarded in the regular course of financing and delivering medical services. The disconnect between personal values, particularly traditional moral beliefs, and the reigning ethos is no more clearly demonstrated than in today's government-controlled health care programs. In these programs, the ethos governing health care reflects the values of the bureaucrats, professional organizations, industry lobbyists, and the administrators of big hospitals that embody the health care establishment.

Generally speaking, the representatives of these groups share a commitment to allowing children to receive sexual and mental health services without their parents' knowledge, consent, or involvement. While they may publicly warn legislators not to impose traditional moral values in the formulation or execution of public policy, they see no contradiction in the forcible imposition of their own moral perspectives throughout the health care system in every state in the country, overriding state laws and the protection of parents' rights. They can do this because the government programs that they control and influence are, practically speaking, the only health care options for many people.

Only Fundamental Health Care Reform will Restore Parents' Rights

The experience with Medicaid, SCHIP, Title X, and other government-funded health insurance programs illustrates the adage, "He who pays the piper, calls the tune." If someone other than the patient controls how the doctor is paid, someone other than the patient controls the moral decisions embodied in the financing and delivery of care.

For this reason, broad health care reform cannot simply tinker with the current system in which employers and the government officials retain the key levers of control. A federally administered national health insurance plan, based on a set of moral values determined by "experts," would be particularly threatening to parents, families, and all those who do not share the moral values of the health care establishment or of the reigning political party.

Parents have the primary responsibility for the welfare of their children, and policy-makers must respect their right to make decisions for their children. A central goal of any health care reform, therefore, must be to allow parents to own and control their family's health insurance. This would allow them to make key moral decisions that affect their children, restoring them to the role that is naturally and rightfully theirs.

Eroding Patients' Rights

In a write up in *The Tribune* dated Nov. 27, 2008 Himmat singh Gill justifies the right of life and right of death to any individual. In USA this debate is going on for quite some time. If you've been admitted to a hospital any time in the last five years, you've been asked whether you have an "advance directive". The Patient Self-Determination Act of 1990, which went into effect in December of 1991, requires all hospitals, nursing homes, and hospices to inform patients upon admission of their right to sign such a document. All of us have heard of a living will or durable power of attorney for health care. I venture to guess that most of us do not know what they really are.

What we are told we want to avoid at all costs in this day of high-tech health care is "being hooked up to a bunch of tubes and machines" should we become very ill. To be thus treated is appallingly undignified. In order to protect ourselves from being degraded in this manner, we are told, we should sign a living will or appoint a power of attorney for health care. If we don't, we may find ourselves the recipients of treatment we don't want (P.J King, RN Chairman, Bioethics Committee, Pro-Life Wisconsin).

It is vitally important to understand this: There is no law, no medical society, no religion, no church, and even no pro-life organization which insists on forcing a dying person to be kept alive by heroic or burdensome means. You need no advance directive to protect yourself from unwanted treatment. You (or your family members if you are unable) need only refuse it. The American Medical Association Code of Medical Ethics says that "physicians are not ethically obligated to deliver care that, in their best professional judgment, will not have a reasonable chance of benefiting their patients."

At least two things need to be understood about living wills. First, they are not about giving patients control over their health care; they are about taking away decision-making authority and giving it to the physician. A standard living will focuses on just one option—the rejection of medical care.

Secondly, we need to be aware that living wills do not protect patients; they protect doctors. A living will gives the physician immunity from civil or criminal liability for withholding or withdrawing treatment. Repeatedly court cases have illustrated that, once freed from liability, some doctors are willing to deny ordinary care—even food and water—to severely handicapped people who are not dying.

On the surface, a living will seems harmless enough. Below is the declaration from one such document:

If I should have a terminal illness and if I am no longer able to make decisions regarding my medical treatment, I direct my attending physician to withhold or withdraw treatment that only prolongs the dying process and is not necessary to my comfort or to alleviate pain.

This is the only part most people see. The laws and policies governing the use of living wills, however, explain how they are to be interpreted. These, few see. The U.S. Veterans Administration [Policy M-2, Part I, Chapter 31, 1991], for example, defines "terminal illness" as a "debilitating condition which is medically incurable . . . and which can be expected to cause death . . . [and] includes but is not limited to conditions where death is imminent, as well as chronic and debilitating conditions from which there is no reasonable hope of recovery." Such a definition would allow for the removal of life-sustaining treatment from persons with heart disease or diabetes. The "attending physician" is the physician responsible for caring for the patient at any given moment. "Treatment" is any intervention performed or ordered by the physician. Such interventions may include food, fluids, antibiotics, or insulin for a diabetic.

Living wills empower physicians, not patients. With a living will, the physician need not even consult with a patient's family regarding a non-treatment decision. Even if he does, he is under no obligation to follow their wishes.

A durable power of attorney for health care (DPAHC) provides for the appointment of another person to make medical decisions should the patient become unable to do so for himself. Because they share many of the features of living wills, they will not be discussed here at length. As with living will legislation, DPAHC laws allow life-sustaining treatment to be withdrawn from incompetent patients (in this case, at the request of their proxies), and protect physicians from civil or criminal liability for following proxies' instructions.

The concept of advance directives did not come about in a vacuum. Nor was it a product of human rights advocacy, as we are often led to believe. The living will was the brain child of the euthanasia movement and continues to be pushed by "right-to-die" proponents.

The first living will document was developed in 1967 by Luis Kutner for the Euthanasia Society of America (now called Choice in Dying) for the purpose of gaining public acceptance of euthanasia. A living will bill was first introduced to the Florida state legislature in 1975. The bill's author argued that the law could save Florida $5 billion if 90% of the state's mentally ill and mentally retarded were "allowed" to die. The Association for Retarded Persons and other groups defending the mentally impaired fought the bill, preventing its passage at that time. After a few years the offensive argument was forgotten, and a living will bill passed.

Choice in Dying (CID) has also been active in strengthening the Patient Self-Determination Act of 1990 (PSDA), working closely with Senators Danforth and Moynihan, the original sponsors of the bill. In 1994 CID staff conducted a briefing for all senators and their staff concerning "the role of advance directives within health care reform." President and Mrs. Clinton have also been active in pressing for people to sign living wills to control health care costs. As the President said in an interview with NBC's Tom Brokaw, signing living wills was "one way to weed some of them out."

The PSDA emerged amidst talk of scarce medical resources, health care rationing, and concern about the "graying" of America. In 1987, Dr. Otis Bowen, Secretary of HHS, testified before the Senate Finance Committee that the only way to attack high health care costs was to encourage Americans to write living wills. In 1990 the PSDA was passed as part of the Omnibus Budget Reconciliation Act.

Even supporters of living will legislation acknowledge problems. In the 12/5/92 issue of The New England Journal of Medicine (pp. 1666-1671) sixteen living will advocates reported "Sources of Concern about the Patient Self-Determination Act." Among these are:

1. Discussion of advance directives takes too much time and requires special training and competence [from physicians];
2. Treatment directives are not useful, because patients cannot really anticipate what their preferences will be in a future medical situation and because patients know too little about life-support systems and other treatment options;
3. Treatment-directive forms are too vague and open to divergent interpretations;
4. The incompetent patient's best interests should take precedence over even the most thoughtful choices of a patient while competent; and
5. Even if a directive is valid in all other respects, it is not a reliable guide to treatment because patients may change their mind.

The sixteen signers also criticized appointment of proxies:

1. The appointed proxy may later seem to be the wrong surrogate decision-maker;
2. The proxy may make a treatment choice contrary to the patient's treatment directive, claiming that the proxy appointment takes precedence over the directive; and
3. The proxy [or, for that matter, the treatment directive itself] may make a decision with which the physician or institution disagrees.

The PSDA has created some confusion regarding interpretation. American Medical News, in its 5/17/93 issue (pp. 1, 46), reported two such cases:

In one, staffers at a New Hampshire nursing home were chastised by relatives of a patient whom staffers saved from choking to death. . . . The other case involved a Yakima, Wash., nursing home resident who died after being accidently given medication intended for another patient. The error was discovered almost immediately. But the patient's physician refused to correct the mistake, citing the woman's advance directive barring the use of 'heroic measures' to keep her alive. . . . Some intensive care specialists say they've seen colleagues interpret the mere existence of a living will as authorization to stop treatment or provide only minimal care.

In view of the dangers inherent in living wills, some well-intentioned folks have written Christian or pro-life versions. The result can be likened to tying a string around a rattlesnake's snout before you take it to bed with you. The nature of this beast is to sabotage informed consent, taking rights to reasonable medical care away from patients. Living wills were never intended to serve patients. They are driven, rather, by the "needs" for physician immunity, cost containment, and legalized "aid in dying."

The most obvious alternative to signing a living will or appointing a durable power of attorney is to do nothing. This is, in my opinion, a viable option . . . at least until some future time when a living will or DPAHC might be required of all of us. (Already, suggestions have been made in high places that they be required of certain categories of people.)

Another option is to have a frank discussion with someone you trust and with your physician, in which answers to questions about treatment options are asked and answered. In addition, you might communicate your values and desires in a letter, giving a copy into the keeping of a trusted relative or friend and another to your physician to be kept on file and referred to as needed. There are at least three disadvantages to this choice. No protection from liability for carrying out your choices is guaranteed to the physician, and some may be unwilling to follow the directions of a letter.

Secondly, health care providers may not be comfortable accepting and following directives in an "unofficial" document such as a letter. Finally, this option may be unattractive for a person who has difficulty constructing a written account of his values and preferences.

At least two organizations which do not support euthanasia provide prepared documents that are not living wills, and which may simply be signed after reading and entrusted to the persons mentioned above. The Center for the Rights of the Terminally Ill (CRTI) distributes a "Patient Self-Protection Document" (PSPD). Quoting from their literature:

This is not a living will. Like a Durable Power of Attorney for Health Care, it enables the signer to name a trusted family member or friend as the 'agent' to make medical decisions if he/she is unable to do so. But it differs from other DPAHCs in that it: (1) explicitly defines and prohibits euthanasia, (2) specifies that nutrition and hydration are to be provided unless one is unable to assimilate food and fluids, (3) specifies that the signer is to be provided with ordinary nursing care and medical care, including pain relief and comfort care, and (4) does not confer immunity on any physician, health care provider or institution who will not honor these instructions."

Doctors' have a duty to protect human rights

The tenets of medical ethics are justice, fidelity, beneficence, non-maleficence, and autonomy. Hall clearly shows the link among health, human rights, and justice via the example of Pinochet's ultimate acquittal. by a group of four UK doctors—one for every 10,000 tortured people. That doctors can be coerced into practicing unethical medicine by government should cause shame to the UK home secretary.

Medical students' examination of anesthetized patients concerns autonomy and beneficence. Jennifer Leaning cites article 1 of the Universal Declaration of Human Rights to show that all people are born free and equal in rights and dignity. Her choice of reference is supreme; article 25, which deals with health, is not needed.

The rights of women and atrocities related to war finish off Hall's links. Khassan Baiev, a Chechen doctor who treated casualties from both sides of the Russian-Chechnyan conflict, might better elucidate non-maleficence and beneficence related to conflict medicine. He cared for all sick and wounded, regardless of what cause they were fighting for. His actions in upholding the Hippocratic oath and helping all in need drew threats and accusations from both sides. His practice of linking health, human rights, and ethics eventually forced him to flee the arena and seek asylum in the United States.

Hall correctly asserts that governments have a role in protecting human rights, and cites lack of action on the part of the United Nations regarding Rwanda in 1994. Genocide continues in Sudan today. With sadness but without shock, history yet again repeats itself.

Louis Virchow said, 'If medicine is to fulfil our greatest task, then she must enter the political and social life'. Hall's multiple examples of doctors failing in this regard should be yet another rallying cry for all health professionals and students to protect the health and human rights of all people. There will always be more questions than answers in the complementary yet often-nebulous realm of health, ethics, and human rights. As humans, we have yet to answer all the questions that even two of these principles share, never mind all three together. Yet asking the questions, working on the patient's behalf, and constantly striving to better delineate and improve; humanity's moral compass is not only the role, but the responsibility, of a doctor.

This document should be read in the light of the provisions of the South African Constitution and the ethical duties placed on doctors by the Health Professions Council of South Africa.

DOCTORS		*PATIENTS*	
Rights	*Responsibilities*	*Rights*	*Responsibilities*
To equal treatment and equal benefit of	To treat all his/ her patients equally and	To equal treatment and equal benefit of	To pay for the level of care received or to

the law in all applications by and dealings with government, the private sector and others. Substantive equality means that family responsibility, rural areas, historic disadvantage, etc. are relevant factors.	provide them with the same level of concern.	the law, including provisions relating to medical care, medical schemes, etc	receive assistance in accordance with relevant legislation and policy.
Not to be unfairly discriminated against by any patient, medical scheme, medical faculty or school, government, employer or any other person or institution on the basis of their race, gender, origin or any other ground. Doctors have the right not to be harassed.	Although a doctor has the right to choose his/her patients, such choices may never amount to unfair discrimination and emergency treatment may never be refused. Doctors have the duty not to harass patients, colleagues or others on the basis of sex, gender, sexual orientation, race or any (presumed) group characteristic.	Not to be unfairly discriminated against directly or indirectly on the basis of their race, origin, gender, or any other ground. Patients have the right to be free from harassment.	Not to discriminate against any health care worker or the employees of any doctor. Patients have the duty not to harass doctors, their employees or other health care workers.
To have his/her life protected which includes the right not to be placed in disproportional life-threatening situations.	To protect life, within the confines of a patient's right to physical autonomy and decision-making power.	To have his/her life protected by means of the benefits of medicine, when available and when she/he so wishes.	To ensure that his/her illness or incapacity does not endanger the lives of others.
To freedom and security of the	To ensure that patients are not	To freedom and security of the	To respect the physical and

person which includes the right to physical autonomy and the right to be free from violence.	subjected to cruel, inhuman or degrading punishment or treatment and to report instances where such occur, especially within the spheres of prison, detention, etc, as well abuse of children and the elderly. Doctors have to ensure that patients parttake in all types of research with their full and informed consent.	person which includes freedom from cruel, inhuman or degrading treatment; to be free from violence and not to be subjected to medical experiments without informed consent.	psychological integrity and autonomy of others and not to subject others to any form of violence.
To privacy which includes protection of personal information, communication, family and property.	To protect the privacy and confidentiality of his/her patients and to only disclose health care, treatment, diagnostic and other health information with the patient's informed and written consent or when authorised by law or a court to do so.	To privacy which includes respect by those to whom they entrust such information, as well as other health care workers and intermediaries who deal with their health care information.	To respect the privacy of others, including those of their children of 14 years and older, as well as the privacy of their spouses and partners. Patients should also respect the privacy and family life of their doctors.
To freedom of religion, belief and opinion which includes the right of doctor to act in accordance with their beliefs. Doctors have the right to reasonable	To respect the religion, beliefs and opinions of their patients, even if it differs from their own, and not to force any patient or colleague to prescribe to any religious	To have their freedom of religion, belief and opinion respected by doctors. This includes indigenous belief systems, religious dress and rules in	To respect the religion, belief and opinion of doctors and others and not to force any doctor or other person to act according to a certain set of beliefs.

accommodation of their religious beliefs, short of undue hardship to others. Doctors also have the right to clinical independence.	practice, belief or opinion. Doctors have the responsibility to respect the clinical independence of their colleagues and not to succumb to pressures of dual loyalty.	relation to modesty, as well as certain medical procedures, such as blood transfusions.	
To freedom of expression which includes the right to express themselves and their opinions without victimisation. Doctors have the right to notify their patients of their services according to the rules of the HPCSA.	Not to practice hate speech or to subscribe to expression that is harmful to others or is aimed at inciting harm or violence. Doctors have a responsibility to listen to their patients and take their views into considera-tion. Doctors have the responsibility not to advertise in an unrofes-sional or comparative manner.	To express themselves freely and to have their freedom of expression respected especially where their health care is concerned. This includes the right of patients to complain.	Patients have the responsibility to follow the advice given by their practitioners and to regularly and openly communicate with their doctors on matters affecting their health care.
To freedom of assembly demonstration, picketing and to present petitions, without victimisation.	To exercise their rights to assembly, demonstration, picketing and petitions to such an extent that it does not affect the health care of their patients.	To assemble, demonstrate, picket and present petitions in relation to health care issues.	To exercise their rights to assembly, demonstration and picketing in such a manner that it does not affect health care delivery and that it does not violate any law.
To freedom of association which includes the right to	Not to exercise his/her association in such a manner	To freedom of association with any group, club, scheme or	To respect the rights of doctors and others to associate and to

voluntarily form, join and participate in any association or to disassociate. It includes the unfettered right to choose life partners and friends.	that it discriminates against any other person, amounts to supporting any scheme providing perverse incentives or to a denial or exclusion of the rights or enefits potentially due to other doctors or others.	project, as long as it is within the boundaries of the law. To freedom and security of the person	respect the duties flowing from their own free association.
To make political choices and participate in political activities without any victimisation.	To ensure that any political affiliation and activities does not interfere with his/her duties to good patient care.	To make political choices and to participate in political activities without victimisation or detriment in terms of health care.	To tolerate the political activities and viewpoints of others.
To freedom of movement and residence which includes not to be subjected to unreasonable limitations in terms of where doctors must live and work.	Not to interfere with the rights of movement and residence of others and to, as far as possible, accommodate patients whose residence may cause difficulty in accessing health care.	To freedom of movement and residence.	To permit others freedom of movement and residence and to respect regulation by law in this regard.
To freedom of trade, occupation and profession including choices in relation to specialisation where positions exist. This	To ensure that they exercise their occupation within the limits set by the HPCSA and the law. This also means that economic	To suitably qualified doctors in respect medical treatment in every aspect of their health care.	To respect the occupation of medicine.

includes the rights of doctors to take part in economic endeavours.	endeavours should not amount to perverse activities, or undermine good patient care.		
To fair labour practices including fair dispensations of overtime, leave and working conditions and the right to have their grievances taken up at appropriate forums. Doctors have the right to be assisted in disciplinary enquiries, to state their side of the case and to an impartial chairperson. Doctors have the right to work in an environment that is not hostile in terms of sex, gender, sexual orientation or (presumed) race or ethnicity. Doctors have the right to post-exposure prophylactics in cases of occupational exposure to HIV.	To fulfil their employment duties. The heads of facilities have the responsibility to facilitate and harmonise the employment rights of doctors employed by them. Doctors who are HIV positive have the duty to modify their practice of medicine to such an extent so as not to endanger the lives of their patients.	Not to have their employment relationships jeopardised by unlawful disclosures or any unauthorised participation in any aspect of their employment relationship with an employer.	To respect doctors exercising their employment rights in, for example, the form of leave. Employers have the duty not to place doctors in ethically difficult positions in relation to their employees who are patients as such doctors.
To an environment that is not harmful to their health or well-being, including	To ensure that medical waste are disposed off appropriately and that appropriate	To an environment that is not harmful to their health or well-being, including a	To create an environment that is not detrimental to the health and well-being of

appropriate management of stressful situations and supervision/ assistance of junior doctors.	protocols are followed in terms of infectious disease control. Doctors have the responsibility to inform their patients of the harmful effects of medicines and how to store and use it properly.	setting that is conducive for recovery.	others, by ensuring that medicines are stored safely and used correctly, as indicated by their doctors.
To property, which includes the right to be paid a fair remuneration for services rendered and not to have any unlawful interference with these and other property rights. Doctors have the right not to be taxed more or targeted exclusively based on their assumed financial status.	To pay their dues, to fairly remunerate their own employees and to respect the property of others.	To pay a fair amount for services rendered by doctors, not to be over-serviced or overcharged and to make enquiries in relation to accounts.	To pay for services rendered by doctors and to take personal responsibility for accounts, even where a medical scheme is involved. Where a patient is unable to pay immediately, s/ he has to make appropriate arrangements with the doctor so as to repay any debts.
To access to housing especially where doctors are fulfilling training requirements, community service, or contributing to alleviate the plight in rural areas.	To take care of state housing provided to them and not to refuse housing (to let or sell) to any person based on a prohibited ground of discrimination.		
To access to health care	Not to unreasonably	To access to health care and	To pay for health care

where reasonably possible within the state's available resources. The duty to realise this right rests on the state that has to proof the reasonability of their measures and laws in that regard. The state has to ensure that appropriate systems are in place for medico-legal work, such as cases of rape, domestic violence, abuse, assault, drunken driving, etc.	refuse a patient's access to health care, especially where there are no state facilities available to assist patients. Doctors may not refuse emergency treatment to patients. Doctors have a responsibility to assist in realising the right of access to health care, which may include issuing prescriptions ensuring access to the best available treatment.	to obtain a second opinion. This includes access to the best available treatment and medicines, which have to be progressively realised by the state. The state has to ensure that everybody has at least access to primary heath care facilities in their immediate vicinity.	services received, where such services cannot be provided for free in terms of the public or a charitable system. Patients have the duty to follow the advice of their doctors and to fully inform their doctors of their health status.
Of access to social security which includes access to insurance and social assistance. Social security institutions have to remunerate doctors fairly and timely.	To ensure that medical reports are fair and accurate and that only particulars that are authorised by law are disclosed to insurance and assistance agencies.	To access to social security, including occupational health schemes, medical schemes, private insurance, road accident funds, social grants, etc.	To make provision for their own social security, to ensure that their dependants are covered and to pay the required premiums or contributions, where applicable.
To education and further education which includes access to CPD activities. Private institutions must maintain standards not inferior to that of public institutions.	To ensure that s/he is informed about the latest developments in their fields and take part in educational activities.	To seek and receive education on public and private health matters.	To act in accordance with public and private education received.

To language and culture which includes the right to converse in the language of one's choice, where practicable.	To tolerate and respect linguistic and cultural diversity. Doctors have to recognise that language and culture may serve as barriers in health care.	To language and culture which includes the right to converse in the language of one's choice, where practicable. Patients also have the right to take part in cultural practices.	To tolerate and respect linguistic and cultural diversity and to speak out when these constitute barriers to good health care. Authorities and individuals have the responsibility to ensure that their cultural practices are not detrimental to the subjects thereof.
To access to information held by the state and/ or private institutions.	To provide access to information requested by their patients and to ensure that health data is stored safely and not sold or passed on without the patient's informed consent.	To obtain copies of all health information held on him/her.	To respect the privacy and information belonging to others, including family members. Patients have to deal with their health information in a responsible manner and realise that they may need expert advice on the interpretation thereof.
To just administrative action which includes the right to reasons in writing where a doctor's rights or interests are affected/ threatened. This includes action taken by the HPCSA and government.	To ensure that the principles of administrative justice are adhered to if they are in positions of authority, policy-making and decision-making that affects people.	To receive reasons where their rights/ interests in relation to health care benefits, such as by medical schemes, are affected.	

To access to the courts which includes the right to have their justifiable disputes heard in a court of law or other appropriate forum. Doctors who act as witnesses in cases have the right to be fairly remunerated for their services.	To assist in legal proceedings when called upon as expert witnesses. Doctors have a particular responsibility in relation to crimes such as child abuse, domestic violence and abuse of the elderly.	To take legal action to enforce their rights in the health care setting.	Not to be vexatious in taking doctors to court.
Not to be arrested, detained or accused in contravention with section 35 of the Constitution. Doctors have the right not to be forced to take part in any unlawful (bodily) search or seizure and have the right to enquire as to the status of the subject brought to them, as well as the legislation in terms of which this is done.	To assist in the realisation of the right of access to health care of all arrested, detained and accused persons and to bring to the attention of the authorities or inspecting judge any irregularities or needs in relation to health care.	To medical care when in detention and to raise concerns in relation to health issues, either to the relevant health care workers or to the authorities, and to have such concerns addressed expeditiously.	To look after his/her own health and to ensure that s/he is not endangering the health of others when in detention

Codes, laws and declarations about patients' rights

There are many national and international documents that declare, enact, or contain proposals for patients' rights. At the national level, France was one of the first European countries to adopt a charter on the subject. The 1974 Charter for hospital patients was not a legally binding text, but an annex to a ministerial circular. Amongst current EU Member States to have adopted legislation are: Finland (in 1992), The Netherlands (in 1994), Greece, Hungary, Lithuania, Latvia and Portugal (in 1997), Denmark (in

1998), Belgium, Estonia and France (in 2002) and Cyprus (in 2005). At the international level, prominent examples of documents about patients' rights include:

- The Declaration on the promotion of patients' rights in Europe of March 1994. This resulted from an initiative of the World Health Organization Regional Office for Europe;
- The Ljubljana Charter on Reforming Health Care of 1996 (also a W.H.O. initiative);
- The Council of Europe's 1997 Convention on Human Rights and Biomedicine. Despite its name, this Convention also deals with patients rights in general; and
- The European Charter of Patients' Rights, drafted under the auspices of an Italian-based NGO called the Active Citizenship Network.

Varieties of rights

In contemporary legal and political debate, the language of rights is increasingly used to assert and to recognize the legitimacy of a wide variety of claims and interests. Look, for example, at a modern document such as the Charter of Fundamental Rights of the European Union. The Charter was proclaimed at the Nice summit of the European Council in December 2000 and forms Part II of the Constitution Treaty for Europe. It constitutes the European equivalent of a Bill of Rights. In the Charter, we find not only individual rights, but also statements of principle that could imply group or collective rights, such as prohibitions on making the human body and its parts a source of financial gain, and on reproductive cloning. These prohibitions are included in Article 3 of the Charter on the right to the integrity of the person.

That is not because I consider these questions as unimportant, but because the issues are different from those involved in individual rights. The introduction to the 1995 version of the French Charter for hospital patients expresses well the approach that I am adopting: [a] hospital patient is not just someone who is sick. He is first and foremost a person with rights and duties. I should add: that goes for all patients, not just those in hospital.

Categories of individual rights

In my view, the individual patient's rights fall into three categories:

- Rights to redress, including compensation;
- Rights of access to medical care; and
- Autonomy rights.

These three categories of rights are best understood as the concretization of certain fundamental human rights. I will briefly discuss the first two categories before focusing on the autonomy rights and the doctor-patient relationship.

Rights to redress

The most fundamental right to redress is the right to bring proceedings in a court of law. This is a traditional civil right associated with the principle of the rule of law. It can be found in Article 6 of the European Convention on Human Rights and Article 47 of the Charter of Fundamental Rights.

In the medical context, the right to go to court provides the most fundamental guarantee of the autonomy rights that I shall discuss later. It may also be an appropriate way to enforce certain rights of access to medical care.

The right to compensation if medical care falls below an acceptable standard also comes under this heading. I will not discuss this complex question in detail, but only to point out that there are basically two legal pathways to the provision of compensation, each of which has its own particular costs and benefits.

The first is litigation. As already mentioned, this is the traditional and fundamental pathway to justice. As the example of the United States illustrates, however, lawsuits about medical negligence can become big business, not always to the benefit of patients.

The second pathway is a compensation scheme, which may be based on no-fault liability. Such a scheme may be offered to patients as an alternative to court proceedings. From my perspective as an Ombudsman, I will add that rights to redress are not just about damages or compensation. Complaints provide complex organizations, such as hospitals and public health care systems, with essential feedback on the quality of services. Justified complaints are an opportunity not only to apologize for mistakes and provide compensation if appropriate, but also to help avoid similar problems from arising in the future. Proper handling of a complaint, with a fair procedure, provides an opportunity to explain what has been done and can often satisfy the complainant.

Rights of access to medical care

As regards rights of access to medical care, the first point to note is that the general right not to be discriminated against applies in the field of medical care. Non-discrimination does not require any particular level of service, but forbids unjustified variations. In the European legal order, the substantive right to medical care is a social right, which requires government to ensure, directly or indirectly, the availability of adequate provision.

The right can be found in the European Social Charter (Article 13) and the United Nations' International Covenant on Economic, Social and Cultural Rights (Article 12), but is set out most clearly in the Charter of 255 Fundamental Rights

The first sentence of Article 35 of the Charter states: that "everyone has the right of access to preventive health care and the right to benefit from medical treatment under the conditions established by national laws and practices."

How government is to secure this right to citizens, and the general level of service to be provided, are matters of debate.

In this connection, I would like to draw your attention briefly to the case-law of the European Court of Justice concerning the conditions under which patients may claim re-imbursement in their own Member State for treatment obtained in another Member State. Although the legal basis of this case law is the freedom to provide services, it also has great significance for rights of access to health care in the European Union.

Autonomy rights

The third category of rights, and those which I propose to devote most attention to, are what I call autonomy rights. To talk about autonomy in the context of medical care may seem at best a polite fiction. The paradigm of the patient is a person who is suffering from an illness, or dysfunction, and who needs treatment in order to become well. The process of treatment is in many cases almost the opposite of what we normally understand by autonomy. Think, for example, of an anaesthetised patient undergoing an operation.

Furthermore, there are many different conceptions of autonomy. Some of them have even been used to justify coercion, as Isaiah Berlin, the great Oxford political philosopher who recently passed away, pointed out in his famous 1969 essay on liberty.

To explain what I mean by autonomy and why the autonomy rights are fundamental to the idea of patients' rights, we need to examine the doctor-patient relationship. In doing so, we shall draw on two well-known pieces of published work. The first is by Professor Edward SHORTER, holder of the Hannah Chair in the History of Medicine at the University of Toronto, on the history of the doctor-patient relationship. The second is by Linda and Ezekiel EMANUEL (respectively now Professor of Medicine and Director of the Buehler Center on Aging at Northwestern's Feinberg School of Medicine and Chair of the Department of Clinical Bioethics at the National Institutes of Health, Bethesda, Md), presenting four ideal-typical models of that relationship.

Periodisation of the doctor-patient relationship

Shorter divides the history of the doctor-patient relationship since the 18th Century into three periods, which he calls traditional, .modern and post-modern. For reasons that need not detain us, I prefer to label the third period as contemporary or "late modern".

The traditional period was characterized by an unscientific and largely unfounded therapeutic confidence on the part of doctors, which met with considerable skepticism among patients. As a result, doctors had a relatively modest social status during this early period.

The modern period begins with the gradual arrival, during the 19th Century, of a scientific basis for medicine, founded on the proper physical examination of patients, accurate diagnosis and finally the success of the germ theory of infectious disease.

Although unable to offer cures for many of the conditions that he could diagnose and explain, the doctor became, as Shorter puts it, a demi-god possessed of boundless authority over patients. The doctor's authority as a man of science was the foundation for what the Emanuels call the paternalistic model of the doctor-patient relationship.

In this model, the doctor determines what is in the patient's interests, including how much the patient should know and indeed whether the patient should be told the truth about his or her condition and prognosis.

The patient's role is, in essence, to follow the doctor's orders.

The paternalist model thus focuses on the inequality of expertise in the relationship as a reason for giving the doctor, rather than the patient, autonomy in making decisions about what should happen to the patient.

The contemporary or late modern period began when scientific advances made it possible for doctors to cure patients with drugs, such as the sulphonamides in the 1930s and antibiotics after the Second World War.

Paradoxically, this spectacular therapeutic success has been accompanied by a decline in medical authority. In Shorter's view, this results from the effect of the media on patients' knowledge of medicine and medical procedures.

I am persuaded that the phenomenon should also be seen as part of a more general development in contemporary societies. Science and expertise are no longer accepted as constituting, by themselves, the legitimate basis for decisions that also involve values, or individual and social preferences.

This development is in turn connected to the wider cultural and political context defined by the growing ascendancy in the world of late modernity of democracy and especially of its liberal variant with its emphasis on both equality and liberty as fundamental to the ordering of our lives.

Two models of the contemporary doctor-patient relationship

In any event, the era of the doctor as a demi-god has passed and with it has gone the basis for the paternalistic model of the doctor-patient relationship, in which the doctor's knowledge and expertise justifies authority over the patient.

A model for the contemporary period must be built on equality in the relationship and on respect for the autonomy of the patient.

I will put forward two possible models of the contemporary doctor-patient relationship, each of which is based on a different idea of what equality and autonomy should mean in this context.

For reasons that I shall explain in a moment, I call the first model "consumerist."

The consumerist model

Its main characteristics are the same as those of what the Emanuels called the .informative model. The essence of their model is that the doctor's role is to supply full information to the patient about his or her condition and about the available treatment options. The patient then decides which, if any, of the treatments to choose.

The doctor is thus a technical expert; on tap, but not on top.

The implications of this model are that the inequality of knowledge and expertise can be fully corrected through the supply of information and that autonomy for the patient consists of making an unconstrained choice on the basis of his or her own values and preferences.

The Emanuels criticized this model mainly on the grounds that it fails to capture an essential part of the doctor's role, which is to care for the patient. Nor does it reflect most patients' wants and expectations of their relationship with a doctor.

Even from a purely technical perspective, and I wish to stress the word "technical", making choices about medical treatment is not like choosing between different models of car or washing machine. The complexity involved makes it more like choosing financial services, a field in which even the most liberal European states recognize that consumers (and this is why I call the model 'consumerist') need protection. For this reason, I think the most likely outcome of the consumerist model would not be patient autonomy in the doctor-patient relationship, but that forces external to that relationship would establish new forms of paternalism. This could take the form of public regulation of the doctor-patient relationship, in which a State bureaucracy sees itself as responsible for making decisions about patients' best interests.

Alternatively, or perhaps additionally, there could be legal paternalism, in which lawyers and judges pursue their version of the patients' best interests. This is likely to produce a more adversarial context for the doctor-patient relationship, with an excessive focus on rights of redress.

This in turn could lead to 'defensive medicine', in which the doctor's actions are focused on avoiding liability rather than treating the patient. In other words, a model that is based on a purely economic approach and on the logic of the market only ignores, and therefore does violence to, an idea of autonomy that is linked to the ethical dimension of the patient as a whole person, as a human being and not a mere economic agent.

The communicative model

In this model, the doctor does not merely provide information but communicates with the patient and is willing to engage in a genuine dialogue.

Equality in this model is not equality of knowledge and expertise achieved through the flow of information, but equality at the fundamental level of the right to be an autonomous agent making choices about one's own life.

Respect for the patient's right to be an autonomous agent implies that the patient has the right to choose the balance in his or her relationship with the doctor between paternalism, information, advice, guidance and deliberation.

In practice, the doctor is the party who presumptively starts out with more power, based both on expertise and knowledge, and on the vulnerable situation of the patient who is possibly suffering from illness or dysfunction.

The burden should thus be on the doctor to take the initiative to explore how the patient wishes the relationship to function and to respect those wishes.

In doing so, the doctor should begin from the paradigm of the patient as an autonomous agent with the right to make informed choices about his or her medical treatment.

Equality and autonomy

It is against the background of this model of the doctor-patient relationship, not the consumerist model, that we should understand the emerging international consensus that patients have certain fundamental autonomy rights.

These are: the right to give or withhold consent to treatment; the right to know the risks and benefits of proposed treatment; and the right to privacy.

The right to give or withhold consent to treatment.

The right to give or withhold consent to treatment is perhaps the most fundamental of the autonomy rights.

In France, the principle of obtaining the consent of the patient before an operation was first clearly set out in the Teyssier decision of the Cour de Cassation in 1942, in the name of respect for the patient as a human being.

More recently, this right has been tested in cases on the so-called 'right to die' and 'living wills', which usually state the patient's wishes to be allowed to die in certain future circumstances. The converse situation is currently before the Court of Appeal in the United Kingdom, in which Leslie Burke, a patient with a degenerative brain condition, insists that he should not be deprived of food and drink when his situation deteriorates to the point that he can no longer communicate his wishes. The legal and ethical complexities of this kind of situation and of other special cases, such as children and psychiatric patients should not, however, obscure the paradigmatic case of the right of a conscious and competent patient to give or refuse consent to treatment.

The right to information

The right to information is the natural counterpart of the right to give or withhold consent to treatment. Put together, the two rights constitute the principle of informed consent.

This principle can itself be expressed as a right, as for example in Article 3 of the Charter of Fundamental Rights, which contains—as part of the right to the integrity of the person—the requirement to respect the free and informed consent of the person concerned in the fields of medicine and biology.

The right to control the flow of information about oneself

The right to control the flow of information about oneself is an aspect of the fundamental right of privacy.

As the European Court of Justice has expressed it: The right to respect for private life (...) is one of the fundamental rights protected by the legal order of the Community.(...) It includes in particular a person's right to keep his state of health secret.

This principle was also applied in 1998 by the European Ombudsman in a case where a European Commission official had contacted without permission a trainee's doctor in order, as the official put it, to .clarify the situation. as regards a medical certificate issued by the doctor.

The requirements of privacy as regards the handling of personal information are made more concrete by European Union laws on data protection.

These laws require special protection for certain categories of personal data, including information about a person's health.

The Physicians for Human Rights (PHRs)

Colleagues at Risk Program advocates on behalf of many brave health professionals around the world who attempt to treat all types of patients or speak out on behalf of persecuted groups, often at great personal and professional cost. PHR sends letters to government officials, reaches out to the media, and urges its members and the general public to write letters on behalf of health professionals in danger. In the case of Libya, PHR mobilized 30 prominent physicians and scientists from 10 countries including the United States, several European nations, Iran, Egypt, and the West Bank and Gaza, to sign a letter to Libyan authorities calling for the release of the health workers, who are appealing their sentences at the time of this writing. In 2003, PHR monitored, publicized, and provided advocacy support for colleagues in South Africa, Pakistan, Cuba, Burma, Iran, Malaysia, Azerbeijan, China,Vietnam, Egypt, Colombia, and Turkey.

PHR's efforts have contributed to the dismissal of charges, release from prison, improved treatment, and even saved lives of health professionals, as well as improved government policies on human rights and health. Following advocacy on behalf of Dr. Mollendorff, for example, the South African Department of Health agreed in March of 2003 to pay his back salary and benefits for 12 months and compensate him for his legal costs. The government unconditionally withdrew the charges against Dr. Mollendorff and offered him the opportunity to reclaim his job.

Physicians for Human Rights was also successful in helping Dr. Khassan Baiev safely leave Chechnya in 2000 and gain asylum for himself and his family in the United States. For many other colleagues at risk, however, Physicians for Human Rights and others are still advocating. The more individual health professionals and medical associations that support our Health Professional Colleagues At Risk Program, the larger and louder will be the collective voice we have to help our brave colleagues throughout the world practice medicine and speak their minds safely. It is also through this advocacy that we are able to improve national and international human rights policies, which inevitably affect the health and well-being of all people.

Our society is very concerned with endowing and protecting people's rights and the existence of a National Health Service in this country has allowed such concepts to be applied to medical care. It is not clear, however, whether the concept of rights helps either doctors or patients, and it may in fact be misleading or even damaging. A discussion of the suitability of rights and ethics to the health care context is a matter of debate. The way in which rights create corresponding duties and responsibilities, and the particular problems that this creates for our health service needs to be addressed. The background of the welfare state, of which the NHS is a central part, protected such projects and further encouraged individual endeavor. In medical ethics, this has been paralleled by the fall from grace of the paternalistic principles of beneficence and non-maleficence, and the apparently inexorable rise of autonomy as the 'trump card' in the ethical pack. As autonomy has become more and more important to us, we have found a new language with which to defend it, and talk of 'rights' to and within health care (inconceivable before the existence of the NHS) is increasingly commonplace.

Rights and responsibilities in the NHS

Positive rights will also conflict not just in principle but in daily practicalities, when the number of hours in the day will mean that not everything that one or other of our patients has a 'right' to, can be physically achieved. This is a reality that the use of the term 'right' rather denies. Again, the negative rights (to be free from unwanted interference) seem to be the easiest to establish and exercise in practice. It is much less clear what positive 'rights' truly exist. When a positive duty is created by a proclaimed right, an additional complication arises, in that it is not always clear how such a right is to be enforced or implemented. This is particularly true in the current NHS structure where the doctor–patient relationship may be less prominent than the hospital—or practice—patient relationship.

As mentioned above, the increasing importance attributed to rights ethics has naturally flowed from the rising importance of the individual in today's society. It is not clear, however, whether such considerations are well suited to the work of a communal/societal institution such as the NHS.

For whilst on one level we do exist to protect individuals (the first duty of a doctor being to 'make the care of your patient your first concern'), we also have responsibilities outside this one doctor-patient encounter and are bound to consider the well-being of other members of the public, resource allocation, waiting lists, etc. before we spend all the tax-payers' money in securing the rights of the patient we happen to be treating. This restriction on resources and the communal nature of the NHS will certainly limit the positive rights that can be granted. Current best practice sets the doctor and patient as partners in decision-making. Both bring particular knowledge to the encounter. The physician holds technical knowledge, data and experience; the patient holds the knowledge of their own particular symptoms, the problems they are causing them, and contextual detail that make one therapeutic option more desirable in their situation than might at first be obvious to the treating physician.

Perhaps we are reaching a time when this contract should become just that—the doctor and patient both signing upto an agreed action plan and each being held to it. How such a scheme could be implemented is, however, far from clear. It does seem important to understand, though, that rights and responsibilities go hand in hand and that as more power is gradually handed over to patients and their representatives (for whose benefit after all, the NHS exists), so we will have to somehow ensure that our health care resources continue to be used responsibly and equitably, and that those for whom the protection of rights was really necessary do not end up becoming more disenfranchised than they already are.

Doctors Rights and Responsibilities

It is incumbent on a physician to treat all his/her patients equally and provide them with the same level of concern. To equal treatment and equal benefit of the law, including provisions relating to medical care, medical schemes, etc. To pay for the level of care received or to receive assistance in accordance with relevant legislation and policy. Not to be unfairly discriminated against by any patient, medical scheme, medical faculty or school, government, employer or any other person or institution on the basis of their race, gender, origin or any other ground. Doctors have the right not to be harassed. Although a doctor has the right to choose his/her patients, such choices may never amount to unfair discrimination and emergency treatment may never be refused. Doctors have the duty not to harass patients, colleagues or others on the basis of sex, gender, sexual orientation, race or any (presumed) group characteristic. Not to be unfairly discriminated against directly or indirectly on the basis of their race, origin, gender, or any other ground. Patients have the right to be free from harassment. Not to discriminate against any health care worker or the employees of any doctor. Patients have the duty not to harass doctors, their employees or other health care workers. To have his/her life protected which includes the right not to be placed in disproportional life-threatening situations. To protect life, within the confines of a patient's right to physical autonomy and decision-making power. To have his/her life protected by means of the benefits of medicine, when available and when s/he so wishes. To ensure that his/her illness or incapacity does not endanger the lives of others. To freedom and security of the person which includes the right to physical autonomy and the right to be free from violence. To ensure that patients are not subjected to cruel, inhuman or degrading punishment or treatment and to report instances where such occur, especially within the spheres of prison, detention, etc. as well abuse of children and the elderly. Doctors have to ensure that patients part take in all types of research with their full and informed consent. To freedom and security of the person which includes freedom from cruel, inhuman or degrading treatment; to be free from violence and not to be subjected to medical experiments without informed consent. To respect the physical and psychological integrity and autonomy of others and not to subject others to any form of violence. To privacy which includes protection of personal information, communication, family and property. To protect the privacy and confidentiality of his/her patients and to only disclose health care, treatment, diagnostic and other health information with the patient's informed and written consent or when authorized by law or a court to do so. To privacy which includes respect by those to whom they entrust such information, as well as other health care workers and intermediaries who deal with their health care information. To respect the privacy of others, including those of their children of 14 years and older, as well as the privacy of their spouses and partners. Patients should also respect the privacy and family life of their doctors. To freedom of religion, belief and opinion which includes the right of doctor to act in accordance with their beliefs. Doctors have the right to reasonable accommodation of their religious beliefs, short of undue hardship to others.

Doctors also have the right to clinical independence, but to respect the religion, beliefs and opinions of their patients, even if it differs from their own, and not to force any patient or colleague to prescribe to any religious practice, belief or opinion. Doctors have the responsibility to respect the clinical independence of their colleagues and not to succumb to pressures of dual loyalty. To have their freedom of religion, belief and opinion respected by doctors. This includes indigenous belief systems, religious dress and rules in relation to modesty, as well as certain medical procedures, such as blood transfusions. To respect the religion, belief and opinion of doctors and others and not to force any doctor or other person to act according to a certain set of beliefs. To freedom of expression which includes the right to express themselves and their opinions without victimization. Doctors have the right to notify their patients of their services according to the rules of the HPCSA. Not to practice hate speech or to subscribe to expression that is harmful to others or is aimed at inciting harm or violence. Doctors have a responsibility to listen to their patients and take their views into consideration. Doctors have the responsibility not to advertise in an unprofessional or comparative manner. To express themselves freely and to have their freedom of expression respected especially where their health care is concerned. This includes the right of patients to complain. Patients have the responsibility to follow the advice given by their practitioners and to regularly and openly communicate with their doctors on matters affecting their health care. To freedom of assembly demonstration, picketing and to present petitions, without victimization. To exercise their rights to assembly, demonstration, picketing and petitions to such an extent that it does not affect the health care of their patients. To assemble, demonstrate, picket and present petitions in relation to health care issues. To exercise their rights to assembly, demonstration and picketing in such a manner that it does not affect health care delivery and that it does not violate any law. To freedom of association which includes the right to voluntarily form, join and participate in any association or to disassociate. It includes the unfettered right to choose life partners and friends. Not to exercise his/her association in such a manner that it discriminates against any other person, amounts to supporting any scheme providing perverse incentives or—to a denial or exclusion of the rights or benefits potentially due to other doctors or others. To freedom of association with any group, club, scheme or project, as long as it is within the boundaries of the law. To freedom and security of the person, To respect the rights of doctors and others to associate and to respect the duties flowing from their own free association. To make political choices and participate in political activities without any victimization. To ensure that any political affiliation and activities does not interfere with his/her duties to good patient care. To tolerate the political activities and viewpoints of others. To freedom of movement and residence which includes not to be subjected to unreasonable limitations in terms of where doctors must live and work. Not to interfere with the rights of movement and residence of others and to, as far as possible, accommodate patients whose residence may cause difficulty in accessing health care. To freedom of movement and residence. To permit others freedom of movement and residence and to respect regulation by law in this regard. To freedom of trade, occupation and profession including choices in relation to specialization where positions exist. This includes the rights of doctors to take part in economic endeavors. To ensure that they exercise their occupation within the limits set by the law. This also means that economic endeavors should not amount to perverse activities, or undermine good patient care. To suitably qualified doctors in respect medical treatment in every aspect oftheir health care. To respect the occupation of medicine. To fair labour practices including fair dispensations of overtime, leave and working conditions and the right to have their grievances taken up at appropriate forums. Doctors have the right to be assisted in disciplinary enquiries, to state their side of the case and to an impartial chairperson. Doctors have the right to work in an environment that is not hostile in terms of sex, gender, sexual orientation or (presumed) race or ethnicity. Doctors have the right to post-exposure prophylactics in cases of occupational exposure to HIV. To fulfil their employment duties. The heads of facilities have the responsibility to facilitate and harmonize the employment rights of doctors employed by them. Doctors who are HIV positive have the duty to modify their practice of medicine to such an extent so as not to endanger the lives of their patients. Not to have their employment relationships jeopardized by unlawful disclosures or any unauthorized participation in any aspect of their employment relationship with an employer.

To respect doctors exercising their employment rights in, for example, the form of leave. Employers have the duty not to place doctors in ethically difficult positions in relation to their employees who are patients as such doctors. To an environment that is not harmful to their health or wellbeing, including appropriate management of stressful situations and supervision/ assistance of junior doctors. To ensure that medical waste are disposed off appropriately and that appropriate protocols are followed in terms of infectious disease control. Doctors have the responsibility to inform their patients of the harmful effects of medicines and how to store and use it properly. To an environment that is not harmful to their health or wellbeing, including a setting that is conducive for recovery. To create an environment that is not detrimental to the health and well-being of others, by ensuring that medicines are stored safely and used correctly, as indicated by their doctors. To property, which includes the right to be paid a fair remuneration for services rendered and not to have any unlawful interference with these and other property rights. Doctors have the right not to be taxed more or targeted exclusively based on their assumed financial status. To pay their dues, to fairly remunerate their own employees and to respect the property of others. To pay a fair amount for services rendered by doctors, not to be over-serviced or overcharged and to make enquiries in relation to accounts. To pay for services rendered by doctors and to take personal responsibility for accounts, even where a medical scheme is involved. Where a patient is unable to pay immediately, s/he has to make appropriate arrangements with the doctor so as to repay any debts. To access to housing especially where doctors are fulfilling training requirements, community service, or contributing to alleviate the plight in rural areas. To take care of state housing provided to them and not to refuse housing (to let or sell) to any person based on a prohibited ground of discrimination.

To access to health care where reasonably possible within the state's available resources. The duty to realize this right rests on the state that has to proof the reasonability of their measures and laws in that regard. The state has to ensure that appropriate systems are in place for medico-legal work, such as cases of rape, domestic violence, abuse, assault, drunken driving, etc. Not to unreasonably refuse a patient's access to health care, especially where there are no state facilities available to assist patients. Doctors may not refuse emergency treatment to patients. Doctors have a responsibility to assist in realising the right of access to health care, which may include issuing prescriptions ensuring access to the best available treatment. To access to health care and to obtain a second opinion. This includes access to the best available treatment and medicines, which have to be progressively realized by the state. The state has to ensure that everybody has at least access to primary heath care facilities in their immediate vicinity. To pay for health care services received, where such services cannot be provided for free in terms of the public or a charitable system. Patients have the duty to follow the advice of their doctors and to fully inform their doctors of their health status. Of access to social security which includes access to insurance and social assistance.

Social security institutions have to remunerate doctors fairly and timely. To ensure that medical reports are fair and accurate and that only particulars that are authorized by law are disclosed to insurance and assistance agencies. To access to social security, including occupational health schemes, medical schemes, private insurance, road accident funds, social grants, etc. To make provision for their own social security, to ensure that their dependants are covered and to pay the required premiums or contributions, where applicable. To education and further education which includes access to CPD activities. Private institutions must maintain standards not inferior to that of public institutions. To ensure that s/he is informed about the latest developments in their fields and take part in educational activities. To seek and receive education on public and private health matters. To act in accordance with public and private education received.

To language and culture which includes the right to converse in the language of one's choice, where practicable. To tolerate and respect linguistic and cultural diversity. Doctors have to recognise that language and culture may serve as barriers in health care. To language and culture which includes the right to converse in the language of one's choice, where practicable. Patients also have the right to take part in cultural practices. To tolerate and respect linguistic and cultural diversity and to speak out when these constitute barriers to good health care. Authorities and individuals have the responsibility to ensure that their cultural practices are not detrimental to the subjects thereof. To access to information held by the state and/or private institutions. To provide access to information requested by their patients and to ensure that health data is stored safely and not sold or passed on without the patient's informed consent. To obtain copies of all health information held on him/her. To respect the privacy and information belonging to others, including family members. Patients have to deal with their health information in a responsible manner and realise that they may need expert advice on the interpretation thereof. To just administrative action which includes the right to reasons in writing where a doctor's rights or interests are affected/threatened. This includes action taken by the HPCSA and government. To ensure that the principles of administrative justice are adhered to if they are in positions of authority, policy-making and decision-making that affects people. To receive reasons where their rights/interests in relation to health care benefits, such as by medical schemes, are affected. To access to the courts which includes the right to have their justifiable disputes heard in a court of law or other appropriate forum. Doctors who act as witnesses in cases have the right to be fairly remunerated for their services.

To assist in legal proceedings when called upon as expert witnesses. Doctors have a particular responsibility in relation to crimes such as child abuse, domestic violence and abuse of the elderly. To take legal action to enforce their rights in the health care setting. Not to be vexatious in taking doctors to court. Not to be arrested, detained or accused in contravention with section 35 of the Constitution. Doctors have the right not to be forced to take part in any unlawful (bodily) search or seizure and have the right to enquire as to the status of the subject brought to them, as well as the legislation in terms of which this is done. To assist in the realization of the right of access to health care of all arrested, detained and accused persons and to bring to the attention of the authorities or inspecting judge any irregularities or needs in relation to health care. To medical care when in detention and to raise concerns in relation to health issues, either to the relevant health care workers or to the authorities, and to have such concerns addressed expeditiously. To look after his/her own health and to ensure that s/he is not endangering the health of others when in detention.

References

Abate T. Doctors charge three HMOs with racketeering. The San Francisco Chronicle. 2000.

ACT WorkCover (2000), Guidance on Workplace Violence (available through www.workcover.act.gov.au).

Alderson P, Goodey C. Theories of consent. BMJ. Nov 7 1998;317(7168):1313-5. [Medline].

AMA. Code of Medical Ethics. Council on Ethical and Judicial Affairs. Available at www.ama-assn.org/ama/pub/category/2498.html. Accessed 1997.

Amdur RJ, Biddle C. Institutional review board approval and publication of human research results. *JAMA*. Mar 19 1997;277(11):909-14. [Medline].

Anthony T. Child abuse. In: Rosen P, Barkin RM, eds. Emergency Medicine. 4th ed. St. Louis, Mo: Mosby; 1998.

Asser SM, Swan R. Child fatalities from religion-motivated medical neglect. Pediatrics. Apr 1998;101(4 Pt 1):625-9. [Medline].

Baiev K. The Oath: A Surgeon Under Fire. New York: Walker & Co.; 2003.

Beauchamp T, Childress J. Principles of biomedical ethics, 5th edn. Oxford: Oxford University Press, 2001.

Breakaway courses: www.basistraining.co.uk/BreakAway SelfDefence.htm.

Calman K. The profession of medicine. *BMJ*. Oct 29 1994;309(6962):1140-3. [Medline].

Convention for the Protection of Human Rights and Dignity of the Human Being with regard to the Application of Biology and Medicine: Convention on Human Rights and Biomedicine, 1997, CETS No. 164.

Council of Europe Recommendation Rec (2000)5 for the development of institutions for citizen and patient participation in the decision-making process affecting health care, Adopted by the Committee of Ministers on 24 February 2000 at the 699th meeting of the Ministers' Deputies.

Davis K. Incremental coverage of the uninsured. In: Lee PR, Estes CL, eds. The Nation's Health. 5th ed. Sudbury, Mass: Jones and Bartlett Publishers; 1997:407-8.

Delaney J (2001), Prevention and Management of Workplace Aggression: Guidelines and Case Studies from the NSW Health Industry, Central Sydney Area Health Service, Sydney (available through www.workcover.nsw.gov.au).

Donelan K. Whatever happened to the health insurance crisis in the United States?, In: Lee PR, Estes CL, eds. The Nation's Health. 5th ed. Sudbury, Mass: Jones and Barlett Publishers; 1997:283.

Emanuel EJ, Wendler D, Grady C. What makes clinical research ethical?. *JAMA*. May 24-31 2000;283(20):2701-11. [Medline].

Estes CL, Close L. Public policy and long-term care. In: Lee PR, Estes CL, eds. The Nation's Health. 5th ed. Sudbury, Mass: Jones and Bartlett Publishers; 1997:177.

Excerpts from court's ruling on suing HMOs. *New York Times*. 2000.

General Medical Council. Duties of a doctor. London: GMC, 1995.

Gerstenzang J. Clinton takes GOP to task on health care. *Los Angeles Times*. 1999.

Isaiah Berlin, 'Two Concepts of Liberty', in Four Essays on Liberty, London: Oxford University Press 1969.

Job Watch and WorkSafe Victoria (2003), Workplace Violence and Bullying: Your Rights, What to Do, and Where to Go for Help (available through www.workcover.vic.gov.au).

Journal of the American Medical Association. World Medical Association declaration of Helsinki. Recommendations guiding physicians in biomedical research involving human subjects. *JAMA*. Mar 19 1997;277(11):925-6. [Medline].

Klein R. The new politics of the NHS, 4th edn. London: Pearson Education Ltd., 2001. 28. Melissa Smith, 502, *Clinical Medicine*, Vol 5, No. 5, September/October 2005

Lee NG. Update on EMTALA. *Am J Nurs*. Sep 2000;100(9):57-9. [Medline].

Mayhew C (2000), Preventing Client-Initiated Violence—A Practical Handbook, Research and Public Policy Series, No. 30, Australian Institute of Criminology, Canberra (available through www.aic.gov.au).

Mayhew C and Chappell D (2001), Prevention of Occupational Violence in the Health Workplace, Working Paper Series no. 140, UNSW, Sydney (available through www.health.nsw.gov.au).

Moreno J, Caplan AL, Wolpe PR. Updating protections for human subjects involved in research. Project on Informed Consent, Human Research Ethics Group. *JAMA*. Dec 9 1998;280(22):1951-8. [Medline].

National Commission for the Protection of Human Subjects of Biomedical and Behav. Report and recommendations: research involving those institutionalized as mentally infirm. Government Printing Office; 1978. 58.

NSW Department of Health (2003), Zero Tolerance Policy and Framework Guidelines, NSW Government (available through www.health.nsw.gov.au).

NT WorkSafe (2000), Work Environment—Violence in the Workplace (available through www.worksafe.nt.gov.au). 36. QLD: The Queensland Workplace Health and Safety Board is developing a Workplace Violence Advisory Standard which is expected to be issued during 2004.

Physicians for Human Rights. Bulgarian and Palestinian health professionals in Libya sentenced to death by firing squad. July 1, 2004; Nature, 430:8. Accessed July 20, 2004.

Physicians for Human Rights. Dr. Thys Van Mollendorff—charges dropped! Accessed July 20, 2004.

Physicians for Human Rights. Update: six Cuban physicians sentenced from 13 to 25 years. Accessed July 20, 2004.

Rice MM. Legal issues in emergency medicine. In: Rosen P, Barkin R, eds. Emergency Medicine. 4th ed. St. Louis, Mo: Mosby; 1998:77, 217, 235-36, 242-45.

Trials of War Criminals before the Nuremberg Military Tribunals. Trials of war criminals before the Nuremberg Military Tribunals under Control Council Law No. 10. Vol 2. Government Printing Office; 1949. 181-182.

Witman AB, Park DM, Hardin SB. How do patients want physicians to handle mistakes? A survey of internal medicine patients in an academic setting. *Arch Intern Med*. Dec 9-23 1996;156(22):2565-9. [Medline].

WorkCover Authority of NSW (2002), Violence in the Workplace: Guide 2002, WorkCover NSW, Sydney (available through www.workcover.nsw.gov.au).

WorkCover Corporation of South Australia (2002), Guidelines for Reducing the Risk of Violence at Work (available through www.workcover.com).

WorkCover Tasmania (2003), Violence at the Workplace (available through www.workcover.tas.gov.au).

WorkSafe Western Australia (1999), Code of Practice: Workplace Violence (available through www.safetyline.wa.gov.au).

APPENDIX

PERSONAL SAFETY AND PRIVACY FOR DOCTORS

(A Statement of American Medical Association—2005)

I. Preamble

The AMA recognizes that violence against doctors is a growing concern. This Position Statement is provided in an effort to reduce the vulnerability of medical practitioners to physical harm in all locations or settings in which they practice or may be exposed to personal danger arising from their professional work as doctors. It is recognized that there will be wide variation in the level of risk, the practicality of protective measures for prevention of threats to personal safety and the availability of emergency help when such threats do arise.

The statement is framed within a risk management approach, focusing on risk identification, risk assessment, risk control and evaluation of the effectiveness of risk management strategies. It is intended to guide the violence management efforts of hospitals, practice managers and individual doctors—these parties should also keep up to date with current literature on the subject.

1.1 Scope

Standard workplaces for doctors include public and private hospitals, other health and aged care facilities and private practices. Many doctors work shifts and many provide after hours services and home visits to patients in the community. Some doctors attend accident scenes and other locations requiring travel by vehicle, boat or aircraft. There is obviously a wide range of workplaces. Some of these workplaces, such as major hospitals, are able to provide formal protective measures in terms of both prevention of and responses to violence against doctors and other staff. Others, such as small hospitals and private practices, cannot provide the same sorts of formal protective measures, but they should apply the principles set out in this statement in regard to the personal safety and security of doctors. In these smaller workplaces the risk of violence may be lower, but the impact of it is likely to be higher when it occurs because of the lack of immediate response and assistance from security staff or police. This also applies where doctors are working on their own, particularly outside static workplaces, for example on home visits or emergency callouts. In addition, there are times when the process of consultation and treatment of medical conditions can involve the transmission of deeply sensitive information regarding both the patient and other individuals. Such information generally remains private between the parties, but in some circumstances statutory obligations will require the doctor to convey appropriate information to the relevant authority. This can include information regarding infectious diseases, fitness to drive motor vehicles, etc. The repercussions of these obligatory disclosures can be profound for the patient and, where there is emotional or psychological instability, for others. Doctors involved in these work situations may find themselves faced with threats to their personal safety even while at home or otherwise going about their private business. Thus occupational safety strategies for doctors may need to address risks outside the workplace.

1.2 Managing Risk

Every State and Territory has occupational health and safety (OH&S) legislation that places on employers a general duty of care to provide and maintain a safe and healthy workplace. The legislation also assigns to each employee a duty to take reasonable care for their own health and safety, as well as for the health and safety of others who may be affected by that employee's acts or omissions at the workplace. Violence risk management needs to take into consideration the work environment as a whole. To be successful it requires the commitment of management through sufficient investment of time, money and personnel. This includes commitment to regular audits of the organization's vulnerability to violence to inform risk management planning. Consultation with staff is essential for violence risk management planning to be effective. A risk management methodology can be used in conjunction with the detailed knowledge of staff in the local work environment to develop tailored solutions to violence problems. It may be appropriate to assemble a working group of staff to develop a violence risk management plan.

2. AMA Position

2.1 Risk Identification

2.1.1 The identification of risks in relation to violence should take into account information from workplace inspections and security assessments, incident and accident reports/investigations, Workers' Compensation records, complaints, and other information obtained from staff and users of health care facilities.

2.1.2 A system should be in place for reporting violent incidents and staff should be encouraged to report all violent or aggressive incidents that have endangered, or have had the potential to endanger, a staff member's safety.

2.2 Risk Assessment

2.2.1 Assessments of identified risks should be undertaken to arrive at ratings of both the likelihood of each risk occurring and its impact. These ratings should be used to ascertain the level of each risk so that the relative priority of actions to deal with these risks can be determined.

2.3 Risk Control

The resourcing and timing of steps to control (eliminate or minimize) risks should reflect the level of each risk as identified through risk assessment. Risk control should include, but not be limited to, the following:

2.3.1 Policy on Violence

2.3.1.1 The organization should develop a zero tolerance policy regarding the management of violence and ensure that staff understand it.

2.3.2 Complaints Mechanism

2.3.2.1 A complaints mechanism should be available for staff and users of health care facilities in order to encourage problems to be addressed in a non-violent manner.

2.3.3 Physical Environment

2.3.3.1 Surroundings should be made as comfortable as possible for users of health care facilities to help lower distress amongst those with health concerns.

2.3.3.2 There should be sufficient lighting inside and in the immediate vicinity of the hospital to provide a safe and secure working environment.

2.3.3.3 External doors should be locked at night with only the main entrances, which should be under staff surveillance, left open for public access.

2.3.3.4 Staff should have access to secure lockers in which valuables can be stored while working.

2.3.3.5 Sufficient car parking spaces should be available to provide for all doctors rostered on at any particular time or likely to be called in, including specific doctors' parking for on call/after hours work. These spaces should be within close proximity of the area of the building in which the doctor is working, sufficiently well lit to provide secure access at night, and reserved for staff use only.

2.3.3.6 Staff only areas (including staff office areas, staff common rooms, and other restricted areas) should be accessible only via restrictive access devices such as card keys with photo identification.

2.3.3.7 Video surveillance in appropriate areas should be considered and, where implemented, signs should be prominently posted advising of its presence to maximise its deterrence value.

2.3.4 Personal Protection

2.3.4.1 Duress alarms should be provided where practicable for doctors exposed to higher-risk situations, including doctors working in mental health treatment areas, emergency departments and in settings where there is little organizational backup or delays in getting emergency help, such as after hours surgeries. Duress alarms should also be provided in Resident Medical Officer quarters and in hospital corridors assessed as dangerous.

2.3.4.2 Where doctors are required to walk significant distances to their cars or walk to their cars at night, an escort should be available upon request to facilitate a safe passage.

2.3.5 Protecting Personal Privacy

2.3.5.1 Employers must ensure that the personal privacy of doctors is protected; particularly sensitive details such as private address and contact numbers. This is particularly important in situations where the nature of doctors' work places them at risk of harassment and violence from unstable or maladjusted patients.

The AMA's position in relation to the personal privacy of doctors is as follows:

- It is a fundamental right for the occupational health and safety of medical practitioners providing services to patients, in any setting, for the personal private details of doctors, including residential address, to remain strictly confidential.
- OH&S principles, as they relate to medical practitioners, require strict observance of the doctor's need for personal privacy. Further, under no circumstances should a doctor's contact address provided to an employer or Medical Board be made publicly available or be included in publicly accessible databases by medical practitioner registration boards or similar authorities unless the doctor has expressly consented to have the information made available.
- Any disclosure of a doctor's private personal information, including private residential address, by an individual, agency or authority, from either the public or private sector, is a clear breach of OH&S principles as they relate to medical practitioners.

2.3.6 Education and Training

2.3.6.1 Doctors, other health care staff, patients and their visitors should be provided with information regarding behaviour expected of them in a health care setting.

2.3.6.2 Staff should be provided with a copy of the organisation's policy on violence and understand what action they should take to address concerns that may arise.

2.3.6.3 Staff should be given appropriate training to assist with the management of violence. Preventative approaches should be covered as part of such training, including the skill of projecting a pleasant manner to help prevent feelings of resentment and alienation on the part of users.

2.3.6.4 Staff should be provided with information regarding the identification and assessment of risks in relation to violence in their work environment, as well as control measures to address the risks.

2.3.7 Home Visits

2.3.7.1 Guidelines should be in place to protect doctors undertaking home visits. These may include, for example, providing security escorts upon request, keeping timetables recording details of doctors' client visits, reporting in at the end of each visit, following predetermined procedures if doctors become uncontactable or do not check in when expected, and ensuring that they carry a duress alarm and/or mobile phone (GPS-linked if necessary) during visits.

2.3.8 Additional Security Measures

2.3.8.1 Additional security measures should be taken to protect doctors working late hours (for instance, in after hours surgeries), in settings where they are on their own or where emergency help is not quickly available and in places where drugs are stored or being distributed. An example in relation to the latter would be to reposition drugs cabinets so that they are within view of as many staff as possible during the course of their work to deter violent incidents.

2.3.9 Post-incident Management

2.3.9.1 Post-incident management activities should include post-incident support (such as first aid, medical attention, and incident debriefing), incident reporting, and incident investigation activities which include recommendations to help prevent future recurrence.

2.4 Monitoring and Evaluation

2.4.1 Continuous monitoring and evaluation of outcomes needs to be undertaken to assess the effectiveness of the risk management strategies that have been implemented. The outcomes of such evaluation should be reflected in updates to violence risk management plans.

5

Promoting Health through Hospitals

The Ottawa Charter for Health Promotion (WHO, 1986) has led to the development of a series of health promotion initiatives based on settings. These settings have included cities, villages, schools, workplaces and hospitals. Settings approach to health promotion is about much more than introducing a variety of opportunities for individuals using the hospital to change their behavior. To be health promoting in any meaningful sense a hospital has to be committed to instituting a process of organization development and change. The pressures on hospitals to broaden their role from the focus on treating diseases towards health promotion has been felt for more than a decade. It has been argued that hospitals should not continue to function in isolation from the community around them and that they 'must develop a community conscience rather than an institutional loyalty'. Despite such calls, hospitals have been ignoring the pressure to embrace a more health promoting role. The general attitude is 'let somebody else do it; we already have too much to do'.

There is a need for a significant re-orientation of the way in which hospitals operate. Given the strong institutional focus of modern hospitals with their very heavy reliance on high technology medicine, such a re-orientation would not be possible without significant and organization-wide commitment to the re-assessment of the hospital's role and function.

WHY PROMOTE HEALTH THROUGH HOSPITALS?

Hospitals are in a strong position within the health care system to be advocates for health promotion. They represent the main concentration of health service resources, professional skills and medical technology. Communities readily identify with hospitals. They generally have substantial prestige and their staff are well respected. They are seen as credible sources of advice and expertise on health issues beyond their responsibilities for sick care services. So although hospitals are the high temples of sick care, the extensive resources they command mean that even a small shift of focus has the potential to bring about an increase in resources dedicated to health promotion and, in time, health benefits to a community.

Health promoting hospitals

The basic premise of the notion of a health promoting hospital is to put into practice the fifth strategy of the Ottawa Charter for Health Promotion, that is the re-orientation of health services. Using the hospital as a setting also means implementing the Ottawa Charter's other strategies of devising healthy public policy, creating environments that are supportive of health, involving community people, and developing personal skills for promoting the health of staff and community members.

In practice, since the emergence of the health promoting hospital concept in the late 1980s, there have been many different interpretations of the concept and many of these have not incorporated the range of strategies suggested by the Ottawa Charter. Some examples of health promoting hospital practice have simply relied on behaviour change strategies and little else. The varying methods of implementation and differential interpretation of the concept of a health promoting hospital have led a number of commentators to call for a more consistent approach to the concept. The main focus of health promotion activity during the period of the case study at the Adelaide hospital was on disease management and prevention, activities oriented towards 'patients and their families'. This was through using the strategies of health education and health counselling, and developing partnership-in-care relationships between staff and patients and their families. The coordination of care and linking of patients and their families to community supports were also emphasized.

There were several 'community'-oriented health promotion activities implemented by staff at the Adelaide hospital. The staff developed working relationships with consumers and a range of community groups and organizations, both within the health sector and other sectors. These relationships had the purposes of improving hospital to community support; collaborating to develop health education resources; collaborating to undertake health promoting projects to impact on the health to targeted groups of the community, e.g. 'Never Shake a Baby', 'Folate before Pregnancy', 'Partnerships with Youth', 'State Food and Nutrition Health Promotion Program', 'State Asthma Program', 'Stop the Rot' (prevention of dental caries in toddlers), 'Safe Eating for the Under 4s', 'Safe Sleeping in the Under 2s', and 'Lock Up and Away! Poison Prevention Project'. Community education activities such as monthly health seminars, a hospital awareness programme for children <7 years of age, the infant cardio pulmonary resuscitation programme; and health information available through the Internet and health information centre were also introduced. An emphasis was also placed by the hospital on increasing by amount of information about health and illness provided to the community through the mass media. Health promotion activities directed at staff and developed during the case study period were as follows: staff immunization; women's health clinic; nutritious hospital food for staff; lunchtime walking groups; and staff aerobics classes. Health promotion activities may include organization-wide programmes that primarily relate to the occupational health and safety programme; an infection control programme; and the implementation and maintenance of the no-smoking policy. These programmes also meet legislative requirements. Activities in this area tend to come under the banner of continuous improvement projects as part of the quality management programme, rather than being described as health promotion activities.

Heath promotion through 'Physical environment' include activities related to the waste management programme to reduce the amount of medical and general waste and improve recycling, and the different strategies used within the hospital to reduce energy consumption and green house gas emissions. As with the 'organization' activities, the 'physical environment' activities are quality management programmes that have an impact on the health of the organization (setting), and, in the instance of 'physical environment' activities, also on the broader physical environment of the community. Both of these areas involve a significant number of staff at all levels of the organization and have potential to result in significant cost savings to the organization. The development of a hospital health promotion programme is central to supporting these different types of health promotion activities. The key elements of a hospital health promotion programme should include:

- strong leadership at different levels of the organization (especially from the Board of Management, Chief Executive Officer, Assistant Chief Executive Officer, Health Promotion Consultant and several champions from corporate and clinical areas);
- incorporation of health promotion into the hospital's vision and strategic role statements, policies, service agreements with divisions, and job descriptions for staff, as well as a specific health promotion policy;
- strategic, operational and evaluation plans for health promotion;
- staff development and education; and
- resources allocated (human, physical facilities and financial).

Unless each of these key elements is present and supportive of health promotion within a hospital, a significant organizational re-orientation to health promotion is unlikely.

Two factors affect the outcome of organizational arrangements for health promoting hospital initiatives. These two factors are: (i) the degree of organizational commitment made by hospitals; and (ii) the types of health promotion activities undertaken.

The types of health promotion activities undertaken by hospitals could be grouped into five categories.

- patients and their families;
- staff;
- the organization as a whole;
- the physical environment; and
- the community that is served by the hospital.

When the various types of health promotion activities are combined with the level of organizational commitment to health promotion observed in various hospitals, four distinct approaches to health promotion emerge.

- doing a 'health promotion project';
- delegating it to 'the role of a specific division, department or staff';
- being a 'health promotion setting'; and
- being a 'health promotion setting and improving the health of the community'.

It is evident that the first two of these approaches do not necessarily require an organizational commitment towards health promotion. Health promotion is often marginalized to the role of specific staff, departments or divisions, and is not integrated into the practice of staff throughout the organization. The last two approaches, 'being a health promotion setting' and 'being a health promotion setting and improving the health of the community', require an organizational commitment to extend its role to be more health promoting. To create a support hospital environment for staff, and for a hospital to succeed in developing a more sustainable approach to becoming more health promoting, a hospital health promotion programme needs to be in place and health promotion needs to be integrated into the practice of staff throughout the organization. The following section describes each of the four types of health promoting hospitals suggested by the authors as being of relevance to understanding how different hospital approach implementing the concept of health promoting hospitals.

Doing a project

The 'doing a health promotion project' approach does not generally challenge hospitals to re-orient the whole organization and the roles of staff to health promotion. In this approach, health promotion projects are usually *ad hoc* isolated events. The projects are not part of a strategic approach to re-orient the hospitals' role in the community towards improving the health of the population, or develop the 'setting' to improve the health and well-being of patients and their families and staff. In this approach, the projects can be oriented towards all the five categories and patients and families, staff, organization, physical environment, or community.

A health promoting hospital has health promotion as a core value within the organization. It is not simply a hospital with a few health promotion projects' [(Rushmere, 1996), p. 11]. However, despite this criticism of the 'doing a health promotion project' approach, it may have an important place in the evolution, rather than transformation, or a hospital to become more health promoting. For example, it may be an appropriate starting point for staff who are interested in their hospital becoming involved in health promotion, but do not have the support of senior management for an organizational commitment at that stage. Implementing and evaluating an individual health promotion project may serve as a catalyst for gaining or organizational commitment. However, sustainability becomes a key issue if an organization continues to undertake *ad hoc* health promotion programmes without developing an organizational infrastructure to support the health promotion efforts of staff.

Delegating health promotion to the role of a specific division, department or staff

This approach has been observed in hospitals that have a health promotion unit, have designated health promotion workers, or have established community-oriented visions or departments who 'do health promotion' or 'have a community orientation' for the hospital. If health promotion is restricted to particular divisions, departments or staff it remains a marginalized activity and does not necessarily challenge the whole organization to re-orient its role in the community, or for health promotion to be integrated into the roles of staff throughout the organization. A common phenomenon observed in organizations with this orientation is that staff working in these roles, departments or divisions often became limited in the impact they can have on re-orientation of the broader hospital, as health promotion was often seen as 'their job'. When hospital becomes a health promotion 'setting'. The organization is committed to health promotion in the form of a hospital health promotion programme and health promotion activities directed at the health of patients and their families, staff, organization, and the physical environment of the hospital. However, there is no broader commitment to improve the health of the community served by the hospital. The approach is also consistent with the 'get our own house in order' philosophy expressed in some hospitals. This philosophy is based on the premise that until such time as the hospital is a healthy environment and has addressed the health needs of patients, their families and staff, the hospital cannot broaden their approach to improve the health of the community.

Being a health promotion setting and improving the health of the community

Health Promotion through hospitals . approach signifies an organizational commitment to re-orient the hospital to be a health promotion 'setting', as well as improving the health of the community.

Within this approach there is a hospital health promotion programme and there can be health promotion activities in all five categories. Vang supports this approach and states that it is important for hospitals to improve the balance between projects that are oriented towards the 'setting', and projects that are aimed at improving the health of the community (Vang, 1995). What is significant about this approach is that the hospital has to systematically develop effective and collaborative working relationships with patients and their families, other service providers and the broader community to achieve the best outcomes. Table 5.1 represents a typology of the four types of hospital organizational arrangements for health promotion identified through this study. The four orientations towards being a health promoting hospital provide a framework to analyse how a hospital and its staff may perceive their health promotion role and responsibilities. For example, if a hospital approaches the concept of health promoting hospitals as type one or two, staff would view health promotion very differently to staff in a hospital that chooses to integrate health promotion into practice to 'be a health promotion setting' (type three) or to 'be a health promotion setting and improve the health of the community' (type four). With the first two types, staff would view health promotion as a marginal role for the hospital and externalize it as 'someone else's role' or the role of specific staff. The staff working in a hospital that adopts either type three or four would see health promotion as integrated into their own role as being part of the core business of staff throughout the hospital. There can be a variety of interpretations of the meaning of a health promoting hospital initiative.

Hospitals in the United States are increasingly positioning themselves as the leading provider of health promotion services within the community. As consumer demand for health information and preventive services intensifies, hospitals are re-evaluating their traditional focus on sick care, and considering optional ventures that will mobilize and satisfy an expanding market of health-conscious, apparently well people. Traditionalists argue that hospitals should maintain their long-established role as centres for acute care, relegating the responsibility for to the public health sector and other community agencies. Progressive hospital leaders, however, are establishing integrated health care systems as a strategy for long-term survival. By diversifying and expanding their traditional revenue base, hospitals can increase their revenue from diversified services assuring sufficient capital to provide high-technology, labour-intensive and costly acute care. Hospitals are targeting health promotion and wellness services as a viable diversification strategy. In addition to the potential for generating revenue, health promotion activities contribute positively to patient satisfaction, the hospital's image within a community and relations with medical staff. Hospitals can benefit by taking an active and leading role in ensuring the good health of the community they serve. In a statement on health promotion in 1979, the American Hospital Association recommended the following:

In addition to their primary mission of providing health care and related education to the sick and injured, hospitals have a responsibility to work with others in the community to assess the health status of the community, identify target health areas and population groups for hospital-based and cooperative health promotion programs, develop programs to help upgrade the health in those target areas, ensure that persons who are apparently healthy have access to information about how to stay well and prevent disease, provide appropriate health education programs to aid those persons who choose to alter their personal health behaviour or develop a more healthful lifestyle, and establish the hospital within the community as an institution which is concerned about good health as well as one concerned with treating illness. In today's health-conscious environment, physicians continue to be perceived as the primary source of useful and reliable health information, but few people are satisfied with the information they receive from their physicians. Most people associate hospitals with physicians and transfer this perceived reliability and credibility to hospital-based activities. In many communities the hospital is identified as a centre for health. It seems likely, therefore, that people would want hospitals to take a leading role in health promotion. In order to provide quality health information and guidance, hospital-based health promotion services should be multidisciplinary, relying on the expertise of a variety of health professionals, typically physicians, nurse, physiotherapists, physiologists and nutritionists. Each member of the health care team may work with individuals as inpatients, outpatients or in the community to assist them in achieving their health-related goals.

The professional practice standards established by many professional organizations specifically refer to the role and responsibilities of hospital-based practitioners in promoting health as an integral component of quality care. Many institutions include health education and health promotion responsibilities in performance standards, and evaluations, promotions and salary increases are then based on compliance with these standards. Because hospitals have not emphasized prevention and health promotion in the past, these standards serve as important reminders and incentives to the staff to look beyond treatment protocols. Hospital-based health promotion programmes typically include patient education and counseling services, clinical rehabilitation programmes, and community and corporate wellness services. All the activities in each programme area are consistent with the goals of health promotion and are designed to (4): foster awareness, influence attitudes, and identify alternatives so that individuals can make informed choices and change their behaviour in order to achieve an optimum level of physical and mental health and improve their physical and social environment. Hospital-based health promotion programmes support individual efforts to achieve a state of optimal health and physical, mental and emotional well-being.

Patient Education

One of the earliest health promotion initiatives within a hospital was the establishment of formal programmes for patient education. The Joint Committee on Health Education Terminology defined patient education as: the health experiences designed to influence learning which occurs as a person receives preventive, diagnostic, therapeutic and/or rehabilitative services, including experiences which arise from coping with symptoms, referral to source of information, prevention, diagnosis and care, and contacts with health institutions, health personnel, family and other patients. Patient education services include a variety of activities designed to inform patients about their illness and the effect of those illnesses on their daily lives, to prepare patients for diagnostic and treatment procedures and the experience of being in hospital, to assist patients in managing their diseases after discharge, and to modify their behaviour to promote optimal health and prevent further illness. The goal of patient education is to foster an active partnership between patients, their families and their health care providers so that collaborative decisions can be made about care, treatment plan, and lifestyle after discharge.

Many social factors led to the increased interest inpatient education observed in the late 1960s and 1970s including: the increased prevalence of chronic diseases requiring long-term and continuous management, often self-administered; a growing social concern about containing costs, the utilization of health services, and quality care; the consumer movement, public demand for influence in medical care decisions, and frustration with the complexities of the health care delivery system; documented evidence that patient education helps attain treatment goals; legislation related to informed consent; and malpractice issues. In response to these factors and others, supportive documents, mandates and guidelines have evolved to further entrench patient and family education as an integral component of quality care and professional practice in hospitals. Patient education programmes are typically planned and coordinated at three levels within hospitals: the institutional level, involving the entire facility or hospitals; the programmatic level, targeting specific patient populations or groups having a similar disease, in hospital experience, or demographic characteristic; and the patient level, involving direct contact and interaction with the patient. The activities at each level directly affect people at the other levels. For example, an institution-wide policy that specifies the role of nursing service personnel. Inpatient and family education can greatly support the bedside teaching activity conducted by nurses. Lesson plans developed for specific patient groups enhance the consistency of the patient teaching provided by a variety of care givers working with any one patient. Programme planning at all three levels enhances the quality and quantity of patient education and decreases the likelihood of duplication of effort and inefficient use of resources.

Developing and designing a comprehensive inpatient education programme encompasses four sequential and interrelated steps: assessment of need, planning and objective setting, implementation and evaluation. Each step of this process has a different focus for each level of programming being considered.

In assessing the needs of institutions, existing policies, roles and responsibilities, resource allocation and the strategic goals of the organization must be assessed. At the programmatic level, disease profiles, staff capacities and medical staff idiosyncrasies must be analysed. At the patient level, the learning needs of patients and their families should be assessed, focusing on their current knowledge, skills and attitudes. A comprehensive needs assessment at any level of programming becomes the foundation and justification for the activities being planned. After the needs of the institution, patient population or individual are assessed, a plan of action with specific and measurable objectives should be established. The objectives may be short- or long-term and should guide subsequent programme evaluation. Throughout implementation, teaching must be documented in the medical record and evidence of learning must be monitored. Effective communication, both written and verbal, is critical. For institutions, communication between work groups and between providers such as physicians, nurses and pharmacists enhances receptivity to innovative programming strategies and new or revised policies and procedures. Skill in lading groups and communicating concepts and information is an essential part of teaching patients effectively.

Evaluation at the institutional level measures the success of the overall plan. The parameters often monitored are the satisfaction of patients, medical staff and providers, and quality audits related to documentation and compliance with predetermined standards of practice. For patients, behavioural outcome prior to discharge is the measure of successful intervention. At all levels of programming, the objectives of the plan form the basis for an effective evaluation system. Many studies have demonstrated the benefits that patients realize from a planned and coordinated approach to patient education. Reductions in length in stay, reductions in complications, and reductions in admissions and readmissions to hospital are the benefits to patients most widely documented in research on patient education.

Clinical Rehabilitation

Clinical rehabilitation programmes that incorporate exercise therapy and health education enhance the continuity of care and treatment of people moving from the inpatient unit to the outpatient unit or home treatment. Following the treatment and stabilization of an illness, a rehabilitation programme is designed to return the person to a level of health equal to or greater than the level before the illness. The goal of clinical rehabilitation programmes is to improve stamina and strength, return people to their homes and activities of daily living, and at the same time prevent recurrence of the illness or injury. Clinical rehabilitation programmes typically provided by hospitals include: cardiac rehabilitation and pulmonary rehabilitation; exercise therapy to rehabilitate mental health patients and those suffering from substance abuse and eating disorders; and sports medicine.

Clinical rehabilitation programmes begin with inpatients and continue when they become outpatients. These programmes provide a continuum of supervised care and treatment until the patient is trained in self-care skills and ready for discharge from the programme.

All patients must be referred to the clinical rehabilitation programme by their attending physician. Typically, the referring physician prescribes exercise and education. The success of clinical rehabilitation programmes depends on the patient's relationship with the referring physician. Physicians frequently resist referring their patients to rehabilitation programmes for fear of losing control of the treatment plan. The personnel of the rehabilitation programme are responsible for revolving referring physicians in the rehabilitation process. Encouraging the physician to prescribe graded levels of exercise and education for the period of rehabilitation, and assuring periodic feedback and consultation with the physician encourage medical staff to support the programme.

Patient entry into rehabilitation usually begins with a physiological and medical evaluation. For example, in cardiac rehabilitation programmes, the patient undergoes a battery of tests that can include a graded exercise test, blood chemistry analysis, determination of body composition, and nutritional analysis. This information offers a baseline for developing an individualized prescription for exercise and education. Similar assessments are made for patients entering other types of rehabilitation programme. An exit evaluation is compared with initial test results, documenting the progress made.

Outpatient rehabilitation programmes vary in length. The period of time depends on: the physician order, the type of rehabilitation, the patient's response to the rehabilitation, the patient's motivation and interest, and the patient's ability to pay for the service.

To participate in a medically supervised programme, people must live within a reasonable distance of the rehabilitation site. Accessibility is a critical factor in adherence to the rehabilitation regimen. Often people live an unreasonable commuting distance from the hospital or rehabilitation centre. It is best to refer these people to a home rehabilitation programme.

Self-directed, home rehabilitation programmes are prudent alternatives to structured hospital-based programmes. Typically, the guide for the home programme is provided on discharge from the hospital. Rehabilitation professionals carefully educate people in exercise and lifestyle modification. Home programmes require frequent follow-up to evaluate progress, encourage adherence, and provide support.

Since professionals are not in direct contact with the patient, home programmes are less effective than supervised programmes in achieving rehabilitation. The disadvantages of home programmes are the risk of non-adherence, reliance on self-motivation, and the patient's fear of unsupervised activity. Peer camaraderie and the sense of security provided by trained personnel are strong advantages of participating in hospital-based rehabilitation programmes. Discharge criteria are established collaboratively by the patient, the physician and the rehabilitation team. These criteria depend on the type and severity of the patient's initial illness. Continuous documentation of patient progress is essential to determine appropriate discharge points. Clinical rehabilitation is a systematic and progressive process that assists individuals in making the transition from acute illness through recovery to an optimal state of health and fitness.

Community and Corporate Wellness

Motivated by changes in the market and potential new revenue, hospital decision-makers are targeting community and corporate wellness services as a form of diversification. As hospitals capitalize on growing consumer interest in health practices and fitness, they target the apparently well population for a variety of hospital-based health promotion services.

Wellness programmes are designed to educate and motivate individuals to reduce their risk of preventable diseases. By adopting healthy lifestyle practices, the individual decreases the risk of premature death and disability, and the costs associated with medical care. The enhanced community relations and direct revenue resulting from providing health promotion services can justify entry into the wellness arena for many hospitals.

Hospital-based programmes are typically directed at three audiences: apparently well groups or individuals within the community, employees of local businesses and industries (and their dependants), and the health professionals and other staff employed by the hospital. The programmes encompass a broad spectrum of activities and services, and are planned to address the health-related needs and interests of the target population.

Many hospitals with well established inpatient education and clinical rehabilitation programmes have moved quickly into the market for apparently well people. Inpatient education programmes focusing on disease management, self-care skills, and prevention have great appeal to non-patient groups. By 1984, 67% of all hospitals in the United States offered some type of wellness programme for the community. This number is expected to increase as more hospitals recognize the potential benefits of a community-wide campaign.

The motives for hospitals to initiate a community wellness programme are varied and are based on the institution's outreach objectives. The objectives that can be attained include: improving the hospital's image, promoting specific services, recruiting physicians and marketing their services, and establishing a presence within a target service area.

Most community wellness services are marketed to individuals within the primary service area of the hospital. Many hospitals are segmenting their market, as they focus health promotion activities on specific groups such as women, old people and young people. Once the target population is identified, its health needs can be more precisely assessed. Segmenting the community in this manner facilitates advertising the promotional efforts, and enhances the meaning and value of the activity for the target audience.

A study by Miaouli profiled the health-seeker segment of the disease prevention and health promotion market. Health-seeking individuals actively participate in fitness programmes and frequently use preventive medical services. They tend to be opinion leaders for health-related issues, and thus stimulate positive health behaviour among other people. They are usually well educated and have high incomes. Designing hospital-based health promotion services for health-seekers helps to nurture a socially and medically desirable attitude among large numbers of people and leads to improved public health via word of mouth. In addition, it increases the satisfaction of health-seekers and prevents them from abandoning the traditional health care delivery system for alternative services that may be of questionable benefit.

Participation in these programmes also appears to be related to individual health status and how recently care was received at a hospital. People in fair or poor health and those who have been in hospital within the last three years are most likely to participate in hospital-based health promotion programmes.

The needs and interests of the target audience determine the components of the programme. Nutrition education, stress management, smoking cessation, cardiopulmonary resuscitation, aerobic exercise and prenatal education are a few of the typical popular offerings in the wellness market.

Activities and services of health promotion should be designed to achieve three objectives: assessing the risks to the health of the individual or group, intervening appropriately, and providing continuing support to maintain healthy behaviour. Assessment is most often accomplished through appraisals of health risk. These are screening tools or programmes that identify individual health risks before illness or symptoms of disease become apparent. Assessment is based on a quantitative measurement of a variety of physiological, spiritual, psychological and sociological parameters related to health habits and lifestyle. These are combined to present a composite of the individual's risk of illness. Aggregate data for groups compiled from the assessment of health risks can be used to set priorities among intervention strategies.

A myriad of intervention strategies are used to modify unhealthy behaviour and practices. Health education classes and fitness activities, typically led by health care professionals, are designed to inform, motivate, and substitute healthy forms of behaviour for unhealthy ones. Health professionals from the hospitals, such as physiotherapists, nutritionists, exercise physiologists, nurses and counsellors, contribute their expertise in planning and developing wellness curricula. All intervention strategies are based on the results of the assessment, focusing on reducing risk factors and modifying behaviour.

Continuing support is crucial. In the past decade, 500,000 self-help groups have been formed in the United States, reaching more than 15 million people. More than half of all American hospitals currently sponsor or co-sponsor support or self-help programmes for individuals and their loved ones. Self-help groups provide education, counselling and peer support over an extended period of time, services that hospital departments typically cannot offer to patients whose stays are limited.

Hospitals can obtain several benefits by associating closely with such groups as Alcoholics Anonymous and Overeaters Anonymous (for people with substance abuse and eating disorders), Mended Hearts (for people recovering from open-heart surgery), and Resolve (for people afflicted with life-threatening illnesses). Some of the cost-effective ways that a hospital can support the work of a self-help organization are by offering space at the hospital for meetings, assigning health professionals on the staff to be guest speakers, and initiating referrals for episodic care. In return, the hospital realizes many benefits in its relations with patients and the public, inpatient referrals, and visibility in the community. Hospitals can thus redirect their resources to narrow the gap between patient needs and available medical services.

Many hospitals are able to reach their target groups through existing networks in the community. Local YMCAs, churches, community agencies, and racket and health clubs offer promising opportunities for joint ventures with hospitals. The medical expertise and resources within a hospital are an attractive incentive for existing fitness programmes conducted through local agencies. Facilities that are suitable for recreational activities are often an investment too expensive for hospitals. Hospitals can join community agencies in offering health promotion programmes at locations that are convenient and accessible to the target population, decreasing duplication of service and reducing needless competition between other provider groups.

More and more employers are demonstrating a commitment to promoting the health of their employees, in the hope of reducing the spiralling costs associated with acute inpatient care. Many employers lack the number of employees needed to justify an in-house department of occupational medicine and health promotion, and are therefore contracting with local hospitals to provide the necessary medical expertise and resources to create a safe and healthy workplace environment.

Corporate health promotion programmes are designed to protect the health and safety of employees at the workplace, prevent work-related illness and injury, and create an environment that promotes healthy living. Services hospitals often provide to employers include: environmental assessment of health hazards, screening for health problems related to specific work tasks, and education focused on preventing accident and injury. Other typical services include diagnosis and emergency care for work-related accidents, disability evaluation, and processing workers' compensation claims.

A combination of occupational health and wellness services provided by hospitals at the workplace is a highly attractive alternative for employers considering offering a health promotion benefit to their employees.

Companies view health promotion initiatives as a strategy to reduce costs. Combining occupational health and wellness services addresses the employees' perception that the company is interested in their well being, and the employer's needs to cut the cost of episodic care. The goal of all health promotion programmes marketed to employers is to improve the relations between the hospital and employers, a critical need in today's health care marketplace. The private sector is demanding that health care costs be more effectively controlled. By promoting prevention, self-care and outpatient treatment, hospitals can actively help in containing health care costs, which is highly appealing to insurance companies and employers.

The hospital work environment presents unique challenges to health promotion programmes that target hospital workers. Burnout, inferior working conditions, rotating shifts, and frequent exposure to communicable diseases increase the hospital employee's risk of stress disease and on-the-job injury.

Successful workplace health promotion programmes within hospitals are often linked directly to employee benefits, as the employee benefit plan provides incentives for participation. Top management must assure release time for participation and implement institution wide policies that create a healthier working environment for the programme to be successful. The typical workplace health promotion activities provided to non-hospital employees can be supplemented by: banning smoking in designated areas of the hospital, educating staff about preventing back injury and controlling infection, and providing counselling services to employees so that they can better cope with grief, stress and burnout. A model initiative schedules activities around the clock, reaching all staff with risk-reducing activities that target the unique needs of hospital employees.

Benefits to Providers

Hospitals can realize numerous benefits by providing comprehensive health promotion services. It is essential, however, that the goals of the health promotion programme are linked to the goals of the hospital. Health promotion programmes can improve the profitability of a hospital by generating new revenue.

Health promotion programmes also improve the community's image of the hospital. Historically, this was the primary reason for hospitals to enter the health promotion arena. Hospitals provided free education and preventive services in an effort to fulfil their leadership role as providers of health promotion services. The out-reach programmes continue to enhance awareness of the hospital and its medical staff.

Health promotion services help hospitals to obtain patients. Highly popular community screening programmes (health fairs) identify varying percentages (2.6-47.9%) of participants with abnormal test results. These participants are typically referred to their physicians or to a physician on the staff at the sponsoring hospital. One hospital found that 1.5% of the participants screened at a health fair used hospital services or were admitted to the hospital within five months of the fair. This is applicable to the hospitals where the attendance is low.

Relations with medical staff are often improved through health promotion programmes. In areas with a surplus of physicians, hospitals have used community education and other health promotion services to market staff physicians' practices. Collaborative ventures between physicians with a preventive orientation and hospital-based health promotion programmes are becoming more common.

CONCLUSION

Hospitals need to re-evaluate their mission for inclusion of disease prevention and health promotion services. Prompted by people frustrated with the cost and complexities of the traditional system of health care delivery, many hospitals are instituting non-traditional services oriented towards consumer education, self-care, rehabilitation and wellness.

Because hospitals have been slow to enter the health promotion arena, there has been little research to support the benefits of diversification. Early indications, however, are that hospital-based health promotion initiatives can save money and improve the quality of health care.

The long-term effect of the commitment of hospitals to health promotion will only be realized if health care professionals begin to enter hospitals oriented towards prevention. The success of a programme directly depends on the values and skills of the physicians, nurses and other health professionals who provide the services. Hospitals that actively recruit this new breed of practitioner, and that manage the programmes in a customer-oriented way will be leaders in the health care system of the future.

A particular difficulty is associated with the varying usage of 'health promotion'—at times describing a total package of education, health care and policy, at other times specific health education activities. The differential use may not always matter but it can be significant if it leads to failures in communicating about and developing effective practice.

In examining health promotion in health care settings as a totality, different strands of activity can be identified. In addition to preventive and curative health care we can identify three strands of activity as shown in Table 5.1.

Early work in health care contexts, especially in hospital settings, was oriented towards education specific to the immediate condition and only later was general health education given more attention. The use of 'patient' rather than 'client' is also open to criticism. The former term is said to carry connotations of the passive recipient of whatever aspect of health care is under consideration and 'client' is preferred. The term 'client', notwithstanding the growing consumerism in many health services, may also be challenged as not fully reflecting the relationship between users and providers of health services. Hence the term 'patient education' remains widely used in the literature.

TABLE 5.1

Health promotion in health care

Patient education	*General health education*	*Health promotion policy*
Condition specific education with patients. Frequently focused on tertiary levels of prevention but includes activities directed to primary and secondary prevention	Aimed at primary prevention and promotion of positive health. For hospital patients and hospital workers. For patients in GP consultation in primary care. For all people on GP practice lists	General or specific health promotion policies. Focused on health care institutions or local communities

As in other contexts, a diversity of approaches to education exists in health care contents. Until comparatively recently education in hospitals was largely a condition specific activity with patients and strongly influenced by a preventive medical model. Much of the health education in primary care was also oriented to achieving lifestyle change. With the development of conceptions of the patient as an active rather than as a passive participant in health care, elements of educational and empowerment approaches have been more apparent. Much of the debate about approaches has centred on the activity of 'patient education'.

In sum the call for patient education or information comes from two different directions—a patient centred one in which autonomy is the key word and a medico-centred one in which compliance still reigns. There have been advocates of both preventive and educational approaches throughout the history of patient education. Early demands for education were a response to the acknowledged lack of compliance with prescribed medical regimens and to the perceived need to secure behavioural change in the prevention of contemporary chronic diseases. The term 'compliance' fitted in with the classic Parsonian model of the patient role—passive, dependent, co-operating with the doctor and an unequal partner in the relationship.

With the recognition that in many chronic conditions the individual needed to be more fully involved in the working out of lifestyle changes and in planning adherence to complex regimens, a development from the guidance/co-operation model to a mutual participation model was proposed. Although this model may appear to use more patient centred language its underlying implication is that patients will comply with rational beahviour as defined by the professional. Health services were first persuaded of the value of patient education because of its reported successes in improving compliance, increasing patient satisfaction and contributing to reducing costs of care. From the 1960s onwards a number of social movements led to a challenge to compliance oriented patient education. These included the women's, consumer, primary health care (WHO, 1978) and self-care movements. Although the focus of their concerns with health issues varied they shared a commitment to self-determination and active participation in health care. Rights to information and to an active role in health decision-making were central concerns and the language of compliance was rejected.

In 1991 the WHO issued a Health Promoting Hospital declaration and hospitals have been identified as one of the key settings in The Health of the Nation. The latter document affirms that hospitals exist to provide treatment and care but they also offer unique opportunities for more general health promotion of patients, staff and all who come into contact with them. Prior to this focus on general health promotion policy, there had been a slow development of specific health promotion policies in this setting—'nutrition and smoking being common targets in some countries, joined more recently by breast-feeding. The recent WHO/UNICEF Baby Friendly Hospital Initiative asks every health care facility where babies are born to re-examine their policies in the light of current knowledge and to implement the Ten Steps to Successful Breastfeeding'. The health promotion developments in hospitals represent a broadening out from the emphasis on specific patient education.

Reorientating the health care system to the maintenance of good health and prevention rather than primarily to the treatment of acute illness.

Patient education services should enable patients and their families, when appropriate, to make informed decisions about their health, to manage their illnesses and to implement follow-up care at home.

Education is viewed by some primarily as a means to increase patient adherence to regimens and the management of conditions while for others it is a tool for enhancing patient participation in care and diminishing the power differential between patients and professionals.

Health Promoting Hospitals Initiative Network was established in Europe in the late 1980s in affiliation with the Healthy Cities network and by 1991 included 24 hospitals in 12 countries (Ashcroft and Summersgill, 1993). The notion of a health promoting hospital provides an appropriate context within which effective health education can take place. The constituent elements have been identified (Baric, 1992) as the:

1. Creation of a healthy environment for staff and clients;
2. Integration of health promotion into all the activities of the institution (prevention, treatment, education, rehabilitation, etc.);
3. Creation of 'healthy alliances' between the hospital and other institutions resulting in a 'health promoting community' in which all the institutions are health promoting.

Five main principles have been proposed for use in assessing whether or not a hospital is 'health promoting' (Ashcroft and Summersgill, 1993):

1. Health must appear on the agenda of policy makers in all sectors and at all levels of the hospital;
2. Work carried out in the hospital must be organized so as to create a healthy hospital environment;
3. Hospital personnel and patients must be empowered and enabled so that together they can have control of the elements that influence their health while in the hospital;
4. Personal and life skills of personnel and patients must be developed; and
5. The hospital must extend its activities in the health care system beyond merely providing clinical and curative services.

For each of these principles specific indicators will need to be developed to monitor progress and achievement. The reports of evaluations from the early hospitals to join the network will be followed with interest.

A number of factors are known to have a bearing on the overall effectiveness of hospitals where education in concerned. We need to achieve successful activity not only in a few areas of health but across a whole hospital institution and ultimately across the hospital system in total. For institution wide successes we need: policies which specify that educational activity is provided as a total part of care; health workers who are appropriately trained to undertake the educational component of care; organizational arrangements which maximize the possibility of educational success; widescale adoption of educational activities in line with client needs and which are known to be effective and efficient; and widescale availability of appropriate educational resources.

A number of policy documents which have recommended education in hospital care and more recently addressed the whole question of the health promoting potential of hospitals. The extent to which recommendations have been put into effect has varied between countries and the extent to which there have been incentives to undertake such development. Because of its perceived capacity to reduce costs patient education received early support in the USA. In other countries it was slower to develop. In the new market oriented NHS the incentive for purchasers to build health promotion into the contracts which they negotiate ought to provide a major impetus to education in hospital settings. Evidence from some countries of the extent of patient education policies and practice was reported in a series of papers in 1990. In Canada, 37% of hospitals (Bartlett and Jonkers, 1990) had health promotion policies while 21% stated that health promotion was not part of their role. From Australia, Degeling *et al* (1990) reported that most hospitals surveyed 'recognized the importance of patient education, but support was based on individual efforts resulting from initiatives taken in specialty areas rather than reflecting overall hospital policy'. In the USA a number of trends were having an impact on hospital patient education and in particular affecting the 'budget and administrative clout' of the coordinators and the increasing use of management features known to contribute to more successful programmes. As Green comments (1990): 'Hard times have forced a more systematic, coordinated, strategically planned and evaluated patient education program'. Finally, the Netherlands had recently seen a rapid development of the coordinator role with 60% of hospitals now employing people for such a role.

Organization

The first stage in ensuring that the educational component of patient care is met is to ensure that it is specified in the care plans. The next stage is to ensure that the educational needs identified are met. In any period of hospital care patients encounter a number of different professionals, ancillary staff, other patients and also their own families and friends. All can provide contributions to their education, both formally and informally. If such varied contributions go unco-ordinated it is highly unlikely that a coherent programme will result.

At the level of the individual patient the educational component can be recorded alongside all other aspects of care. Since hospital stays are reduced in time and may only form a small percentage of the time of an illness episode it is particularly important that there is coordination of education between hospital and primary care. In addition to coordination of education for specific patients there are other levels at which coordination can take place—at the level of specific conditions or as a general hospital-wide activity.

The institution of patient education coordinators first developed in the USA but has now spread more widely. Evidence of the effectiveness of coordination came from the study in Michigan in the USA. Eighteen criteria for patient education were incorporated into a survey of subject based programmes. Of 281 programmes reported, 21 (78%) had either a fulltime or a part-time coordinator (Pack *et al.*, 1983). The mean number of criteria met by these programmes was 13.8 where there was a fulltime and 12.7 with a par-time coordinator but only 8.3 where there was no coordinator. There was some variation in the number of criteria met according to the type of coordinator. Where education was considered to be the prime responsibility more criteria were likely to be met than where responsibilities were diverse. If the coordinator had received further training, programmes tended to be more comprehensive and met more criteria.

The development of the function of patient education coordinator in the Netherlands was described by Fahrenfort (1990). This is instructive for those countries currently at the early stages of development of patient education. This innovation started with a research project funded for three years (later extended to five) in five hospitals. The hospitals selected had to meet certain criteria: agreement to appoint a patient education coordinator for the duration of the project; to have demonstrated an interest inpatient education prior to applying for the grant; and the hospital management had to be supportive to the experiment and agree to external monitoring, advice and evaluation. The monitoring and evaluation were expected to address the following areas: the benefits to the development of patient education of the coordinator appointment; the qualifications for the coordinator role and the tasks to be performed; the changes in the hospital brought about by the coordinator; the organizational supports and barriers to development; and the long-term necessity of the coordinator function.

At the outset of the project two views of the coordinator role were in evidence: hospital administrators tended to stress the public relations aspect of coordination and the actual coordinators were more interested in exploring organizational change. The coordinator job was not defined in detail and the people appointed had to negotiate positions for themselves—a task that took at least two years. The project reported successes in combining aspects of organizational change and the education of members of the medical staff about communication with patients.

During the period of the research project other hospitals appointed coordinators and by 1990 Fahrenfort estimated that 60% of the general hospitals in the Netherlands had, as noted above, fulltime or part-time coordinators. She commented on positive influences on the development of patient education and noted two particular trends: the emergence of the belief inpatients' rights to autonomy and the development of a greater market orientation to the provision of health care. Patient education was seen to be compatible with both although Fahrenfort noted that the 'government support for patient emancipation veered towards supporting emancipation as consumerism'. She commented on potential conflicts which resulted in developing the coordinator role. The easily visible promotion aspects of the role can take priority over the slower and more difficult, but more important work of organizational development and change leading to: improved procedures for health professional-patient contacts; better understanding of the patient education process; support for professionals in changing their professional image; and educating patients to real autonomy. Through the institution of patient advice counters the hospital can 'show its good intentions towards patient education without actually changing anything in the way patients are informed about their own condition'. The skills of the coordinator will need for the longer-term organizational change, recognizing in the process that the former can frequently trigger support for the latter.

Whether or not hospitals appoint specialist patient education coordinators, it is necessary to monitor the progress to meeting educational needs in all areas of service. Hospital care is typically only an element in a 'patient career' which began with consultation in primary care, was followed by referral to hospital and subsequent admission and is followed up by further contact with primary care. The educational needs begin from the point of first referral to primary care and it makes sense therefore to respond to these needs from this point. A mechanism for enhancing the autonomy of the patient in the educational process would be the use of a patient held record care (Dickey, 1993). This would record the process of eliciting needs at different stages and also the nature and timing of all educational responses. Ideally the card wòuld record, at the same time, medical interventions, etc. Use of such a device could make a contribution towards improving articulation between education in the primary and hospital sectors.

Facilitating the educational process

Educational and counselling needs have to be defined through dialogue with patients, possibly with the use of diagnostic tools such as Patient Learning Needs Scales (Bubela *et al.*, 1990) and normative needs also taken into account before educational activities can be specified and organized. In deciding on these activities, in addition to needs, account has to be taken of other characteristics of patients and facilitators and the particular constraints of the context in question.

A few issues which have a bearing on meeting the educational needs of all patients across all hospital settings: timing and delivery of education; choice of educational methods; choice of educators; use of mass media.

Timing and Delivery

It is a truism to say that education and counselling are most effective provided as near as possible to the time when need arises. In a study by Wallace (1988) patients expressed a consistent preference for preparation (including booklets) prior to hospitalization rather than after admission. With the use of individualized care plans and the encouragement of active participation of patients in their care, there ought to be a continual monitoring of educational need and organization of appropriately timed response. Much of this response may take place on a one-to-one basis in association with other ongoing activities. In addition, there may be needs which could usefully, and cost effectively, be met through group methods.

Although the intention in many situations is to integrate education within total care it can also be organized on a separate basis or through 'hybrids' of integrated and separate elements. Bartlett (1991) cites as an example of separate educational provision the Patient Learning Centre at the University of Michigan in the USA where cancer patients are taught to perform high technology procedures. Patient self-help groups, consumer libraries and telephone information lines are also educational inputs which can be accessed without formal legitimation by caregivers. The New York University Cooperative Care Unit which employs both educational and clinical nurses is cited as an example of hybrid care. Educational nurses provide most of the formal teaching and counseling to patients and their families although clinical nurses are expected to answer patients' questions and to reinforce informations and skills.

Since many countries now give high profile to the educational skills of nurses a development of hybrid forms of organization of the educational component of care might be opposed. Given the time commitment needed however, to develop a full understanding of the educational process and competence in diagnosing and meeting educational needs in a crowded nurse training, it may be worth considering some development of both general and specific nursing contributions education.

Educational Methods

There are a variety of ways in which cognitive, affective or skills learning objectives can be met. Some may, on the basis of evaluated studies, be more effective than others but not necessarily the most cost efficient methods or popular ones with particular groups. A cheap and simple educational methods which can be available to all patients and their families may be preferred to a more complex one which requires heavy investments of health professional time and can only reach a proportion of people. An instructive example was provided by Wilson-Barnett (1988).

She discussed a study of Ozbolt Goodwin (1979) which evaluated a programmed learning booklet for use by patients following pulmonary surgery according to individual abilities and recovery rates. Adherence to this approach was shown to have significantly positive effects with patients experiencing fewer infections and periods of hospitalization.

Given the reductions in length of time of hospital stay the potential for bringing together groups of patients with equivalent needs at one point in time will be limited for many aspects of health care. There are conditions, however, where use of groups is convenient and a good way of meeting needs. An example can be offered from diabetes education. An interesting study by Basso (1991) reported on the use of structured fantasy group activity as part of education for children with diabetes. The study was not an experimental one or exposed to long-term follow-up but it reported that the group activity helped children to express their feelings about diabetes and its management and their concerns about stresses in their family and peer relationships.

Choice of educators

The question of whether people other than health professionals should be involved in the educational process can be addressed. Clearly if we have a model of the autonomous patient we also accept that this goes along with some opportunities for choice of educational contacts. A common activity is to join self-help groups which can draw on a variety of non-professional input in line with members' needs.

Within institutional contexts where there is a provision of integrated patient education, there has been some assessment of the role of peer educators. These are defined by Bartlett (1985) as people who currently or formerly have experienced the illness or condition in question and have been specially recruited to participate in educational activities. The Reach to Recovery programme for women who have experienced mastectomy is a specific example of the use of peer educators. Van den Borne *et al.* (1987) reviewed studies of the effects of contacts between patients with cancer. Of the 18 studies identified, most did not meet methodological conditions necessary to draw conclusions. Four of the six studies with sound methodological design showed positive effects of contacts including: more knowledge about (breast) cancer; better movement of the arm after mastectomy and more use of breast prostheses; greater improvements in perceptions of general health and greater reductions in negative feelings. In his review, Bartlett said that early experience with the use of peer educators was encouraging but limited empirical research had been undertaken. Based on findings from existing programmes he suggested that peer educators could be used most effectively when the illness was chronic; the illness was socially stigmatizing due to physical handicaps; and/or impairment of self-concept or body image existed.

Use of mass media

They have an important part to play in education in health care settings. The provision of informational leaflets and booklets is a relatively cheap and easy way of meeting informational need, either through the professional-patient encounter or through education 'shops'. Some hospital and primary care settings have introduced the use of video and there has been a small growth of patient libraries in primary care.

Two things are important: generating informational materials appropriate to the range of client groups and providing opportunities for discussion of content when required. Parrinello (1984), in an evaluation of an arterial bypass booklet, said that over 90% of respondents found the booklet helpful but those who had the opportunity to discuss it with a health worker found it of greater value.

CONCLUSIONS

The educational component of health care has developed at varying pace in different countries and in many remains underemphasized and underfunded. However, the growing health promotion movement has led to a new focus on the health promoting nature of hospitals and communities in which primary care is located. It is hoped that this will lead to significant achievements across the range of indicators incorporated into health promotion audit.

At the same time there has been a shift towards a greater market orientation in the provision of health care. As happened earlier in the USA, patient education fits in with a consumerist model of the patient and is seen also to be a means to reducing costs. Some years ago Bartlett (1985) discussed some of the issues pertaining to seeing patient education as a cost saver:

In this cost conscious environment, it is very tempting for patient educators to advocate the need for patient education primarily as a cost savings tool. In economics jargon, patient education is being justified less as a consumable service which is valuable in its own right and more as a social investment which will reduce net costs.

Bartlett saw this strategy as perilous on two grounds. First, it undermines aspects of patient education which do not save money and may well increase costs. He believed that it would, in fact, be difficult to demonstrate a direct relationship between most informal educational activity in hospital and subsequent cost savings. Second, the emphasis on cost containment condoned a double standard. Newly proposed medical treatments and procedures may be routinely approved on the basis of medical necessity while patient education must demonstrate both its effectiveness and capacity to cut costs. Since some patient education activities are associated with cost saving it is worth making this known but education as in integrated component of every patient's care may not necessarily lead to cost saving in either the short or long-term. The danger of an increasing focus on costs is to increase pressure to set educational goals which are more easily and cheaply achieved. The specific behavioural and medical outcomes associated with preventive medical approaches to health education may, therefore be preferred to the more diffuse and probably more difficult ones associated with empowerment models.

We have noted the need for more results of evaluation in some places because development are new and we await evaluation, in others because there has been insufficient evaluations or those undertaken have has methodological shortcomings. At the same time the increasing availability of meta-evaluations has demonstrated effective interventions. On the basis of existing knowledge proven interventions were routinely applied across health care settings as a whole, significant gains could be achieved. The statement made in 1985 by Bartlett still holds good: The answers to many research questions remain cloudy and other questions remain to be formulated. Yet a considerable body of knowledge now exists upon which effective, practical and acceptable patient education programs can be developed. More research attention now needs to be directed to the question. 'Why aren't we applying the knowledge we already have?'

For some, health promotion is an activity synonymous with health education; for others it is a related but substantially different process having different goals and values. Since health education is not a unitary process having a universally accepted philosophy and clear goals, it therefore follows that it is not possible to provide an unequivocal definition of what constitutes success without first examining the values upon which different approaches to health education are based. And since there still appears to be some confusion between health education and health promotion it would seem appropriate to try to resolve this demarcation dispute prior to considering the nature of different health education approaches.

A HISTORICAL PERSPECTIVE

Many publications have provided definitions of and perspectives on health promotion during the last few years (Anderson, 1984; Tones, 1985; Green and Raeburn, 1988; Minkler, 1989). It has been used to distinguish attempts to foster positive health or 'well-being' as contrasted from initiatives designed primarily to prevent disease, i.e. 'health protection' and 'preventive health services'. Indeed, the concept of health promotion is rather like virtue: it means all things to all people—who are united only in their agreement that it is rather desirable.

The origins of health promotion may be found in WHO's original and classic definition of health (WHO, 1946) with its holistic emphasis and its accentuation of the positive. More recently, a major impetus was provided with the launch of 'Health for All by the Year 2000' (HFA, 2000) at the 30th World Health Assembly in 1977. Interestingly, in the context of developing indicators of performance, this new movement included a more realistic definition of health than the classic 1946 version. As the then Director General of WHO pointed out:

'The challenging constitutional objective of the World Health Organization: the attainment by all peoples of the highest possible level of physical, mental and social well-being, is now being transformed into the dynamic notion of a Health for All movement. With this change in emphasis, public health is reinstating itself as a collective effort, drawing together a wide range of actors, institutions and sectors within society toward a goal of a 'socially and economically productive life'. This social goal . . . moves health from being the outcome measure of social development to being one of its major resources.

Kickbusch (1986) describes health promotion as '. . . a new forcefield for health (which) integrates social action, health advocacy and public policy'. It incorporates:

> . . . diverse, but complementary, methods or approaches, including communication, education, legislation, fiscal measures, organizational change, community development and spontaneous local activities against health hazards. It offers new challenges to existing professional groups, commercial and corporate bodies, cultural norms and the inertia of health institutions . . . it reiterates the Health for All components of intersectoral action and advocacy for health, stressing the need to go beyond health care and equity in access to a healthy life.

The Ottawa Charter (WHO, 1986; Health Promotion, 1986) provided an international clarion call for action towards a new public health. It embodied the principles of health promotion; its major thrust was for social change and political activity. Although it urged the development of personal skills its paramount recommendation was the need to 'build healthy public policy'. In so doing, it could be said that it marginalized health education—dislodging it from the center stage position which Alma Ata bestowed on it.

THE ANATOMY OF HEALTH PROMOTION

Tannahill has developed an elegant model in which health promotion is viewed as a number of different combinations of prevention, health protection and health education (Downie, Fyfe and Tannahill, 1992). The model however, differs in its concern to emphasize and explicate the contribution made by education; its structure represents a development of the familiar health field concept (Figure 5.1).

FIGURE 5.1

The Health Field Concept

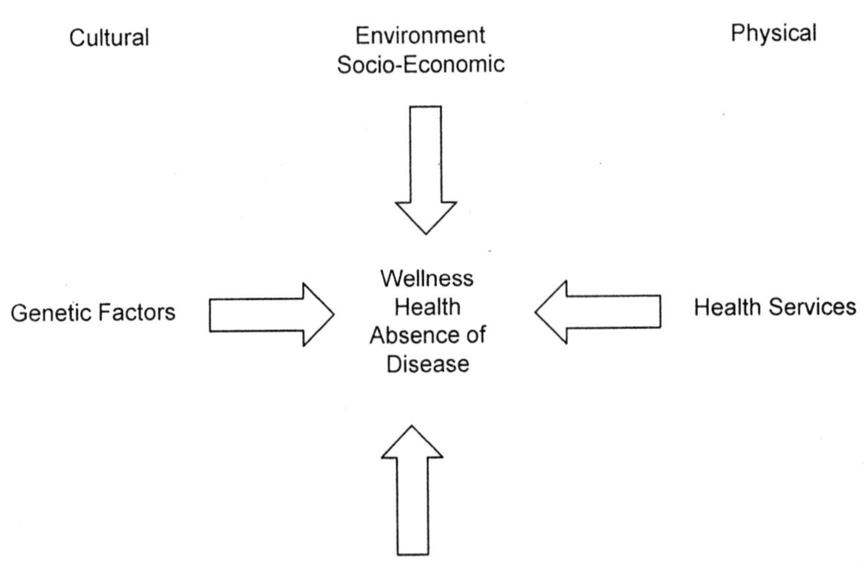

The health field concept was popularized in a working document on the health of Canadians which became widely known as the Lalonde Report (Lalonde, 1974). In fact, this derived from a conceptual schema outlined by LaFramboise (1973) which provided a simple map of 'health territory'. Health and illness are considered to result from the interplay of four key influences: genetic factors, the environment, lifestyle and medical services. Although this formulation was hardly novel, it acquired a special status when endorsed by a government agency!

Nonetheless, the health field concept identifies the key influences on health and, therefore logically, health promotion might be described as any deliberate or planned attempt to foster health or prevent and manage disease by achieving some judicious mix of the four 'inputs'. Since the genetic aspect is not effectively amenable to intervention (except perhaps by genetic counseling), the concerns of health promotion would in practice center on the remaining three factors. Apart from the exhortation to 'reorient medical services' as part of a more general trend to demedicalization, curative medicine has (rather churlishly perhaps) often been excluded from the health promotion field, leaving lifestyle and environment as the main areas of interest. This formulation of health promotion as any measure which promotes health is, of course, consistent with WHO's approach which accepted that health promotion was a '. . . unifying concept for those who recognize the need for change in the ways and conditions of living, in order to promote health' (WHO, 1984). Dennis *et al.* made a similar point in 1982, seeing health education as operating within a broad framework of policy.

Before considering how the health field concept might usefully be expanded, two incidental points should be made: first, health is defined both in terms of the prevention and management of disease and also as having 'positive' or 'wellness' aspects. Second, both health promotion and health education are considered to be planned activities. Of course, serendipitous events may result in health gain just as health learning may occur without any deliberate attempt to influence. Organization of learning experiences (i.e. teaching) and the intentional planning of policy initiatives are more likely to result in a positive outcome than reliance on happenstance. Clearly, it is assumed that the superiority of planned interventions will depend on the skills of the health promotion practitioner although we must, however, regrettably accept that not all intentional attempts at health promotion will be in competent hands! 'Anatomical' analysis of health promotion. The three central elements of the health field concept (i.e. those which are potentially amenable to influence) may be readily identified. They comprise first of all, environmental influences, which are depicted as under the control of 'healthy public policy'. Second, we may note the impact on health of individual choice of lifestyle and, third, an expanded health services input may be seen in Figure 5.2.

In addition, two deliberate strategies for producing change are—'lobbying' and 'education'. Of the two, education is considered to have potentially the more powerful and multifaceted role. Lobbying may, nonetheless, make a major contribution to health promotion and its function is primarily that of bringing about 'healthy public policy'. Indeed, both education and policy are central to the achievement of individual, community and national health status. According to this conceptualization, it is possible to distil the concept of health promotion into an essential 'formula'—as follows: Health Promotion × Health Education × Healthy Public Policy.

Health is substantially influenced by environmental factors: physical socio-economic and cultural. The influence may, of course, be positive or

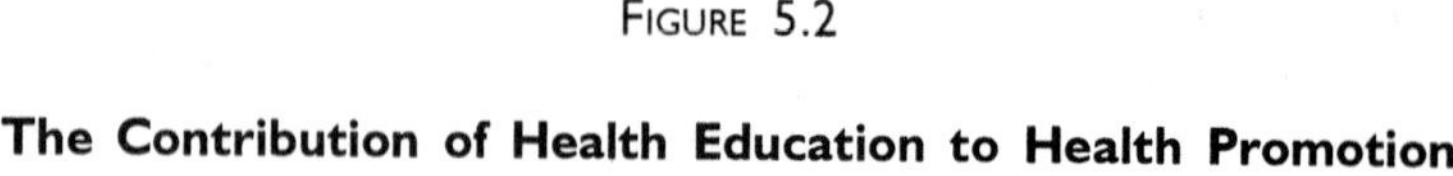

FIGURE 5.2

The Contribution of Health Education to Health Promotion

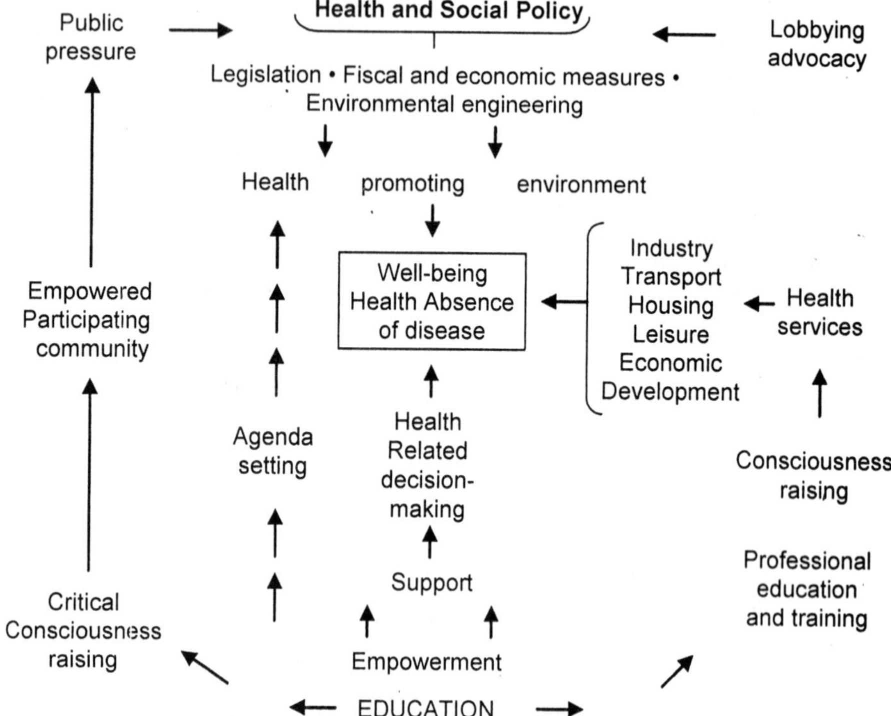

negative. One key aim of health promotion is to 'engineer' these various environmental factors in order to maximize opportunities for health and the avoidance of disease and disability. In so doing, 'healthy' decision-making is potentiated: the healthy choice becomes the easy choice. The process of social engineering may literally involve environmental engineering—for instance, the construction of cycle tracks within 'healthy cities'. It may, on the other hand, require fiscal or economic measures. Legislation may or may not be involved in both of the instances cited above. Again, legislation, financial commitments and the like require the formulation of health policy—or broader social policies which have implications for health. Healthy public policy, then, is necessary for environmental change. Clearly, a health promoting environment may operate at a macro-level: for example, at national and international level. Additionally, the development and implementation of health policies will operate at local levels—and at the level of organizations; for instance, the importance of having no smoking and healthy food policies within hospitals has long been acknowledged.

Healthy public policy is at the heart of an ecological approach to health promotion. It includes: food and education; shelter; a stable ecosystem and sustainable resources; peace; equity and justice. Central to the attainment of all these policy goals is the imperative of redistributing economic resources.

I. Health Promotion

Health promotion is the process of enabling people to increase control over, and to improve health. It is not directed against any particular disease, but is intended to strengthen the host through a variety of approaches (interventions). The well-known interventions in this area are:

(i) health education
(ii) environmental modifications
(iii) nutritional interventions
(iv) lifestyle and behavioural changes

(i) Health education

This is one of the most cost-effective interventions. A large number of diseases could be prevented with little or not medical intervention if people were adequately informed about them and if they were encouraged to take necessary precautions in time. Recognizing this truth, the WHO's constitution states that the extension to all people of the benefits of medical, psychological and related knowledge is essential to the fullest attainment of health. The targets for educational efforts may include the general public, patients, priority groups, health providers, community leaders and decision-makers.

(ii) Environmental modifications

A comprehensive approach to health promotion requires environmental modifications, such as provision of safe water; installation of sanitary latrines; control of insects and rodents; improvement of house, etc. The history of medicine has shown that many infectious diseases have been successfully controlled in western countries through environmental modifications, even prior to the development of specific vaccines or chemotherapeutic drugs. Environmental interventions are non-clinical and do not involve the physician.

(iii) Nutritional interventions

These comprise food distribution and nutrition improvement of vulnerable groups; child feeding programmes; food fortification; nutrition education, etc.

(iv) Lifestyle and behavioural changes

The conventional public health measures or interventions have not been successful in making inroads into lifestyle reforms. The action of prevention in this case, is one of individual and community responsibility for health, the physician and in fact each health worker acting as an educator than a therapist. Health education is a basic element of all health activity. It is of paramount importance in changing the views, behaviour and habits of people.

Since health promotion comprises a broad spectrum of activities, a well-conceived health promotion programme would first attempt to identify the target groups or at-risk individuals in a population and then direct more appropriate message to them. Goals must be defined. Means and alternative means of accomplishing them must be explored. It involves organizational, political, social and economic interventions designed to facilitate environmental and behavioural adaptations that will improve or protect health.

The First International Conference on Health Promotion in Ottawa concisely captured the essence of the earlier definitions by defining health promotion as the process of enabling people to increase control over and to improve their health. Most governments adopting a health promotion policy have based their approach on the identification of a finite number of life-style areas—such as smoking, alcohol abuse, diet, and exercise—shown to account for the major causes of disease and disability in their societies. These behavioural risk factors can be quantified and specifically targeted for strategic planning.

Some critics of this approach advocate a system view, where system stands for the social, economic, political, institutional, cultural, legislative, industrial, and physical-environmental milieus in which behaviour takes place (e.g., Minkler, 1989). The advocates of the system view argue that interventions aimed at changing the behaviour of individuals are inadequate because the system is a more powerful and pervasive determinant of behaviour and of health than decisions made by individuals operating in a supposedly free-choice situation. Also, say the system advocates, a focus on individual behaviour is too appealing to conservative governments; it allows them to evade their responsibility for social change. It also tends to leads to a brand of health promotion most suitable for the middle class and to charges of victim blaming, wherein ill-health resulting from faulty life-styles (such as smoking) is seen as the responsibility of the individual rather than the result of the social pressures under which individuals live. As with the other side of the continuum, the systems side has its shades and variations of theory, philosophy, ideology, and strategy. Critics of the system view argue that the life-styles of people implicated by epidemiological and medical research as responsible for a large proportion of the leading causes of death and disability are undeniably under at least some control by those at risk. To deprive them of access to the information and skills needed to take some action would be unethical. Furthermore, the system changes some seek to make unilaterally affect other aspects of life besides health, so the public will insist on having a role in the decision-making about their social systems and environments. Thus, we will be required to educate or persuade individuals in order to make changes in systems.

How we look at health promotion depends in part on the way we define health, at least on how the word is used in the term health promotion. What are we trying to promote?

The Alma Ata declaration and some of the newer policies in health promotion can be seen as a reaction against traditional Western health systems ministering to individual sick patients in clinical settings, where the professional rules supreme. Increasingly, health policy initiatives seek to work with people in the context of their everyday environments—their homes, schools, and work sites—many aspects of which condition their behaviour and their health. This, in turn, leads to more of a bird's-eye view of environments and systems within which people live, so that social and political factors receive more emphasis and public health and policy views of health emerge as complements to the biomedical view. Along with this is a self-help trend seeking to equalize the power balance between 'the people' and 'professionals'. Of course, what the bland repetition of these concepts and words does not convey is the power of the feeling behind many of them. These are more than sociological concepts for many people. They invoke ideologies related to people's rights, professional privilege, distribution of resources, and inequality. People who are associated with 'old' or 'reactionary' views have considerable feeling registered against them. We would argue, however, that any realistic view of the determinants of health and of appropriate health promotion requires a balance of individual, institutional, community, societal, and political perspectives.

The Alma Ata and Ottawa declarations insist that neither people nor health should be seen in isolation. Each is nested in systems that profoundly affect behaviour and health. Health promotion must take this ecological fact into account. Such an ecological view represents a move away from the educationist tendency of biomedical science and some applications of health education in the service of centralized, categorical, and vertical programs, to a broader systems view. This view recognizes the interaction of life-style and environment when health is being considered. In this view, the individual and the context are of equal account. It legitimates both a life-style and a systems approach to health promotion.

An ecological model of health promotion says that health is the product of the individual's continuous interaction and interdependence with his or her ecosphere—this is, the family, the community, the culture, the societal structure, and the physical environment. Characteristic modes of interacting over time constitute a life-style, as distinct from discrete acts or behaivour. The determinants of a life-style must be seen as a combination of intrapersonal and external environmental forces, continuously interacting. In some instances, health promotion programs need to emphasize the individual or behavioural side, in others, the environmental side needs emphasis as the point of intervention. If the individual has a sense of harmony with, or a degree of mastery over, the everyday environment, then his or her health is likely to be good. But with oppression, poverty, limited opportunity, and lack of mastery, health will suffer.

Health, in the Ottawa Charter, is still given the original WHO definition of a state of complete physical, mental, and social well-being, to reach which 'an individual or group' must be able to identify and to realize aspirations, to satisfy needs, and to change or cope with the environment. (WHO, 1986). Such health is viewed as 'a resource for everyday life', which seems to imply that it is equivalent to having sufficient energy, stamina, and physical capacity to meet the demands of daily living. Significantly, the terms life-style and health education seem to have been replaced in the charter with the concept of 'developing personal and social skills through providing information, education for health and enhancing life skills'. How this is similar to, or different from, what has been understood by concepts of health behaviour and life-style change in the past is not clear. But, certainly, it appears that the intention of the charter is to broaden the base of health promotion beyond a personal life-style approach to a more political approach, so that policy, rather than behaviour, now becomes the centre of gravity. Our plea is to include all the dimensions relevant to health promotion, and to build on the past as well as expand into the future. In looking at the past, we are aware that many threads have been woven into the pattern for health promotion as it now appears.

Institutions

The attitude of medical institutions on health promotion and disease prevention issues is an important one. For example, medical institutions make an important statement when they have a cigarette smoking ban on their premises. Such a policy is a clear message to employees, patients, and the general community as to the attitude of the institution regarding the importance of not smoking. It can be viewed as a caring, concerned approach to the problem, particularly when linked to active smoking cessation programs for employees and patients. The encouragement of such environmental programs in health care institutions is an important support to a community program.

To implement such programs, sensitivity to the workings of an individual health care institution is important. Involving hospital or clinic administrators or, if health care is socialized, even local politicians can be particularly helpful. Working from within the system, they have the opportunity to be advocates for new policies and approaches to health promotion/disease prevention. Supporting these individuals with factual material and information that will help convince their colleagues is an important element in the program. Such environmental programs offer wider opportunities than just restrictive policies. For example, the routine measurement of blood pressure, laboratory standards, and appropriate flagging of abnormal values may be addressed. Specific work-site programs for hospital staff, such as time for exercise, healthy cafeteria selections, routine screening, and other health promotion approaches are also valuable. Finally, medical institutions can take a leadership role through collaborative arrangements to support other community organizations, such as schools, parks, and industry, in their own health promotion and environmental programs.

Screening Programs

The involvement in screening for related risk factors for disease is probably the least controversial way that health professionals can support a community health promotion program.

With the present emphasis on patient education for life-style change, the screening program can form an important vehicle for population-oriented health promotion. The concept of screening education means that in the screening situation every individual is seen as an opportunity for individualized health education, related to the patient's own risk factor pattern and life-style (Murray *et al.*, 1986). The opportunity for risk factors measurement will in this case act as the magnet that attracts the subjects to come for education. It can involve larger strata of the population who will not attend more targeted individualized education efforts.

In addition to continuing medical education and the role of institutions in enhancing a community approach, general clinical practice may provide a significant aid to health promotion programs. There is increasing availability of technology and methods for rationalizing preventive practice within a clinical care system. These are frequently taught in modern CME program.

The involvement of health professionals and health care institutions in community-based health promotion and disease prevention programs is essential. Their active support facilitates the development of the program, its implementation, and finally its incorporation into the fabric of the community. In developing such a program, close attention to the involvement of health professionals, particularly physicians, at the outset is crucial. With the active support of community health professionals, the program has markedly increased chances for success.

EVALUATING HEALTH PROMOTION PROGRAMS

Questions for the Planning Stages

- Should this program be developed at all?
- Are the educational materials appropriate?

Questions About Program Operations

- Is the program being implemented as planned?
- Is the program reaching its target audience?
- Who is the program failing to reach, and why?
- Are the program's participants satisfied with their experience?
- Are participants complying with actions requested to them?

Questions About Program Outcomes

- Is the program having the effect it is designed to have?

Besides the foregoing declarations and charters, the notable threads of development that converged to produce contemporary policies in health promotion include (a) the long-standing reliance of public health programs and agencies on health education to gain the cooperation of the public; (b) the community development and mass communications movements and technologies of the 1950s and 1960s, which converted reflecting the public's enlightened self-interests; (c) the self-care, civil rights, and women's movements of the 1960s, which demanded a transfer of authority and resources to people previously beholden to others; (d) the worldwide inflation and cost containment concerns of the 1970s, which led to cutbacks in social programs and caps on expenditures for high-tech medical care; (e) the growing recognition of diminishing returns on investments in medical care and communicable disease control, at least in Western countries, and of increasing chronic diseases attributable to life-style; (f) the strengthening scientific base of social, behavioural, and educational research applied to health; and (g) the growing disillusionment and impatience of the public with conventional medical approaches to health, supplanted by more imaginative (and sometimes ephemeral) concepts encompassing social, mental, and spiritual qualities of life.

Ottawa Charter's definition of health promotion: "Health promotion is the process of enabling people to increase control over and to improve their health."

The principal purpose or *raison d'etre* of the health promotion of the future could be seen to be the increasing transfer of control of important resources in health, notably knowledge, skills, authority, and money, to the community.

The pendulum now seems to be swinging from a technology and institution-based approach to health to a more people-based approach. There could hardly be a total rejection of high-technology medicine and health services—these clearly have many benefits in such areas as infectious disease control and treatment—but the search is now on for those areas in the health and human welfare domain that can be handed back to the people. It is in this context that a new era of health promotion seems to be emerging one that uses the expertise and resources available from professionals and technicians but also involves people at the community level in a fuller and more participatory way. A potential source of tension here is the question, Who will ultimately have control over health promotion? On the one hand, many feel this control should go to the community; on the other, many administrators, professionals, and funding bodies may be reluctant to let this happen. But regardless of this issue, at the heart of the enabling approach to health promotion is the concept of returning power, knowledge, skills, and other resources in a range of health areas to the community—to individuals, families, and whole populations.

Five action areas of the Ottawa Charter—that is, health promotion action involves building healthful public policy, relating supportive environments, strengthening community action, developing personal skills, and reorienting health service.

Health promotion can be defined from an operational standpoint as the combination of educational, organizational, economic, and environmental supports for action conducive to health. So that people can deal effectively with their own health promotion needs and activities, they need information and skills, together with the financial, professional, and organizational resources to put such knowledge and skills to use. It might be thought that the approach to health promotion being outlined here would diminish the role of professionals, but this is not the case. However, the professional will undoubtedly have a different role, that of consultant, advocate, mediator, and supporter, rather than being the one who always controls the situation. This puts professionals and 'the people'. on a more equal footing—as partners rather than in a hierarchical relationship with the professional on top.

The World Health Organization initiated the Network of Health Promoting Hospitals with the aim to reorient health care institutions to integrate health promotion and education, disease prevention and rehabilitation services in curative care. Many activities have been carried out and more than 700 hospitals in 25 European Countries and worldwide have joined the WHO network since the establishment of the network.

Health Promoting Hospitals have committed themselves to integrate health promotion in daily activities, i.e. to become a smoke-free setting, and to follow the Vienna Recommendations, which advocate a number of strategic and ethical directions such as encouraging patient participation, involving all professionals, fostering patients' rights and promoting a healthy environment within the hospital.

Health promotion is defined as 'the process of enabling people to increase control over, and to improve, their health'. (Ottawa Charter for Health Promotion), and is here understood to embrace health education, disease prevention and rehabilitation services. It is also understood to include health enhancement by empowering patients, relatives and employees in the improvement of their health-related physical, mental and social well-being.

Hospitals play an important role in promoting health, preventing disease and providing rehabilitation services. Some of these activities have been an essential part of hospital work, however, the increasing prevalence of lifestyle-related and chronic diseases require a more expanded scope and systematic provision of activities such as therapeutic education, effective communication strategies to enable patients to take an active role in chronic disease-management or motivational counseling.

Changing public expectations, an increasing number of chronic patients requiring continuous support, and staff frequently being exposed to physical and emotional strains require hospitals to incorporate a health promotion focus as a key service for patients and staff.

In addition, hospitals impact on health not only through the provision of prevention, treatment and rehabilitation services of high quality, but also through their impact on the local environment.

The predominant approach to quality management in hospitals is through setting standards for the services. Health promotion is a core quality issue for improving health and sustaining quality of life, however, a review of existing standards for quality in health care for references to health promotion activities yielded little results. Standards for health promotion in hospitals are necessary to ensure the quality of services provided in this area.

As a result, five core standards applicable to all hospitals have been developed in accordance with international requirements established by ALPHA program developed by the International Society for Quality in Health.

The standards are mainly generic with the focus on patients, staff and the organizational management. Disease specific standards are included for groups of patients with evidence for specific needs. The quality goals described in the standards address professional, organizational, and patient-related quality issues.

Standard 1 Demands that a hospital has a written policy for health promotion. This policy must be implemented as part of the overall organization quality system and is aiming to improve health outcomes. It is stated that the policy is aimed at 'patients, relatives and staff.'

Standard 2 Describes the organizations' obligation to ensure the assessment of the patients' needs for health promotion, disease prevention and rehabilitation.

Standard 3 States that the organization must provide the patient with information on significant factors concerning their disease or health condition and health promotion interventions should be established in all patients' pathways.

Standard 4 Gives the management the responsibility to establish conditions for the development of the hospital as a healthy workplace.

Standard 5 Deals with continuity and cooperation, demanding a planned approach to collaboration with other health service sectors and institutions.

Management Policy

Standard 1. The organization has a written policy for health promotion. The policy is implemented as part of the overall organization quality improvement system, aiming at improving health outcomes. This policy is aimed at patients, relatives and staff.

Objective

To describe the framework for the organization's activities concerning health promotion as an integral part of the organization's quality management system.

Substandards

1.1 The organization identifies responsibilities for the process of implementation, evaluation and regular review of the policy.

1.2 The organization allocates resources to the processes of implementation, evaluation and regular review of the policy.

1.3 Staff are aware of the health promotion policy and it is included in induction programmes for new staff.

1.4 The organization ensures the availability of procedures for collection and evaluation of data in order to monitor the quality of health promotion activities.

1.5 The organization ensures that staff have relevant competences to perform health promotion activities and supports the acquisition of further competences as required.

1.6 The organization ensures the availability of the necessary infrastructure, including resources, space, equipment, etc. in order to implement health promotion activities.

Patient Assessment

Standard 2. The organization ensures that health professionals, in partnership with patients, systematically assess needs for health promotion activities.

Objective

To support patient treatment, improve prognosis and to promote the health and well-being of patients.

Substandards

2.1. The organization ensures the availability of procedures for all patients to assess their need for health promotion.

2.2 The organization ensures procedures to assess specific needs for health promotion for diagnosis-related patient-groups.

2.3 The assessment of a patient's need for health promotion is done at first contact with the hospital. This is kept under review and adjusted as necessary according to changes in the patient's clinical condition or on request.

2.4 The patient's needs assessment ensures awareness of and sensitivity to social and cultural background.

2.5 Information provided by other health service partners is used in the identification of patient needs.

Patient Information and Intervention

Standard 3. The organization provides patients with information on significant factors concerning their disease or health condition and health promotion interventions are established in all patient pathways.

Objective

To ensure that the patient is informed about planned activities, to empower the patient in an active partnership in planned activities and to facilitate integration of health promotion activities in all patient pathways.

Substandards

3.1 Based on the health promotion needs assessment, the patient is informed of factors impacting on their health and, in partnership with the patient, a plan for relevant activities for health promotion is agreed.

3.2 Patients are given clear, understandable and appropriate information about their actual condition, treatment, care and factors influencing their health.

3.3 The organisation ensures that health promotions is systematically offered to all patients based on assessed needs.

3.4 The organization ensures that information given to the patient, and health promoting activities are documented and evaluated, including whether expected and planned results have been achieved.

3.5 The organization ensures that all patients, staff and visitors have access to general information on factors influencing health.

Promoting a Healthy Workplace

Standard 4. The management establishes conditions for the development of the hospital as a healthy workplace.

Objective

To support the establishment of a healthy and safe workplace, and to support health promotion activities for staff.

Substandards

4.1 The organization ensures the establishment and implementation of a comprehensive Human Resource Strategy that includes the development and training of staff in health promotion skills.

4.2 The organization ensures the establishment and implementation of a policy for a healthy and safe workplace providing occupational health for staff.

4.3 The organization ensures the involvement of staff in decisions impacting on the staff's working environment.

4.4 The organization ensures availability of procedures to develop and maintain staff awareness on health issues.

Continuity and Cooperation

Standard 5. The organization has a planned approach to collaboration with other health service levels and other institutions and sectors on an ongoing basis. **Objective:** To ensure collaboration with relevant providers and to initiate partnerships to optimise the integration of health promotion activities inpatient pathways.

Substandards

5.1 The organization ensures that health promotion services are coherent with current provisions and health plans.

5.2 The organization identifies and cooperates with existing health and social care providers and related organizations and groups in the community.

5.3 The organization ensures the availability and implementation of activities and procedures after patient discharge during the post-hospitalisation period.

5.4 The organization ensures that documentation and patient information is communicated to the relevant recipient/follow-up partners inpatient care and rehabilitation.

References

Matching Services to needs. Copenhagen, WHO Regional Office for Europe, 2002 (document EUR/RC50/10).

Ottawa Charter for Health Promotion (http://www.who/int/hpr/NPH/docs/ottawa_charter_hp.pdf). Ottawa, WHO, 1986 (accessed 4 March 2004).

The International Society for Quality in Health Care. Alpha and accreditation (http://www.isqua.org.au/isquaPages/Alpha.html). Victoria, Isqua, 2003 (accessed 4 March 2004).

Vienna Recommendations for Health Promoting Hospitals (http:/Iwww.euro.who.int/document/IHB/hphviennarecom.pdf) (accessed 4 March 2004).

WHO Regional Office for Europe. Health Promoting Hospital, (http://www.euro.who.int/healthpromohosp). Copenhagen, WHO Regional Office for Europe, 2002 (accessed 4 March 2004).

WHO Standards Working Group. Development of standards for disease prevention and health promotion. WHO, Meeting on standards for disease prevention and health promotion, Bratislava, 14 May 2002.

APPENDIX

Extension Services as a Part of Health Promotion through Hospitals

Health promotion implies general measures undertaken to improve the health of community at large. It incorporates general measures for improving our living conditions with a view to provide opportunities and settings which are conducive to healthy living. Health promotion measures minimize the chances of disease occurrence by preventive emergence of risk factor, by improving physical environment and by educating the masses. Health promotion generally refers to broad measures undertaken in prepathogenesis phase, i.e. before the occurrence of disease. These measures are not directed towards a particular disease, pathogen or a particular individual, e.g. safe water supply is not directed towards cholera or jaundice only rather provision of safe water is a general measure and a part of quality of life. This measure, if undertaken for the whole community, will prevent the whole gamut of water borne diseases both infective and chemical (pesticide, poison, etc.). Similarly, ensuring provision of safe blood transfusion facilities as a health promotion measure is neither directed towards a particular individual or community nor towards a specific disease (HIV/AIDS). It is meant for all clients using the services and for prevention of all blood borne infections. Health promotion measures are, because they address the whole society, large scale ventures and hence are very costly. However, the returns are quite worthwhile, these measures are real preventive measures rather than fire fighting measures like early diagnosis and treatment (secondary prevention) and rehabilitation (tertiary) which are undertaken after the disease process has started.

In western countries the health promotion role of hospitals is being encouraged to tackle utilization of physicians' time. This plea will not hold good for developing countries like India where hospitals are already overcrowded and physicians overworked. Hence, the health promotion through hospitals has to be advocated on its own merit. In fact, some of HP practices are already in place in Indian hospitals viz. no smoking, no horn signs, BFHI, counseling services, well baby clinics. However, there are not universally practiced.

What is needed is the adequate publicity of the existing HP services and a visible support for development and implementation of new and innovative HP services. Further, mandatory adoption of key HP practices in all government and private hospitals may be enforced (and made a prerequisite for registration of private hospitals).

In our country, we need to encourage HP in hospitals with a view to reduce unnecessary overcrowding,, e.g. reduction in hospital stay and unnecessary visits, enhancing patients and their families' self-care activity.

Patients and their escorts' visit to the hospital should be fully utilized by providing them education counseling. Of special importance is inclusion of yoga in the management of illnesses. Sufficient evidence need to be collected on this aspect so that a scientific basis can be provided to yoga training in hospitals.

Hospitals should be projected as role models for adopting HP practices,, e.g. hygiene, environmental cleanliness, food hygiene, safe water supply, provision of healthy food, clear air.

People's religious sentiments may also be honoured by providing prayer facilities within the premise.

All health promotion measures can be implemented in hospital settings. These serve to improve the image of hospitals in the society. Such measures are likely to yield rich dividends if incorporated in the hospital functioning from the outset, e.g. building design, layout, tree plantation, natural lighting, night shelters, traffic flow, parking space, computerization and above all the policies incorporating HP measures.

The following needs attention.

1. PHYSICAL ENVIRONMENT
   - Traffic
   - Green cover—tree/flowers
   - No dark corners
   - Roads
   - Lighting
   - Model Bio-waste disposal system
   - Model drainage system
   - Model of healthful housing/building
   - Elderly/disable friendly building
   - Mosquito free—elimination of breeding place
   - Quake proof building

2. SOCIAL ENVIRONMENT
   - Sports/games facilities/swimming pool
   - Social events—festivals, bhazans, plays

3. COUNSELLING SERVICES
   - Counselling: HIV/AIDS, sex, marriage, school, de-addition (DDTC)
   - Genetic counseling
   - Diet counseling and health-oriented diet in the hospitals food corners.

4. SELF HELP GROUPS
   - AAA
   - Self-help group: thalassemia, cleft lip/palate

5. HEALTHY NUTRITION
   - Milk birth (milk, and, yogurt, lassi)
   - Juice bar/soup counters
   - Healthy food—fruits, etc.

6. MEETING CENTRE
    - Meetings/days

7. LEGISLATIVE MEASURES
    - Policy—HP-H

8. STAFF WELFARE
    - Welfare clubs/canteen

9. HEALTH PROMOTION SERVICES
    - Yoga Centre

10. GOOD PRACTICES
    - Creche
    - Voluntary blood donation
    - Hotline services
    - BFHI practice
    - Terminal cases—Religious discourse
    - Antenatal clinic—Postpartum center
    - Generic medicines
    - ORS wards
    - Immunization clinic
    - Well baby clinics

11. EDUCATION SERVICES
    - Health education
    - Nutrition education
    - Sex education
    - Physical education
    - Family life education

12. SELF CARE SERVICES
    - Self care ability enhancement services
    - diabetes
    - hypertension
    - post-stroke cases
    - arthritis
    - paraplegia

13. HOME VISIT SERVICES
14. AMBULANCE SERVICES (FLYING SEQUED ON CALL)
15. NATURE PATHING
16. GYMNASIUM
17. FIELD PRACTICE

6

Complementary and Alternative Medicines (CAM): India's Strengths

CAM is described as a set of medical and health care practices that are not currently part of MODERN Western medicine, according to the National Center for Complementary and Alternative Medicine of the National Institutes of Health. Complementary medicine is used with conventional medicine, whereas alternative medicine is used instead of conventional medicine. Newer terms for CAM include *holistic medicine* to describe patient-centered care involving biological, psychological, spiritual, social, and environmental considerations and *integrative medicine* to describe relationship-based care combining mainstream and evidence-based complementary treatment. The AAP convened the Task Force on Complementary and Alternative Medicine in 2000 and the Provisional Section on Complementary, Holistic, and Integrative Medicine in 2005. This report from the task force, with contributions from the provisional section, describes complementary and alternative medicine therapies in children; the medicolegal, ethical, and research issues; education and training for providers; and communication strategies for clinicians to use with patients and families.

Various systems of Indian medicines view the mind and body as unified, and approach healing as an internal process. Of late we have started talking of holistic medicine, recognizing the complementary role of the alternative systems of medicine. For example, in addition to using anti-inflammatory drugs to ease muscle pain, they also use Yoga, massage, chiropractic, and/or osteopathic manipulation. Alternative approaches are generally thought of as being used instead of conventional methods. For example, this might mean seeing a homeopath or naturopath or Ayurvedic doctor instead of your regular doctor. India received over 2 lakhs of health tourists from abroad in the year 2006, mostly in search of CAM. They were not disappointed. Several hospitals set-up as Hospitals of modern medicine and surgery are now including CAM also as an alternative treatment in their premises . Dr. Trehan's medi-city at Gurgaon is a notable example. The proposed Medicity at Chandigarh also carried provision of Ayurveda and other alternative systems of medicine. Thus brief description of CAM as an emerging area in hospital management is relevant.

SOME REASONS PEOPLE CONSIDER CAM

- Belief that Western medicine is not holistic.
- A perspective that the cause of a problem may lie in life experiences, not diseases.
- Concern about the safety of medications and their much publicized side effects.
- Seeing CAM as less invasive and want to try it prior to seeing a medical doctor.
- Objections to what they see as "instant fix-it" or "pill-popping" attitudes.
- Lack of trust in doctors, or fear of medical errors.
- Religious beliefs that preclude drugs or surgery.
- Desire for a sense of spirit, missing in Western approaches.
- Exploring practices that have been popular in India to treat chronic ailments.
- Feeling that Western medicine is too mechanical, dogmatic, or compartmentalized.

There are some important characteristics to be pointed out of the therapeutic modalities offered by these medical traditions.

1. Foremost characteristic is safety

This is because the individual botanicals, minerals and the compound formulae have been established there through an empirical process lasting several hundred to several thousand years. Because of that process many of those treatments have outstanding record of safety and effectiveness. In addition some of the botanicals used in Ayurveda—for example, peppers—are among the first plants to be cultivated by man and have been in use for several thousands years.

2. Broad action on the macro-organism

In fact terms adaptogen and the most recent one bioprotectant were developed on the basis of the mechanisms of action of several plants derived from Ayurveda materia medica. For example, curcuminoids or derivatives of Curcuma longa (turmeric) are being recognized now as versatile phenolic anti-oxidants, providing two-pronged anti-oxidant activity: prevention of free radical formation and intervention to neutralize existing free radicals. This action of curcuminoids exemplifies a new mechanism characteristic of the therapeutical ingredients called 'bioprotectants'.

3. Attention to the digestive processess

The other recognized feature of Aurveda and related arts like Tibetan medicine is its emphasis on proper functioning of the digestive tract, specifically digestion and absorption, or bioavailability, of food, nutrients, and (when necessary) drugs.

Primary care for the digestive tract is approached in Ayurveda by providing a digestive formula to correct the suspected nutritional problem. Secondary care is provided by supplementing various formula with a digestion-enhancing component. Importantly the nutrient for the 'digestive process' is understood in Ayurveda not only as food that we eat, but also air that we breathe and significantly the .food. that feeds our mental and emotional processes.

VARIOUS SYSTEMS OF CAM

Ayurveda is the oldest medical system, where the focus is on energy and balance rather than symptoms that seeks to restore wholeness in the mind-body-spirit system. Each person has a particular combination of physical, mental and emotional characteristics known as Vata, Pitta, and Kapha. Physical and mental health is achieved by balancing diet, exercise, sleep, and sexual activity. Some of the tools of Ayurveda include a variety of stress management techniques, meditation, aromatherapy, yoga, and massage. The four pillars of Ayurvedic health maintenance are: (1) detoxification, (2) palliation, (3) rejuvenation, and (4) spiritual hygiene.

Homeopathic Medicine ("like cures like") was developed in the early 20th century. It does not treat a "disease" by name (such as depression) but rather by symptoms (including things that affect symptoms, such as sounds, smells, tastes, moods, energy, time of day or temperature when symptoms are worse, etc.). Micro-quantities of specific substances are used to cure symptoms, which would actually be caused by larger doses of the same substance? Conventional drugs are usually prescribed in individual capacities to act upon specific parts of the body, so it follows that several different drugs might be prescribed to treat the various symptoms of one individual. Homeopathic medicine offers an alternative. Instead of giving one medicine for a person's headache, another for his constipation, another for his irritability and yet another to counteract the effects of one or more the medicines, the homeopathic physician prescribes a single medicine at a time that will stimulate the person's immune and defense capacity and bring about an overall improvement in that person's health. The procedure by which the homeopath finds the precise individual substance is the very science and arts of homeopathy.

The treatment was discovered some 200 years ago by a German doctor, Friedrich Samuel Hahnemann, who found when he took a dose of quinine. It made him feverish, gave him the symptoms he would have expected to get if he had contracted malaria, then very common. It is the very same principle that was discovered at around the same time in Britain by Dr. Edward Jenner, who proved true the old wives' tale about cowpox protecting against smallpox. He went on to develop the vaccine that made his name in history and which eradicated the disease world-wide. Hahnemann pursued the principle in different direction and found that if the strength of a homeopathic remedy were diluted, its effect was improved. Homeopathic medicine is a natural pharmaceutical system that utilises microdoses of substances from the plant, mineral and animal kingdom to arouse a person's natural healing substances from the plant, mineral and animal kingdoms to arouse a person's natural healing response. Homeopathy is a sophisticated method of individualising small doses of medicine in order to initiate that healing response. Unlike conventional drugs, which act primarily by having direct effect upon physiological process related to a person's symptoms' homeopathic medicines are, thought to work by stimulating the person's immune system, which raises his or her overall level of health thereby enabling him or her to re-establish health and prevent disease. As people develop greater understanding and respect for the body's immune system, homeopathy will gain popularity as a primary pharmacological means to stimulate immune response. Those convenient medical therapies that primarily treat and suppress symptoms will be accepted for their valuable role in health care, but not necessarily as a first course of treatment. Homeopaths have found clinical experience that their medicines often replace conventional drugs and eliminate the need for heroic procedures. Ideally, homeopaths are taking the best of the natural science to create a kind of care that will be commonplace in future. Even a skeptical Edelman agrees that Homeopathy is an unorthodox but no longer crazy way to perform immunotherapy. By homeopathy any ailment, acute or chronic, local or general can be treated except diseases where surgery is unavoidable. Even in cases of enlarged tonsils, kidney stones, warts, piles, homeopathy has received accolades. Moreover good homeopathic prescribing has made many operations unnecessary.

Medical Education in ISM&H

Medical education in Indian Systems of Medicine and Homoeopathy has been a cause of concern. After enactment of Indian Medicines Central Council Act, 1970 and Homoeopathy Central Council Act, 1973, five-and-a-half years Under-Graduate course and three years Post-Graduate course were introduced, provisions for adequate clinical exposure and internship made. The number of Indian Systems of Medicine and Homoeopathy colleges have increased phenomenally to 404. The Central Councils have implemented various educational regulations to ensure minimum standards of education. Depite this, there has been a mushroom growth of sub-standard colleges causing erosion to the standards of education and harm to medical training and practice. Liberal permission by the State

Government, loopholes in the existing Acts and weakness in the enforcement of standards of education have contributed to this state of affairs.

Intellectual Property Rights (IPR) of ISM

Our wealth of knowledge on formulations and medicinal uses of plants available in ancient texts and treatises have been attracting foreign interest and a large number of such medicinal uses have been patented by them claiming as innovations though these are already available in the public domain and therefore can not be patented. This has happened as such knowledge is not available in easily accessible form and in the language generally used by the patent examiners overseas. This has harmed our national interest as the process for retrieval and contesting patents is very costly and time consuming which we can ill-afford. Protection of India's traditional medicinal knowledge would be undertaken through a progressive creation of a Digital Library for each system and eventually for uncodified knowledge leading to innovation and good health outcomes. Relevant International fora would be addressed about the need for fair and equitable sharing of benefits to the custodians of the knowledge and a system of compensating the originators of such knowledge introduced. TRIPS has provided the signatory countries the freedom to choose intellectual property protection of plant varieties either under a patent regime or a *sui generis* system or a combination thereof. A *sui generic* system will be set-up to provide grassroots innovators of plant based knowledge an incentive to disclose knowledge.

Naturopathic Medicine sees physical and mental health as arising from a healing power in the body that establishes, maintains, and restores health. Naturopathic practice may encompass hydrotherapy, botanical medicine, dietary and nutritional considerations, and counseling and lifestyle modifications. learning to relax the mind and body will ease many symptoms. Examples of mind body healing include: Relaxation techniques or deep breathing, Yoga, Hypnosis, Biofeedback, Chiropractic, Osteopathy, and Massage, etc.

Traditional Chinese Medicine (TCM), is based on the flow of vital energy throughout the body. In a healthy state, the yin and yang (negative and positive energies) are balanced, while a disease state results from an imbalance. Thus, the use of herbs, nutrition, meditation, acupuncture, and exercise are intended to restore balance and return the body, mind, emotions and spirit to health.

Energetic therapies are used to describe practices like Reiki, external Qi Gong, therapeutic touch, and bioenergetics that involve non-local interactions viz., interactions in which there is no physical contact between the practitioner and the patient. All of them involve non-tactile, non-contact interactions between practitioner and patient, in which the practitioner uses information garnered from other senses to assess and treat the patient's condition.

Ayurveda's concepts and Studies

All ayurvedic studies conducted on herbal and holistic medicine in ancient India, followed from the fountainhead of the two principle ayurvedic schools. The School of Physicians (Atreya) and the School of Surgeons (Dhanvantari) epitomized the eight main areas of ayurvedic studies and specialization during ancient times.

Kayachikitsa or internal medicine

This natural alternative medicine recognizes that the body of a person is the product of the constant psychosomatic interactions. The imbalances in the three doshas of vata-pitta-kapha occur sometimes by the mind and sometimes by the body's dhatu (tissues) and mala (toxin deposits). Hence, the kayachikitsa branch of this system of herbal and holistic medicine, delves deep into ascertaining the root cause of the illness.

The section of Nidana Sthana of Charaka Samhita deals with etiology, pathogenesis and diagnosis of an illness. Six stages of the development of disease are enumerated as aggravation, accumulation, overflow, relocation, build up in a new site and manifestation into a recognizable disease. One of the significant methods of treatment under kayachikitsa is panchakarma. This is a method of reversing the disease path from its manifestation stage back into its site of original development through special forms of emesis, purgation and enema, etc. Another unique aspect of kayachikitsa is rejuvenation called kaya kalpa.

Shalya Tantra or surgery

It is a significant branch of ayurveda. The name of the sage-physician Susruta is synonymous with surgery. From his treatise Susruta Samhita we come to know that thousand of years ago sophisticated methods of surgery were practiced in India.

The original text of Susruta discusses in detail about an exhaustive range of surgical methods including about how to deal with various types of tumors, internal and external injuries, fracture of bones, complications during pregnancy and delivery, and obstruction in intestinal loop. Susruta was the first surgeon to develop cosmetic surgery. His surgical treatment for trichiasis can be to some of the modern operative techniques used for this eye disease. The long foreign rule in India and lack of promotion stalled the progress of ayurvedic surgery in the middle of the second millennium.

Shalakya Tantra or Eye and ENT

The name of this branch was called Shalakya due to excessive use of 'Shalaka', which means a rod or probe. Though all the three main classics of ayurveda deals on this subject, Susruta Samhita describes more deeply about this branch. Susruta discussed about 72 diseases of the eye. He has stipulated drug therapy for various types of conjunctivitis and glaucoma along with surgical procedures of the removal of cataract, pterygium, diseases of ear, nose and throat besides cosmetic surgery for traumatized nose and ear (rhinoplasty and auraplasty).

Agada tantra or Toxicology

This branch of ayurveda described various methods of cleaning the poisons out of the body as well as recommends antidotes for particular poisons. It deals with a wide range of natural toxins originating from wild lives (animals, birds, insects, etc.), plants/herbs (belladonna, aconite, etc.), vegetables, minerals (leads, mercury, arsenal, etc.) and artificial poisons prepared from poisonous drugs. This branch also deals with air and water pollution, which are basically the causes of various dangerous epidemics.

Kaumarabhritya

This branch deals comprehensively about prenatal, postnatal baby care and gynecology. With the view to achieve its ultimate aim of creating a healthy and disease free society ayurveda strives to make the baby from the time of its conception upto the time of its growth into an adult. Kaumarabhritya has recognized that the mental and physical state of the mother has direct links with the health of the child. It has recommended particular diet, regimen, nutrition and conduct for women during and after delivery. Apart from that kaumarbhritya deals with various disorders concerning children's health such as gastrointestinal diseases, teething disorder, rickets other than midwifery.

Vajkarana

This branch of science explains the art of producing healthy progeny for the creation of a better society. Hence, deals with various diseases like infertility and conditions relating to weak shukra dhatu or the vital reproductive fluids of the body. Apart from prescribing a lot of effective formulations to provide nutrition to enhance the quality of vital body fluids it specifically emphasized to lead a highly disciplined life. This branch of ayurveda highlighted that celibacy is essential for good health. It helps increase the will power, intellect and memory in addition to a healthy body. The shukra dhatu has a direct link with ojas or the immunity of the body. Hence, vajikaran prescribed the therapeutic use of various aphrodisiacs and tonic preparations for enhancing the vigor and reproductive capabilities of men that also strengthens other body tissues like muscles, fats, bones and blood.

Bhuta Vidya

This branch of ayurveda specifically deals with the diseases of mind or psychic conditions, which can be caused by super natural forces. Different experts have explained the word bhuta differently. Some experts say that bhuta means ghosts and similar bad spirits who cause abnormal psychological conditions. Others say bhuta represents microscopic organisms such as virus, bacteria that are not visible to naked eye. Ayurveda also believes in the past karma as a causative factor of certain diseases. Bhuta Vidya deals with the causes, which are directly not visible and have no direct explanation in terms of tridosha.

Rasayana

The rasayana therapy increases the life force (ojas) and immunity of a person and thus there is a regeneration of cells and tissues in the body. Rasayana is a therapeutic process to defer old age. The sages of ancient times led long, disease-free, and vigorous lives with the help of rasayanas. Lord Indra is supposed to have given the knowledge of these panaceas to the sages. Literally, rasayana means the augmentation of rasa, the vital fluid produced by the digestion of food. It is the rasa flowing in the body which sustains life. Rasayana in ayurveda is, the method of treatment through which the rasa is maintained in the body.

The three medicine categories are known in ayurveda as rasayana, vajikarana, and aushadhis, respectively. These categories are complementary to each other. Rasayanas prepared from the herbs and medicinal plants of amalaki, haritiki, triphala, bhringaraja, ashwagandha, punarnava, chitraka and many other herbal medicines have been used from time immemorial and have been instrumental in giving long, disease-free, and vigorous lives to their users. Jewels or ratnas include precious and semiprecious stones, which are used as drugs because of their therapeutic properties. Major jewels or maharatnas include: diamond—hiraka; ruby—manikya; pearl—mukta; topaz—pushparaga; sapphire—neelam; emerald—tarksha; cat's eye—vaidurya; zircon—gomedak; and caulk—vidruma. Uparatnas or minor jewels like sun-stone—suryakant, moonstone—chandrakanta, and crystal—sphatik were in use. Rasayana is held as the culmination of ayurvedic wisdom

According to World Health Organization report, over 80% of the world population relies on plant-based traditional medicine for their primary health care needs.

MILESTONES IN THE DEVELOPMENT OF AYURVEDA

- Divine origin from Lord Brahma—Dates back to origin of human race
- Health, Diseases and Medicinal Plants in Rig-veda and Atharv-veda—5000 BC
- Origin of Attreya and Dhanwantari School of Ayurveda—1000 BC
- Documentation of Charaka Samhita—600 BC
- Documentation of Sushruta Samhita—500 BC
- Advent of Muslim Rulers and start of the Decline of Ayurveda —1100 to 1800
- Resurrection of the system of Medicine under the rule of Peshwas—1800 AD
- Ayurvedic medicine opened in Government Sanskrit College, Calcutta—1827
- Discontinuation of classes in Government Sanskrit College by British—1833

- Dr. Komar Commission; investigation in indigenous system of medicine—1917
- Indian National Congress Convention at Nagpur recommended acceptance of Ayurvedic system of medicine as India's National Health Care System—920
- Mahatma Gandhi inaugurated Ayurvedic and Unani Tibbia College Delhi—1921
- Malviya established Ayurveda college in B. H.U., Varanasi—1927
- Drugs and Cosmetics Act for Ayurvedic/Siddha/Unani medicines—1940
- Bhore Committee or Health Survey and Development Committee recognized past services of indigenous medicines—1943
- Chopra Committee recommended systems of old and modern systems of medicines to evolve a common system of medicine—1946
- Pharmaceutical Enquiry Committee headed by Dr. Bhatia, for intensive research in indigenous drugs of Ayurveda—1953
- Dave Committee for uniform standards of Ayurveda education —1955
- Establishment of Institute of Post-Graduate Training and Research in Gujarat Ayurvedic University, Jamnagar, Gujarat—1956 to 1957
- Udupa Committee set-up. It recommended that there is a need for integrated system of medicine and a training course in Siddha and Ayurveda—1958
- Establishment of Post Graduate Institute of Ayurveda at Banaras Hindu University, Varanasi, Uttar Pradesh—1963 to 1964
- Drugs and Cosmetics Act, 1940 for Indian systems of medicines/drugs—1964
- Central Board of Siddha and Ayurvedic Education—1964 to 1965
- Apex Research Body for Indian medicine and Homoeopathy, 'Central Council for Research in Indian Medicine and Homoeopathy (CCRIMH)'—1969
- Pharmacopoeia Laboratory for Indian medicine, Ghaziabad, U.P. —1970
- Constitution of Central Council of Indian Medicine (CCIM) under an Act—1970
- National Institute of Ayurveda, Jaipur, Rajasthan—1972 to 1973
- Publication of of Ayurvedic formulary containing 444 preparations—1976
- Central Council of Research in Ayurveda and Siddha (CCRAS) —1978
- Amended Drugs and Cosmetics Act regulating import/export of Indian Systems of Medicine—1982

- Setting up of Indian Medicine Pharmaceutical Corporation Ltd. in Mohan, Almora Distt., Uttaranchal—1983
- Silver Jubilee function of Jawaharlal Nehru Ayurvedic Medicinal Plants Garden, Pune. Inaugurated by Shri R. Venkataraman, Vice-president of India—1986
- Second World Conference on Yoga and Ayurveda held at Banaras Hindu University, Varanasi, Uttar Pradesh—1986
- Jawaharlal Nehru Anusandhan Bhawan, Institutional Area, Janakpuri, New Delhi by Hon'ble Vice-President of India, Dr. Shankar Dayal Sharma—1988
- National Academy of Ayurveda (Rashtriya Ayurveda Vidyapeeth)—1989
- Creation of separate Department of Indian Systems of Medicine and Homoeopathy in Ministry of Health and Family Welfare, Government of India—1995
- Introduction of Extra mural Research Programme for accredited organizations with central assistance—1996
- Implementation of Central Scheme in 33 organizations for development of agro-techniques of important medicinal plants—1997
- Maiden participation of Ayurveda alongwith other systems in India International Trade Fair—1998
- Implementation of Central Scheme in 32 laboratories for developing pharmacopoeial standards of Medicinal Plants/ISM Formualations—1998
- Establishment of specialty clinic of Ayurveda in Central Government Hospital (Safdarjung Hospital) New Delhi—1998
- Implementation of IEC (Information, Education and Communication) Scheme for NGOs for propagation and popularization of Ayurveda—1998 to 1999
- Participation in Mystique India—1997 to 1999
- Introduction of Vanaspati Van Scheme for cultivation of Medicinal Plants—1999
- Inauguration of Ayurveda conference at Newyork, USA by Hon'ble Prime Minister of India Sh. Atal Bihari Vajpayee—2000
- Gazette Notification for constitution of Medicinal Plant Board under the Deptt. of Indian Systems of Medicine and Homoeopathy—2000
- Publication of 2nd volume of Ayurvedic Pharmacopoeia—2000
- Introduction of Ayurvedic Medicines in RCH Programme—2000
- Constitution of Advisory group for research in Ayurveda—2000
- Policy Decision on mainstreaming of Ayurveda in RCH programme as per National Population Policy—2000
- Implementation of Central Scheme of assistance for strengthening of State Drug Testing Laborites and Pharmacies—2000 to 2001

- Publication of 3rd volume of Ayurvedic Pharmacopoeia—2001
- Publication of English edition of 2nd volume of Formulary of India—2001
- Maiden participation of ISM tableau on Republic Day—2001
- Exhibition and presentation of Ayurveda during World Health Assembly—2001
- Presentation on evidence based support by Deptt. of ISM&H before House of Lords, U.K. against Sir Walton Committee's Report on · status and nomenclature of Ayurveda among Complementary CAM—2001
- "Made in India" exhibition organized by CII in South Africa—2001

MEDICAL TOURISM AND EXPORT OF ISM PRACTITIONERS

The interest in our systems overseas for gentler and plant based treatment has been growing rapidly. More than that certain therapies are becoming extremely popular and tourists/visitors come to India for therapies like Panchkarma and Yoga. Medical tourism not only popularizes our system but offers good avenue for foreign exchange earning. Little has been done to create a chain of Panchkarma Centres and establish centres of excellence for yoga therapy, meditation and teaching.

Financing ISM

ISM shares only 2-4% of the National Health Budget. This should be raised to 10% of the total health plan at the Central level and further growth should be designed to climb at the rate of 5% in every Five Year Plan. For the first five years of the New Policy, Central Government will directly provide or earmark budgets for consolidation of infrastructure, purchase of drugs and support for opening speciality clinics and ISM services.

Preservation, Promotion and Cultivation of Medicinal Plants and Herbs

Over the last two decades there has been a steady increase in the demand for drugs used in ISM&H. However, the demand for good quality medicinal plants and herbs have not been met. The prices of several plants have increased sharply, making them unaffordable and some species of medicinal plants are also reported to be endangered because of increasing pressure on forests.

The Planning Commission had constituted a Task Force on the Conservation, Cultivation, Sustainable Use and Legal Protection of Medicinal Plants. The Task Force recommended: establishment of medicinal plants conservation areas (MPCA), covering all ecosystems, forest types and sub-types; *ex-situ* conservation of rare, endangered medicinal plants may be tried out in established gardens managed by the Departments of Agriculture, Horticulture or Forests; gene banks created by the Department of Biotechnology should store the germplasm of all medicinal plants; establishment of 'Vanaspati vans' in degraded forest areas; forest areas rich in medicinal plants should be identified, management plans formulated and sustainable harvesting encouraged under the Joint Forest Management System; technically qualified NGOs must be encouraged to take up the task of improving awareness and increasing availability of plant stock and involved in the promotion of agro-techniques for cultivation of medicinal plants; screening/testing/clinical evaluation of herbal products to be taken up and completed; drug testing laboratories for ISM&H products should be established with qualified staff; establishment of a Traditional Knowledge Digital Library so that information on medicinal plants and their use in the country could be accessed readily; and establishment of a Medicinal Plant Board for integrated development of the medicinal plants.

Herbal supplements may be popular, but are they for you? That depends on the herb, your current health and your medical history. Herbal supplements have active ingredients that can affect how your body functions, just as over-the-counter and prescription drugs do. Herbal supplements may be particularly risky for certain individuals and their labels are often vague, confusing and of little help when it comes to making a selection. If you're considering herbal supplements, educate yourself about any products you intend to use before purchasing them, and talk to your doctor about any herbal supplements you're considering taking.

HOW DO YOU CHOOSE AN HERBAL SUPPLEMENT?

The limited amount of regulation makes choosing an herbal supplement of the highest quality a difficult prospect. In order to choose the best herbal supplement brands:

- Look for standardized herbal supplements. The U.S. Pharmacopeia's "USP Dietary Supplement Verified" seal on a supplement indicates the supplement has met certain manufacturing standards. These standards include testing the product for uniformity, cleanliness and freedom from environmental contaminants such as lead, mercury or drugs. Other groups that certify herbal supplements include ConsumerLab.com, Good Housekeeping and NSF International. Although each group takes a slightly different approach, the goal of each is to certify that herbal supplements meet a certain standard. Don't assume that all herbal products on the market are safe. Even the groups that test herbal supplements aren't obligated to report products that fail to live up to their standards.
- Buy only single-herb products. And choose products that clearly show how much of the herb each dose contains. Some products are mixtures of several herbs with unknown proportions of each.

- Beware of claims that sound too good to be true. If a claim sounds outrageous to you, trust your instinct. No one herbal supplement can possibly address a wide spectrum of health concerns.
- Be extremely cautious about herbal supplements manufactured outside the United States. Many European herbs are highly regulated and standardized. But toxic ingredients and prescription drugs have been found in some herbal supplements manufactured in other countries.

Who shouldn't use herbal supplements?

- You're taking prescription or over-the-counter (OTC) medications. Some herbs can cause serious side effects when mixed with prescription and OTC drugs such as aspirin, blood thinners or blood pressure medications. Talk to your doctor about possible interactions.
- A proven medical treatment is available for your medical condition. A traditional medication with an established record for safety and effectiveness will generally be less likely to result in adverse side effects.
- You're pregnant or breast-feeding. As a general rule, don't take any medications—prescription, OTC or herbal—when you're pregnant or breast-feeding unless your doctor approves. Medications that may be safe for you as an adult may be harmful to your fetus or your breast-feeding infant.
- You're having surgery. Many herbal supplements can affect the success of surgery. Some may decrease the effectiveness of anesthetics or cause dangerous complications such as bleeding or high blood pressure. Tell your doctor about any herbs you're taking or considering taking as soon as you know you need surgery.
- You're younger than 18 or older than 65. Older adults may metabolize medications differently. And few herbal supplements have been tested on children or have established safe doses for children.

Are doctors opposed to complementary and alternative medicine?

Most doctors aren't opposed to complementary and alternative medicine. It's true that some doctors may not want to discuss complementary and alternative medicine therapies, but as many as half the doctors in the United States refer people to complementary and alternative practitioners. Your doctor may, in fact, be willing to discuss these options with you. Conventional doctors have good reason to be skeptical when it comes to complementary and alternative medicine. Some alternative medicine practitioners make exaggerated claims about curing diseases, and some ask you to forgo treatment from your conventional doctor to use their unproven therapies. Some forms of alternative medicine can even hurt you.Complementary and alternative medicine may give you additional treatment options, but while some of those options can help you, others can hurt you. When considering complementary and alternative medicine, steer a middle course between uncritical acceptance and outright rejection. Be open-minded yet skeptical at the same time. A growing number of doctors are working to better understand herbal therapies so that they can help you make informed decisions about your health care. If your doctor isn't comfortable discussing herbal supplements with you, ask for a referral to a specialist who is knowledgeable in that field.

Whether CAM has scientific basis?

Many people claim that CAM has no scientific basis and it has failed to evolve on the modern Indian scene due to lack of scientific research. It is well known that physicians with qualification in systems like Ayurveda and homoeopathy trust and practice. Modern medicine more often. A Professor from a US university's department of pharmacology said that homeopathy has barely changed since the start of the 19th Century and was "more like religion than science". He suggested it would be better if courses in aromatherapy, acupuncture, herbal medicine, reflexology, magneto therapy, naturopathy and traditional Chinese medicine and others were taught as part of a cultural history rather than alternative systems of medicine. Let Ayurveda and other systems of CAM invest in research and submit itself for scrutiny to scientific world to emerge as reliable systems of cure.

Investigate complementary and alternative medicine

The Internet offers an ideal way to discover the latest in complementary and alternative medicine. Web sites can be updated at any time to keep up with new products, therapies and advances in the field. But beware—the Internet is also one of the greatest sources of misinformation. According to a study in the Sept. 17, 2003, issue of the "Journal of the American Medical Association," of 433 complementary and alternative medicine Web sites examined, most made misleading or unproven health claims about the herbal remedies they sold.

- *Check out the site sponsor.* Web sites created by major medical centers, national organizations, universities and government agencies are the most credible.
- *Determine the site's objective.* Is the sponsor trying to educate you or just sell you something? Stay away from sites that don't clearly distinguish between scientific evidence and advertisements.
- *Find out if the information is current.* Look for a date. Older material may not include recent findings, such as newly discovered side effects or advances in the field.

- *Red flag words.* The advertisements or promotional materials usually include words such as "satisfaction guaranteed," "miracle cure" or "new discovery." If the product were in fact a cure, it would be widely reported in the media and your doctor would recommend it.
- *Pseudomedical jargon.* Though terms such as "purify," "detoxify" and "energize" may sound impressive and may even have an element of truth, they're generally used to cover up a lack of scientific proof. Watch out for these words.
- *Cure-alls.* The manufacturer claims that the product can treat a wide range of symptoms, or cure or prevent a number of diseases. No single product can do all this.
- *Anecdotal evidence.* Testimonials are no substitute for solid scientific documentation.
- *False accusations.* The manufacturer of the product accuses the government or a medical profession of suppressing important information about the product's benefits.
- *Understand scientific studies.* If you read about studies in journal articles, assess the quality of the research. Look for words such as "double-blind," "controlled" and "randomized."
- *Clinical studies.* These involve studies on human beings—not animals. They generally come after studies that demonstrate the safety and effectiveness of the treatment in animals and in the lab. Studies done solely in test tubes and petri dishes can't prove benefit to humans.
- *Randomized, controlled trials.* Participants in these trials usually are divided into groups. One group receives the treatment under investigation. Another group may be a control group—participants receive standard treatment, no treatment or an inactive substance called a placebo. Participants are assigned to these groups on a random basis. This helps ensure that the groups will be similar.
- *Double-blind studies.* In these studies, neither the researchers nor the human subjects know who will receive the active treatment and who will receive the placebo.

Look for peer-reviewed journals—those that only publish articles reviewed by an independent panel of medical experts.

USA takes a leap forward in CAM

The American Academy of Pediatrics (AAP) has issued a clinical report that addresses the use of complementary and alternative medicine (CAM) in children and has published it in the December 2008, issue of *Pediatrics.* "The National Center for Complementary and Alternative Medicine (NCCAM) of the National Institutes of Health (NIH) defines." CAM as a group of diverse medical and health care systems, practices, and products that are not presently considered to be part of conventional Western medicine," write Kathi J. Kemper, MD, MPH, and colleagues from the Task Force on Complementary and Alternative Medicine and the Provisional Section on Complementary, Holistic, and Integrative Medicine. "Complementary medicine is used in conjunction with conventional medicine; for example, massage, guided imagery, and acupuncture may be used in addition to analgesic medications to help decrease pain. Alternative medicine is used in place of conventional Western medicine; for example, some adolescents use herbs rather than antidepressant medications to treat depression."

Recognizing the increasing use of CAM in children, the AAP also saw the need to provide information and support for pediatricians regarding this field of practice. From 2000 to 2002, the AAP convened the Task Force on Complementary and Alternative Medicine to address issues related to the pediatric use of CAM and to develop resources to educate clinicians, patients, and families.

The aims of the report were therefore to define terms; to review the epidemiology; to list frequently used CAM modalities; to discuss medico-legal, ethical, and research implications; to describe education and training for CAM providers; to offer resources for additional learning regarding CAM; and to suggest communication strategies that clinicians may find helpful when discussing CAM with patients and families.

Now that many CAM modalities, such as guided imagery and massage for pain treatment, have been formally tested and integrated into standard practice, the distinction between CAM and mainstream medicine has become less apparent. The terms *holistic medicine* or *integrative medicine* is being increasingly substituted for *CAM*.

"Holistic medicine refers to patient-centered care that includes consideration of biological, psychological, spiritual, social, and environmental aspects of health," the Task Force writes. "Integrative medicine is relationship-based care that combines mainstream and complementary therapies for which there is some high-quality scientific evidence of safety and effectiveness to promote health for the whole person in the context of his or her family and community. Integrative medicine also reaffirms the importance of the relationship between the practitioner and the patient, emphasizes wellness and the inherent drive toward healing, and focuses on the whole person, using all appropriate therapies to achieve the patient's goals for health and healing."

The Kemper model of holistic care recognizes 4 main components of therapy. Biochemical components include medications, dietary supplements, vitamins, minerals, and herbal remedies. Lifestyle and nutritional interventions include recommendations for exercise and/or rest; environmental therapies including heat, ice, music, vibration, and light; and mind-body treatments such as behavior management, meditation, hypnosis, biofeedback, and counseling.

Biomechanical components include massage and bodywork,

chiropractic and osteopathic adjustment, and surgery. Bioenergetic therapies may include acupuncture, radiation therapy, magnets, Reiki, healing touch, qi gong, therapeutic touch, prayer, and homeopathy. Clinicians caring for children need to advise and counsel patients and their families about appropriate, safe, and effective health services and treatments regardless of whether they are considered mainstream or CAM. Clinicians should specifically ask about all treatments the family is administering to the child because most families use CAM services without spontaneously notifying their clinician.

To provide useful counsel regarding use of CAM and integrating these therapies into the child's treatment plan, pediatricians should stay informed and updated regarding therapeutic options available to their patients. Clinicians should address and counsel their patients' families regarding the safety, appropriateness, and advisability of specific CAM 398 services used by individual patients.

A common-sense approach to advising families regarding use of CAM modalities is that those treatments shown to be safe and effective should be encouraged, those treatments that are safe but ineffective may be tolerated, those modalities that are effective but raise safety issues should be closely monitored or discouraged, and those therapies that are neither safe nor effective should be discouraged.

For patients being treated by a CAM provider, the pediatrician should seek permission of the patient and family to include the CAM provider in the overall management plan.

Helpful communication strategies may include asking about different therapies the patient is using; recognizing and respecting the family's perspectives, values, and cultural beliefs; working together with the parents as a team; and actively listening to families and patients.

The patient's response to treatment should be monitored with use of measurable outcomes, such as specific goals for symptom relief and remembering to "first do no harm."

"A growing number of pediatricians have begun to offer complementary therapies and advice as part of their practice," the task force concludes. "In addition, there is a growing number of academic pediatric integrative medicine programs and new initiatives to promote systematic sharing, support, and dissemination of information to improve collaborative and comprehensive care."

All AAP clinical reports automatically expire 5 years after publication unless reaffirmed, revised, or retired at or before that time. Coauthor Sunita Vohra, MD, has received salary support from the Alberta Heritage Foundation for Medical Research and the Canadian Institutes of Health Research.

STUDY HIGHLIGHTS

- CAM is used in 20% to 40% of healthy children and in more than 50% of children with chronic, recurrent, and incurable conditions, including asthma, attention-deficit/hyperactivity disorder, autism, cancer, cerebral palsy, cystic fibrosis, inflammatory bowel disease, and juvenile rheumatoid arthritis.

- 66% of caregivers did not tell their child's clinician about CAM use.
- CAM is not consistently linked with parent income, sex, or usual source of care.
- Reasons for CAM use include word of mouth, effectiveness, fear of drug adverse effects, dissatisfaction with conventional medicine, and more personal attention.
- Barriers to health insurance coverage of CAM include variable credentialing, accounting issues, and lack of *Current Procedural Terminology* codes.
- Dietary supplements do not need proven safety or efficacy for marketing.
- Biologically-based therapies include botanicals, animal-derived extracts, vitamins, minerals, fatty acids, amino acids, proteins, pre-biotics, pro-biotics, whole diets, and functional foods:
  - Multivitamins are the most commonly used in children (up to 41%).
  - Of teenagers using CAM, approximately 75% use dietary supplements and herbs.
  - The ketogenic diet is an accepted treatment of seizure disorder.
  - Quality is affected by portion of plant, time of harvest, handling, and identification.
- Manipulative and body-based therapies include chiropractic and osteopathic manipulation, massage, reflexology, Rolfing, Bowen technique, and Trager approach:
  - Chiropractors are the most common CAM providers for pediatric patients.
  - Massage is beneficial for preterm infants and alleviates symptoms of asthma, insomnia, colic, cystic fibrosis, and juvenile rheumatoid arthritis.
- Common mind-body therapies in children are meditation, prayer, hypnosis, biofeedback, and progressive muscle relaxation:
  - Guided imagery, hypnosis, and biofeedback complement medical therapy for pain, anxiety/stress disorders, enuresis, encopresis, sleep disorders, autonomic nervous system dysregulation, habitual disorders, attention/learning disorders, asthma, cancer, and diabetes.
  - Two-thirds of parents use prayer for their children.
- Biofield therapies include acupuncture, homeopathy, polarity therapy, magnet, Japanese Reiki and Johrei, qi gong, therapeutic touch, healing touch, and spiritual healing:

  - o Acupuncture is possibly effective for recurrent headaches, nausea, pain, and allergy.
  - o 2% to 10% of children use homeopathic therapies for respiratory conditions, teething, or otitis media.
- Special populations using CAM include adolescents, children with chronic illness or disability, and ethnic and cultural groups.
- CAM research issues include the more likely publication of negative studies in well-known journals and positive studies in foreign-language journals, heterogeneous products and practices, need for more randomized controlled trials in children, few serious adverse effects in children, and lack of priority listing for children.
- Pediatric CAM training for providers and clinicians is variable or lacking.
- Clinicians should understand local and state regulations for CAM provider licensure and specific CAM therapies.
- Ethical issues include need for evidence-based safety and effectiveness information about CAM therapies and therapists, risk/benefit analysis, respect for patient autonomy, non-maleficence, beneficence, and justice.
- Clinicians should routinely ask about specific CAM therapies and stress management; respect the family's values, perspectives, and cultural beliefs; reevaluate treatment if no or negative response; and maintain evidence-based knowledge about CAM therapies.
- Common types of CAM therapies used in children include multivitamins, herbs and other dietary supplements, chiropractic care, massage, prayer, progressive relaxation exercises, meditation, biofeedback, hypnosis, and acupuncture.
- Strategies to use in discussing CAM with children and families include routinely asking whether the child uses vitamins, home remedies, or other services and about stress management; showing respect for values and cultural beliefs; reevaluating therapy if the measured outcome to treatment is inadequate; and maintaining knowledge about CAM therapies.

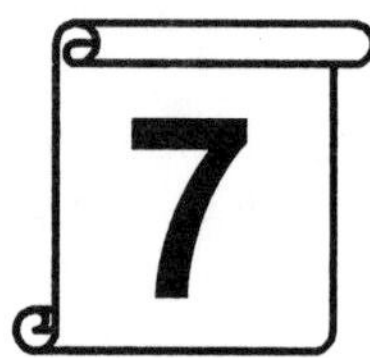

Injuries are a Major Challenge to Health Care: Trauma Hospitals

The planning and development of trauma care systems in India has yet to gain attention and priority from the government or NGOs, even though trauma is a major public health problem. Accelerated urbanization and industrialization have led to an alarming increase in the rate of accidental injuries, crime and violence in India. An unprecedented increase in the number of vehicles has outpaced the development of adequate roads and highways. India has 1% of the motor vehicles in the world, but bears the burden of 6% of the global vehicular accidents. It is well recognized that our health care system is not fully equipped to meet the challenge.

TRAUMA CARE CREATES A PERFECT STORM FOR MEDICAL ERRORS

Trauma care creates a perfect storm for medical errors: unstable patients, incomplete histories, time-critical decisions, concurrent tasks, involvement of many disciplines, and often junior personnel working after-hours in busy emergency departments. Studies in several countries have identified adverse events, including death, that occur in trauma and emergency care. Various studies provide insights into the nature of preventable deaths, including the significance of failure to evaluate the abdomen, delays to treatment, and critical care errors. The estimates of preventable death rates are wide in, ranging from 2% to 50%, indicating the variability of care provided and the need for standardized approaches. These studies also show that trauma surgeons are pioneers in error reduction and quality improvement. In trauma, as in all fields, it is likely that recognizable clinical situations create predictable vulnerability to human error, and the erroneous decision-making that occurs in response to these situations. To reduce errors, institutions need effective means of identifying errors and error-associated deaths. This is all the more difficult in trauma given high baseline mortality rates, often complicated in-hospital care, and the relative paucity of widely applicable management protocols, especially beyond the Golden Hour of initial resuscitation, to which Advanced Trauma Life Support (ATLS) protocols apply. Furthermore, errors that result in death may be relatively infrequent; therefore, opportunities to learn from them may be limited by infrequent attention and lack of institutional memory. In tertiary care hospitals Patients with multi-system injuries are admitted to emergency department under supervision of the general surgery service, as are unstable patients with isolated injuries for resuscitation and stabilization before transfer to other services. An in-house attending anesthesiologist and a full-time operating room staff are present 24 hours per day, 7 days per week. The CT scanner and the angiography suite are adjacent and easily accessible to the emergency department. All trauma deaths are discussed at weekly surgical morbidity and mortality (M&M) meetings. Those identified as being associated with possible or definite errors in care are subsequently reviewed by departmental and hospital quality assurance (QA) officers, and significant cases are presented for discussion at monthly multidisciplinary hospital trauma council meetings.

Need to improve the delivery of trauma care

There is an urgent need to improve the delivery of trauma care for the injured. A chain of trauma care centers is essential in India, since ours is one of the most populous countries in the world, and one with a high incidence of disasters and consequent burden of trauma deaths and disability. Also there is gross disparity between trauma services available, inter se in various parts of the country. Rural India lacks trauma care services almost completely and in urban areas it is a part of emergency department, with inefficient services for trauma care, due to the varied topography, financial constraints and lack of appropriate health infrastructure. There is no national nodal agency to co-ordinate various components of a trauma care. Education in trauma life-support (TLS) skills is hardly available. The doctors trained in super-specialties like orthopedics, plastic surgery, neuro-surgery are not willing to be dumped for the treatment of injured, for the rest of their lives. There is a need to develop a specialty of traumatology to man the proposed centers. Although injury is a major public-health problem; responsible for a large number of deaths, the Government of India has failed to recognize it as a priority area. Some efforts to develop trauma-care systems across the country are seen mainly in the private sector. In the public health system the allocation of funds remains grossly inadequate for any significant impact on the outcome. Chandigarh administration is in the process of setting up its first trauma hospital, though trained manpower in traumatology is a far cry. Presently PGI emergency department is the main stay of trauma management in and around the city of Chandigarh.

In May 2002, Academy of Traumatology (India) undertook a maiden study of trauma systems, one hundred and forty-five institutions across the country of all states in India were invited to participate in the survey. Fifty institutions participated in the survey. The overall data was fairly representative of urban and rural settings, private and public hospitals and facilities across all geographical regions of the country. The following data emerged from the study.

Injury as public health problem

Road-traffic accidents are increasing at an alarming annual rate of 3%. In 1997, 10.1% of all deaths in India are due to accidents and injuries. A vehicular accident is reported every 3 minutes and a death every 10 minutes on Indian roads. During 1998, nearly 80,000 lives were lost and 330,000 people were injured. Of these, 78% were men in age group of 20-44 years, causing significant impact on productivity. A trauma-related death occurs in India every 1.9 minutes. The majority of fatal road-traffic accident victims are pedestrians, two wheeler riders and bicyclists. No credible data is available to ascertain the outcome of trauma victims; it is generally perceived that outcomes inpatients with single system injury (e.g. musculoskeletal trauma) have improved. Unfortunately, the same cannot be said for poly-trauma. There is a high mortality rate amongst those with multi-system injuries, which can be attributed to the primitive state of trauma-care systems, lack of pre-hospital care and inadequate critical care. It is established that the mortality in serious injuries is six times worse in a developing country such as India compared to a developed country.

Despite trauma being a major public-health problem with high morbidity and mortality, the Ministry of Health does not have a designated unit to deal with issues related to trauma. There is no central government agency to integrate policy-making, planning, financing, drafting legislation or establishment of minimum standards for the performance of a trauma-care system. No reliable institutional arrangement exists to lead the development of such a system in any Indian state. In 26% of the systems surveyed, the overall responsibility for leading the system was undefined. The Centralized Ambulance Transport Service (CATS) of the Government of the State of New Delhi is the only noteworthy state initiative in this direction. This is restricted mainly to pre-hospital care. Only 28% of respondents identified the presence of a unified leadership coordinating various components and agencies. The existing systems for trauma care are elementary in nature, predominantly restricted to cities and semi-urban areas, without integration of region or statewide systems. No such systems exist in rural and remote areas to offer prompt life-saving treatment and safe transfer to an appropriate facility. Consequently fatal accident rate (expressed per kilometer of travel) in India is estimated to be sevenfold worse compared to most advanced states. In cities such as Mumbai, Pune, Bangalore, Hyderabad, Ahmedabad and Chennai, the trauma systems are at an embryonic stage, predominantly supported by non-government and private agencies. No law exists to ensure prompt access to life-saving treatment for trauma victims. Statutory provisions to aid national, state, or interstate planning and implementation of trauma-care systems, regardless of jurisdictional boundaries, are yet to evolve. Issues such as the accreditation of trauma centers and critical care units, specialist licensing of health personnel and mandatory training of physicians lack national guidelines. The publication of ISCCM guidelines for ICUs is an important step in that direction. Legislative provisions for the minimum qualification of ambulance personnel, the type and quality of ambulance equipment and essential hospital capabilities are not in place. Available personnel and their skills often do not match the needs of the patients. The optimal number and type of pre-hospital personnel for ambulances is not defined. The concept of a dedicated trauma team is not accepted at all levels. At a majority of hospitals in the public system, the casualty medical officer is the only one to respond to a demand for major resuscitation. This paradox is striking, resulting in the most seriously injured patients frequently being dealt with by the most junior and inexperienced staff. There are no plans for dynamic and flexible responses to the optimal management of trauma patients. The lack of precise and predetermined role allocation during peak periods of activity stresses the fragile current systems and workforce.

Lack of skilled and highly skilled manpower

The state medical and nursing councils control the educational and licensing requirements for physicians and nurses. However, formal education and specialty training (in emergency medicine, trauma surgery and critical care) are not mandatory for personnel involved in trauma care and available only at select private institutions. The standardized education in trauma life-support skills is made available through the efforts of Academy of Traumatology (India) under the 'National Trauma Management Course' (NTMC) with accreditation from the International Association for Surgery of Trauma and Surgical Intensive Care (IATSIC). Currently this training is available mainly in larger centers and is intended for doctors only. The issues of educational standards, certification and continuing education and evaluation requirements for doctors involved in trauma care are yet to be addressed. The National Board of Examinations has recently begun registering courses in trauma care, though in a very limited manner. There are no minimum stipulated educational standards for paramedic and ambulance personnel. Paramedic training programmes are offered in major institutions but there is no accreditation, review or provision for periodic update of skills and knowledge. Gross inadequacy in Pre-hospital Care exists Pre-hospital care is virtually non-existent in most rural and semi-urban areas in India, and implementation of the 'golden hour' concept is still an unachieved goal. The concept of a coordinating agency and a designated authority is restricted mainly to cities where trauma systems are operational in some form. Quite often there is an overlapping of private and public facilities and ambulance services in an urban geographical area.

Gross discrepancy is seen in pre-hospital services between urban and rural settings, as well as between paying and non-paying patients. In the absence of guidelines and trained paramedical staff, decisions about evacuation of the victim and the choice of the destination hospital are made on an individual-case basis. These choices are often made at the behest of patients or their kin. Formal licensing to run an ambulance service is not mandatory. Ambulance services are run by a multitude of organizations including government, police, fire brigades, hospitals and private agencies. Of the facilities surveyed, 12% reported a total absence of any ambulance service. Air ambulance services are not widely available and only 4% of the surveyed systems have even minimal access to air transportation, run by private agencies. The absence of minimal educational and training standards for paramedics brings in unskilled labor to handle the most delicate of tasks. Many private hospitals in large cities offer efficient pre-hospital care, but this covers too small an area and too small a segment of the population. The care is unaffordable for most patients. No national or regional guidelines exist for triage, patient-delivery decisions, pre-hospital treatment plans and transfer protocols. Policies, procedures and regulations governing medical directions are in place only in some city systems. There are recent attempts to provide one-time formal training in pre-hospital care to the ambulance personnel in various parts of the country. Currently, only 4% of the ambulance personnel have any certified formal training. The number of paramedics in the ambulances varies considerably. One-third of ambulances serve only as transport vehicles with no paramedic staff. Only 28% of the ambulances have two or more paramedics. Only 50% of ambulance services have minimal skills and resources for providing airway support and appropriate splintage. The majority of ambulances have the means for intravenous infusion (74%) and blood-pressure measurement (62%). Despite technological advances, communication in trauma systems in India remains rudimentary and inefficient. Only 14% of the systems have a dedicated central telephone number for incident reporting. Some 30% of the trauma systems, mainly in cities, are equipped with wireless communication. Only 4% of systems have a comprehensive network operational between hospitals and ambulances.

Lack of Preparedness is rampant

India is a disaster-prone country with frequent floods, cyclones, landslides and earthquakes. Train accidents and industrial mishaps are not uncommon. Government plans are in place, in general, to deal with disasters. However, regular drills to test preparedness are not carried out. Only 26% of the systems in the survey reported a well-documented disaster management plan. The rest of the systems have plans under development, or no plans. This deficiency has resulted in excessive number of deaths in natural disasters. In 1999, there was an increase of 20.8% in fatalities due to such disasters compared to the previous year. This figure for 2001 is likely to rise even further as a result of a killer earthquake in Gujarat, causing over 12,000 deaths. Many more disasters have occurred since then. Facilities that offer treatment for trauma victims, report 10% to 30% of their beds occupied by people injured in road accidents. Most government hospitals offer free care, but the quality of that care differs from one centre to another. Most medical college hospitals provide a reasonable level of care; these hospitals are able to fulfil the role of tertiary trauma centers but critical care continues to remain the weak link in such settings for a variety of reasons. Private and corporate hospitals, located mostly in large cities, are equipped with modern diagnostic and imaging facilities, good operating environments and intensive-care units. Some of them also run dedicated trauma services. However, there are no norms to govern their standards and their relations with the public trauma system. District hospitals often lack trained staff, adequate infrastructure for management of poly-trauma and supply of consumables. Small hospitals and clinics mushrooming across India are simply unable to cope with poly-trauma. Such small clinics struggle to manage severely injured patients, resulting in substandard care and high mortality. Only 54% of the hospitals have set protocols for triage. In 30% of the hospitals, the casualty medical officers are the only physicians available to provide resuscitation. Their level of training and experience in providing life support is not uniform. The concept and practice of forming dedicated trauma-response teams is yet to percolate beyond tertiary-care hospitals. In acute and elective management of trauma patients, only 36% of the facilities follow NTMC, or locally developed clinical protocols.

There are no dedicated trauma surgeons in India. Orthopaedic surgeons lead the trauma response in 50% of facilities. In the remainder, the responsibility is not clearly defined. Clinical decisions are often delayed, in the absence of clear perceptions of clinical responsibility amongst specialists, putting patients with multi-system injury at a greater risk. Nearly half of the systems surveyed have no protocol for inter-hospital transfers. Linkages between rural and urban facilities do not exist in most regions. The availability of specialist care (for, e.g. spinal trauma, burns, head injuries, childhood injuries, etc.) is restricted to major cities and teaching hospitals. Transfer to such a specialty centre in an emergency is often difficult and time-consuming, resulting in delay in decision-making and management and also unaffordable expenditure. Rehabilitation, though an integral element of any trauma-care system, is a neglected area. It is restricted to physiotherapy centers. Although 76% of the facilities offer physiotherapy services, only a third offer occupational rehabilitation and psychological counseling. The surveyed hospitals failed to demonstrate strong links and transfer agreements between acute facilities and rehabilitation units. The disabled is left alone to fend for herself. The information systems in most places are manual and rudimentary. There is no central trauma registry in any state. Most hospitals have reliable data on trauma admissions, but only 40% have data on the clinical outcome of the trauma patients. This has a negative impact on development and implementation of an effective public policy on trauma care. In the wake of the gross disparity between accessibility and affordability of trauma care; quality assurance is a major casualty. In the absence of a lead agency and with a poor information system, evaluation and research on trauma systems is a difficult proposition. Monitoring of the performance of the system and its individual components, and any quality-improvement programme, is far away. Very little work has been done to evaluate the working of trauma systems in India. CATS New Delhi and CMC Hospital, Vellore have assessed some components of their systems. What lies in store in the future The future appears both daunting and challenging. It is estimated that from its present position of the ninth leading cause of deaths in India, trauma will move up to third position by 2020. It is also estimated that in the developing countries over 6 million will die and 60 million will be injured, or disabled, in the next 10 years. India will have a large share in this, with an estimated economic loss of around 2% of GDP. To meet this challenge several efforts are required: resource creation, education, legislation, upgrading pre-hospital and hospital-based care, public awareness and a change in the attitude of the policy-makers. The public health institutions will also benefit from adopting WHO Essential Trauma Care guidelines for trauma care, which is aimed at low cost improvements to the trauma care. Although the overall picture in trauma care is not as dismal as it used to be three decades ago, 'trauma care for all' continues to remain a distant dream in India. Despite significant overall progress in many other fields, trauma systems in India continue to remain at a formative stage for various reasons. A concerted effort from all the parties involved, as well as the society, is the need of the hour.

A CASE STUDY OF A BIG HOSPITAL IN MUMBAI

In a study, carried out in Lokmanya Tilak Municipal General (LTMG) Hospital in Mumbai, between 1 August 2001 and 31 May 2002, 1074 severely injured patients were included. This study is likely to assist error reduction in 3 important ways. The first is through identification of specific categories of errors that may be targeted. The most commonly identified groups related to airway and hemorrhage control, the ABCs of acute severe trauma management. Several other major error categories were also relatively specific to trauma: inappropriate management of an unstable patient, missed or delayed diagnoses, management of feeding tubes, and over-resuscitation with fluids. The second way this study may help is through considering the type and underlying psychological cause, which may provide insights into the most useful error-reduction strategies. For example, execution errors are addressed through technical training, and ensuring that those performing the tasks are technically competent and appropriately credentialed. Input errors require clinicians to be aware of potential problems and appropriately use and interpret diagnostic tests. The majority of error-associated deaths, however, were intention errors affecting treatment. Indeed, some errors that seemed at first to be execution errors, such as failure to achieve orotracheal intubation leading to anoxic brain injury, may be more appropriately viewed as intention errors, in that one should always be ready to perform a surgical airway in the event of a challenging intubation. Intention errors are greatly reduced by protocols and algorithms that simplify or serve as reminders for particularly complex or time-critical management decisions. The third way in which this study supports error reduction is by demonstrating the likely effectiveness of such evidence-based institutional protocols. In their comparison of major error categories and institutional policies, they instituted new policies that related directly to 4 of the 14 error categories. All 4 policies had emerged after recognition that errors were occurring and that a policy was needed to address them. In all 4 error-associated deaths were less frequent after institution of the policy. It is important to realize that deaths, while the most serious outcome, are just the tip of the iceberg of morbidity associated with errors, and for every prevented death there are probably many patients for whom non-fatal single or multiple organ failure is averted.

Survival analysis was completed for 98.3% of the patients. The majority of the patients were men (84%) and the average age was 31 years. 90.4% were blunt injuries, with road traffic crashes (39.2%) being the most common cause. The predicted mortality was 10.89% and the observed mortality was 21.26%. The average probability of survival (Ps) was 89.14. The M and Z statistics were 0.84 and -14.1593, respectively. The injured in this study were found to be older, the injuries more severe and with poorer outcomes, than in other studies. Sixty-four patients (0.14% admissions, 2.47% deaths) had recognized errors in care that contributed to their death. Important error patterns included: failure to successfully intubate, secure or protect an airway (16%), delayed operative or angiographic control of acute abdominal/pelvic hemorrhage (16%), delayed intervention for ongoing intra-thoracic hemorrhage (9%), inadequate DVT or gastrointestinal prophylaxis (9%), lengthy initial operative procedures rather than damage control surgery in unstable patients (8%), over-resuscitation with fluids (5%), and complications of feeding tubes (5%). Resulting data-directed institutional and regional trauma system policy changes have demonstrably reduced the incidence of associated error-related deaths. This review has identified error patterns that are likely common in all trauma systems, and for which policy interventions can be effectively targeted. Various aspects of errors include:

1. Error Impact, which in this study was death.
2. Error Type, classified as many others have done as errors in diagnosis, treatment, prevention, or other (equipment failures; communication failures; and errors in transfer).
3. Error Domain, for which they were most interested in the phase of trauma management when it occurred, and for which the classifications were: initial assessment and resuscitation

(including prehospital); secondary survey and tests (e.g. CT); inter-hospital transfers; initial interventions (e.g. OR, Angio); ICU; general ward; and rehabilitation.

4. Error Cause, which refers to the psychological cause, that is, it relates to what was probably going on in the mind of the person who erred. Reason has contributed much to this understanding, and they used an internal processing classification, that included: Input error: the input data are incorrectly perceived; therefore, an incorrect intention is formed and the wrong action is performed. Intention error: the input data are correctly perceived, but an incorrect intention is formed, and the wrong action is performed. Execution error: the input data are correctly perceived and the correct intention is formed, but the wrong action is performed; that is, the action is not what was intended.

The occurrence of errors relative to each policy's implementation was then plotted to give an indication of whether or not such policies had been effective in reducing error occurrence. Observations were categorized into whether or not a new policy was implemented during the study period.

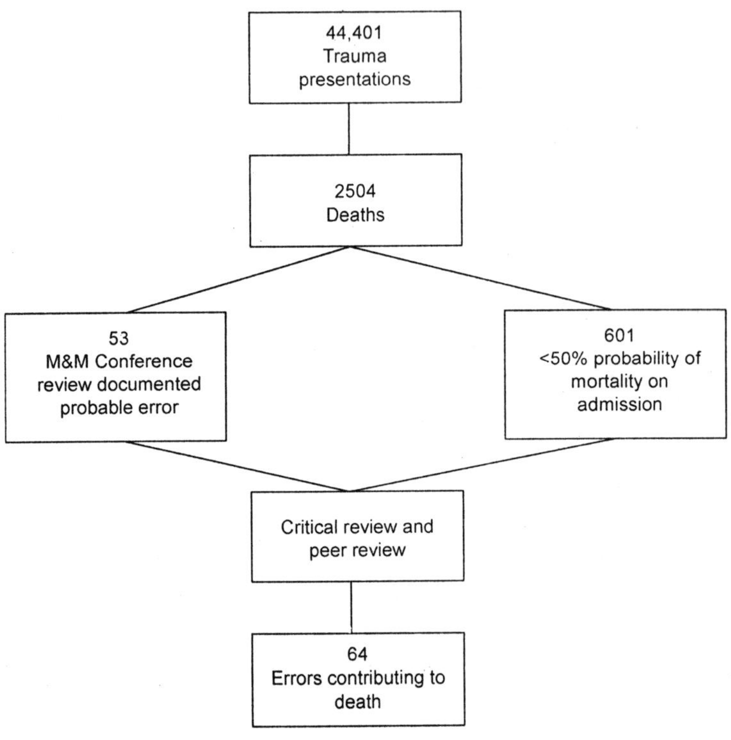

Source: Ann Surg © 2004.

The major clinical groupings of errors included hemorrhage control (28%), airway management (16%), inappropriate management of unstable patients (14%), complications of procedures (12%), inadequate prophylaxis (11%), missed or delayed diagnoses (11%), over-resuscitation with fluids (5%), and other poor management decisions (3%).

Delayed control of abdominal or pelvic hemorrhage using operative or angiographic methods was usually due to delays in the emergency department (ED) assessment of a patient in shock, and occasionally involved the performance of other non-urgent tests or procedures. Delayed control of intra-thoracic hemorrhage was most often a delay in the diagnosis of massive hemo-thorax with inadequate evacuation of blood from the chest, or inadequate recognition of the volume that had already been evacuated. Half of all fatal airway errors involved unsuccessful attempts at endotracheal intubations and failure to adequately gain or regain control using simple maneuvers or a surgical airway. The other airway errors were failure to adequately protect the airway from aspiration during subsequent phases of care. In the operating room, damage-control principles dictate that control of hemorrhage and control of contamination should be prioritized, deferring prolonged surgical interventions and reconstruction until correction of hypothermia, acidosis, and coagulopathy is accomplished in the ICU. They found 5 cases in which these principles were not followed, and the patient subsequently progressed to death due to exsanguination or multiorgan failure. They found 7 cases in which a missed injury or delayed diagnosis led to death. In 4 cases, there was a positive test result that failed to be acted on (a head CT showing subdural hemorrhage, a pericardial ultrasound showing a tamponade, a positive blood culture, and hyperkalemia on blood chemistry). Over-resuscitation is a consequence of aggressive fluid management in the face of hypotension, often due to primary pump failure. The pulmonary consequences of over-resuscitation were fatal in 3 patients.

By phase of trauma management, 34% of errors occurred in the ED (20% during initial assessment and resuscitation, 14% during the secondary survey and initial diagnostic tests), 8% during stabilization and interhospital transport, 11% during initial interventions (surgery and/or angiography), 37% during the intensive care unit stay, and 9% during the general or rehabilitation ward inpatient stay.

Errors of treatment predominated; however, diagnostic errors were particularly evident in the secondary survey and ICU phases, and errors of prophylaxis were most evident after the initial management was completed, in the ICU and post-ICU phases. While half of all errors were intention errors and occurred throughout the hospital stay, input errors and execution errors were particularly prominent in the ICU phase of care, and to a lesser extent, the initial assessment and resuscitation phase.

They have demonstrated that, even in mature trauma systems, errors still occasionally lead to patients' deaths. Among 44,401 admissions and 2594 deaths over 9 years, 2.47% of deaths at the institution were contributed to by errors. This is among the lowest reported preventable death rate in trauma patients. Despite increasing numbers and increasing complexity of cases at the institution, the findings compare favorably with the 23% pedestrian and bicycle fatalities regarded as potentially preventable 18 years ago. As others have suggested, a 2% to 3% error-related death rate may be an absolute baseline in complex trauma systems.

Error reduction cannot be solely attributed to the implementation of policies or protocols, however. Changes in staffing, training, equipment, supervision, and any number of other reasons are likely to also affect error occurrence. Of course, the effect of looking repeatedly for recurrent problems or errors may itself contribute to a reduction in errors through a Hawthorne-type effect of enhanced awareness. Yet by examining the types of errors that occur with some frequency as to constitute a repetitive pattern, we are forced to consider what protocol and policy options might affect real improvement. We have recently recognized overly aggressive resuscitation as a problem causing 3 deaths in the past 3 years. To minimize the risk of over-resuscitation, in 2005 a new protocol was instituted that required early invasive central venous monitoring in the ED, and clear guidelines to limiting fluids, beginning inotropic agents, and obtaining rapid control of bleeding. Challenges emerging from this study that are yet to be addressed include reducing deaths associated with delays to the operating room or angiography for abdominopelvic hemorrhage, employing surgical or other airway maneuvers when faced with a challenging airway, and ensuring damage control principles are followed when necessary.

A GLIMPSE OF THE WESTERN WORLD

In the Western world, trauma is the leading cause of death for individuals under 45 years of age, and it remains the fourth leading cause of death for all ages combined. In 1994, 8,687 people died following accidents in Canada. Approximately four times as many patients suffer severe disability related to accidents each year.

Prehospital care for trauma patients is provided by emergency medical personnel using either Basic Life Support (BLS) or Advanced Life Support (ALS) techniques. BLS (or "scoop and run") consists of non-invasive interventions such as wound dressing, immobilization, fracture splinting, oxygen administration, and non-invasive cardiopulmonary resuscitation. ALS encompasses all of these BLS techniques in addition to invasive procedures, including intubation, initiation of IV access with fluid replacement, administration of medications, and in rare cases application of pneumatic antishock garments (PASG). The rationale for the use of on-site ALS in trauma is that these interventions will reduce the rate of physiologic and hemodynamic deterioration, thus stabilizing the patient before arrival at the hospital. It is expected that this will result in increased chances of survival. The paradox is that on-site ALS increases the amount of time that is spent on the scene and hence increases the delay to definitive in-hospital care. To date, the controversy between the "scoop and run" versus "stay and stabilize" approach to pre-hospital trauma care remains unresolved and has been the subject of a limited number of studies, most of which were based on small numbers of selected patients. Studies supporting ALS have failed to show an association between on-site ALS and increased survival among patients with major trauma. Studies supporting BLS have shown higher survival rates for patients treated using the "scoop and run" approach compared to those treated using on-site ALS. The validity of these studies is often compromised due to the lack of control for confounding variables and appropriate comparison groups.

A 1992 study by Schmidt *et al.* compared trauma patients with equivalent Injury Severity Scores (ISS) transported by helicopter in Germany to patients transported by helicopter in the United States. In Germany, patients received treatment by a paramedic and a trauma surgeon and in the United States by a paramedic and a nurse. They found that the German patients received significantly more advanced interventions, including IV fluids, endotracheal intubations, and thoracic decompressions, than the American group. This led to a decrease in early mortality and improved outcome compared to patients in the Major Trauma Outcome Study (MTOS).

Similarly, the effectiveness of on-site intubations in improving outcome of severely injured patients has not been adequately evaluated. The rationale for on-scene intubations is that this intervention will maintain airway patency and oxygenation. As with IV placement, the argument against intubations is that it causes significant delays to definitive in-hospital care. Unlike IV placement, however, there is some agreement that in certain severely injured and unconscious patients, intubations should be initiated at the scene or en route to the hospital.

The unresolved controversy regarding the on-site management of trauma patients is reflected in the regional variation of pre-hospital patient management protocols. This variation is observed profoundly in Canada, where the type of on-site care available to trauma patients ranges from BLS provided by emergency medical technician (EMTs) to physician-provided ALS. The type of pre-hospital care available to trauma patients is determined by regional policies that are dictated by local political, cultural, and economic factors as well as the influential opinion of local experts.

The objectives of the study were three-fold:

- To compare the effectiveness of three different prehospital trauma care systems-one with only EMTs providing BLS and adhering to the "scoop and run" approach, one with paramedics available to provide on-site ALS (PMD-ALS), and the third with physicians available to provide on-site ALS (MD-ALS)—in reducing trauma-related mortality.
- To evaluate and compare the effectiveness of three different types of on-site management (EMT-BLS, PMD-ALS, and MD-ALS) in reducing trauma-related mortality.

- To evaluate and compare the effectiveness of two different types of on-site care (ALS and BLS) in reducing. trauma-related mortality.

The results of the study show that the use of on-site ALS, in general, does not provide any benefits in reducing mortality inpatients with major trauma. This result is generalizable to patients injured in urban centers served by highly organized trauma care systems with access to a level I trauma center. The data from this study show that when physicians provide on-site ALS to trauma patients, the risk of mortality is significantly increased when compared to both EMT-provided BLS and paramedic-provided ALS. On-site ALS provided by paramedics was not associated with a reduction in mortality when compared to EMTs.

The results of this study are compatible with others in the literature that support the "scoop and run" approach for the pre-hospital management of trauma patients in an urban setting. The lack of effectiveness of ALS in general has often been attributed to the increased time required to perform ALS procedures at the scene. However, there is now a considerable evidence to suggest that certain ALS procedures, such as IV fluid replacement, may be harmful for patients with major trauma. The increased risk of mortality associated with MD-ALS is probably due to the lack of standardized protocols and lack of specific training. The results of this study, in combination with the already existing evidence in the current literature, fail to support the use of ALS in the pre-hospital management of urban trauma patients. These conclusions may or may not apply to rural trauma patients. Resources should be allocated for the establishment of trauma care systems and networks that ensure rapid transport of major trauma patients to highly specialized trauma hospitals. In these systems, emphasis should be placed on minimizing on-scene time and establishing patient transfer corridors to decrease time to definitive in-hospital care and maximize efficiency of the health care resources.

References

Government of Delhi. Evaluation Unit, Planning Department. Report of Evaluation Study on CATS 2001.

Government of India. Ministry of Health and Family Welfare. National Health Policy, 2002.

Joshipura, M.K. Total Trauma Care: International Perspective. *Hospital Today* 1996;11:43-4.

Joshipura, M.K., Mock, C., Goosen, J., Peden, M. Essential Trauma Care: strengthening trauma systems round the world. *Injury*, 2004;35:841-5.

Mock, C.N., Jurkovich, G.J., nii-Amon-Kotei, D., Arreola-Risa, C., Maier, R.V. Trauma mortality patterns in three nations at different economic levels: Implications for global trauma system development. *J Trauma*, 1998;44:804-14.

National Crime Records Bureau, New Delhi. Accidental Deaths and Suicide in India 1999.

Sethi, A.K., Tyagi, A. Trauma Untamed as yet. *Trauma Care,* 2001;11:89-90.

Suresh DS. Trauma Systems in India—the CMC Vellore Experience, *Asian Archives of Anaesthesiology and Resuscitation,* 2002;XLXII:21-3.

Wegman Fred, Road Accidents: Worldwide a problem that can be tackled successfully!, AIPCR Publication No. 13.01.B, 1996.

WHO South East Asia Regional Office, SCN Department, New Delhi—Disability, Violence—Injury, Prevention and Rehabilitation. *Newsletter,* 2001, Vol. 2 No. 1.

Palliative Medicine: An Emerging Concept for the Terminally Ill

According to the WHO, at least a million terminal cases of cancer are diagnosed in India every year. Now, there is some solace for them in the form of palliative care, some comfort in the form of love and care. 'Palliative care is any form of medical care or treatment that concentrates on reducing the severity of disease symptoms, rather than providing a cure. The goal is to prevent and relieve suffering and to improve quality of life for people facing serious, complex illness.' A recent WHO statement calls palliative care "an approach that improves the quality of life of patients and their families facing the problems associated with life-threatening illness." The term "palliative care" is now increasingly being used with regard to diseases other than cancer as well, such as chronic, progressive pulmonary disorders, renal disease, chronic heart failure or progressive neurological conditions. Palliative care improves the quality of life of patients and families who face life-threatening illness, by providing pain and symptom relief, spiritual and psychosocial support to from diagnosis to the end of life and bereavement. In nutshell Palliative care provides the following:

- provides relief from pain and other distressing symptoms;
- affirms life and regards dying as a normal process;
- intends neither to hasten or postpone death;
- integrates the psychological and spiritual aspects of patient care;
- offers a support system to help patients live as actively as possible until death;
- offers a support system to help the family cope during the patients illness;
- uses an approach to address the needs of patients and bereavement counseling;

- will enhance quality of life, and may also positively influence the course of illness; and
- Conjunction with other therapies that are intended to prolong life, such as chemotherapy or radiation therapy, and includes those investigations needed to better understand and manage distressing clinical complications.

HOSPICE AND PALLIATIVE CARE

The need for hospice is the most in India. Hospice is a movement to improve care for people who were dying alone, isolated, in hospitals or dumped in the courtyard of their own homes; totally neglected and discriminated in the Indian conditions. On the other hand in USA, In 2005 more than 1.2 million individuals and their family caregivers received hospice care. It is the Medicare benefit in U.S. that includes pharmaceuticals, medical equipment, twenty-four hour/seven day a week access to care and support for loved ones following a death. The majority of hospice care is delivered at home or in a home-like hospice residence. Hospice care is also available to people in nursing homes, assisted living facilities, veterans facilities, hospitals and prisons. In most countries, hospice and palliative care is provided by an interdisciplinary team consisting of physicians, registered nurses, social workers, hospice chaplains, physiotherapists, occupational therapists, complimentary therapists, volunteers and, most importantly, the family.

The key to effective palliative care is to provide a safe way for the individual to address their physical and psychological distress, that is to say their total suffering, a concept first thought up by Dame Cicely Saunders, and now widely used, for instance by authors like Twycross or Woodruff. Dealing with total suffering involves a broad range of concerns, starting with treating physical symptoms such as pain, nausea and breathlessness. The palliative care teams have become very skillful in prescribing drugs for physical symptoms, and have been instrumental in showing how drugs such as morphine can be used safely while maintaining a patient's full faculties and function. However, when a patient exhibits a physiological symptom, there are often psychological, social, or spiritual symptoms as well. The interdisciplinary team, which often includes a social worker or a counselor and a chaplain, can play a role in helping the patient and family cope globally with these symptoms, rather than depending on the medical/pharmacological interventions alone. Usually, a palliative care patient's concerns are pain, fears about the future, loss of independence, worries about their family, and feeling like a burden. While some patients will want to discuss psychological or spiritual concerns and some will not, it is fundamentally important to assess each individual and their partners and families need for this type of support. Denying an individual and their support system an opportunity to explore psychological or spiritual concerns is just as harmful as forcing them to deal with issues they either don't have or choose not to deal with. Alternative medical treatments such as relaxation therapy, massage, music therapy, and acupuncture can relieve some cancer-related symptoms and other causes of suffering.

Minimizing the pain

The end stages of chronic, progressive, life-limiting diseases bring a host of difficult symptoms and causes of suffering. There are disease-mediated symptoms, such as pain, dyspnea, fatigue, and loss of mobility, and there are the accompanying emotional states, such as depression, anxiety. Of the many symptoms experienced by those at the end of life, pain is one of the most common. The objective at this stage should be limited to giving comfort and a pain free life and not the cure of the underlying ailments. This entails a good nursing care, nutrition and freedom from pain. Palliative care team can play important role in comprehensive pain management. To illustrate the point we bring a case study of Chanderkanta.

Chanderkanta is a frail, 68-year-old woman who lives in the garage of her own house with assistance from a social worker who lives nearby. She was admitted to the hospital with acute respiratory failure due to bronchitis. She has advanced chronic obstructive pulmonary disease (COPD), with general fatigue and a poor appetite, and reports severe, debilitating pain in the midthoracic region from postherpetic neuralgia (PHN). She also struggles with coronary artery disease and attendant angina pectoris that is usually relieved with nitrates. She has been feeling "pretty low" lately and finds herself becoming irritated at small events. She has no options but to suffer pain. She has been allowed to suffer by her own kith and kin, who are enjoying the main house, built by the life time earnings of their parents.

It is important to acknowledge and address the prevalence, high incidence, and serious adverse consequences of pain in the end-stage conditions that affect patients with advanced medical illness, such as controlled and uncontrolled cancer; heart disease; HIV disease; neurodegenerative diseases (e.g. ALS and multiple sclerosis); and end-stage renal and respiratory diseases. More recently, an attempt has been made to characterize the pain experience of those with HIV disease, a disorder frequently seen in palliative care settings. It is also important to take into account common comorbidities, such as sleep disturbances and depression. Patients sometimes complain of pain as a way of expressing other forms of suffering, anxiety, or depression. When this is the case, psychosocial evaluation and intervention will be more effective than analgesics. It is well established that attention and emotion influence pain processing and perception, and conversely, inadequately managed pain can lead to anxiety and depression. There can be two types of pains.

1. Nociceptive pain is typically the result of a musculoskeletal or visceral injury or disease and includes somatic and visceral

mechanisms. This pain is characterized by aching, throbbing, stabbing, and/or a sensation of pressure. Its source is skin, muscle, or bone. Visceral pain is characterized by gnawing, cramping, aching, sharp, and/or stabbing sensations, and its source is the internal organs.

2. Neuropathic pain is caused by lesions or physiologic changes in the nervous system. The pain frequently has qualities of burning, numbness, tingling, touch sensitivity, sharp and shooting sensations (lancinating pain), or electric shocks. Neuropathic pain tends to persist long after the initiating event has resolved. Typical examples include painful diabetic neuropathy, HIV/AIDS neuropathy, postherpetic neuralgia, and cancer-induced as well as post-treatment cancer pain.

CASE STUDY

Banka Ram is a 70-year-old man in the late stages of prostate cancer with severe osteoarthritis in his knees and spine. He lives with her married daughter. He is beginning to experience severe pain from his arthritis, manifest by grimacing, crying, and moaning. The current caregivers are not always sure what he is expressing, but they understand that he is in some distress and are eager to help alleviate it. They meet with their family doctor to talk about options. The objective is to live his last days relatively free of pain and suffering. Banka is a typical patient who responds well to Aspirin intervention. Research suggests that patients with cancer, particularly in the palliative care setting, are increasingly using aromatherapy and massage.

Other kinds of therapies

Acupuncture

These modalities may be effective in selected patients. Similarly, for therapies involving electrical stimulation, awareness of implanted devices (pumps, stimulators, implantable cardioverter defibrillators, or pacemakers) and precautions to prevent malfunction must be taken.

Cognitive Interventions

Simple psychological interventions can have a significant impact on pain. Emotion regulation was found to be prospectively related to pain intensity for both overall emotion and anxiety-specific regulation.

Music Therapy

There is growing interest in the therapeutic use of music. Music is often used to enhance well-being, reduce stress, and distract patients from unpleasant symptoms. Although there are wide variations in individual preferences, music appears to exert direct physiologic effects through the autonomic nervous system.

A combination of treatments is usually most effective when using nonpharmacologic approaches to pain management. Similar to pharmacotherapy, multimodal approaches offer the potential benefit of additive and synergistic effects. Because nonpharmacologic therapies need to be tailored to individual likes, dislikes, and effectiveness, knowledge of the various modalities, management of expectations, open-mindedness, and a "trial-and-error" approach should be embraced.

Case 3: Jai parshad is an 82-year-old man with metastatic colon cancer and diabetes. He sees a geriatric nurse practitioner, in collaboration with a family physician, for ongoing primary care. It has become clear that that there are widespread metastases, and his oncologist agrees that the current goal of care is comfort only.

There are several, possible methods of approaching pharmacologic pain management for patients with advanced diseases. Patients may require several different medications to deal with a variety of pain syndromes and disease- or treatment-related discomfort. For expedient and thorough treatment, it is often wise to adopt a stepwise approach to the use of pain medications. The World Health Organization (WHO) has developed a simple, 3-step model for managing cancer pain that can be applied to many different situations. It has been modified over time to adapt to the evolving fields of pain and palliative medicine. This revised approach recommends that mild pain should be treated with nonopioid pain relievers, such as aspirin, acetaminophen, and non-steroidal anti-inflammatory drugs (NSAIDs), with or without adjuvant therapy. Higher pain intensities indicate the use of non-opioid analgesics along with opiate derivatives, such as codeine, hydrocodone, or tramadol. If pain is not relieved, then titration of opioids, such as morphine, hydromorphone, and fentanyl, in combination with non-opioid analgesics and adjuvants is indicated. Refractory pain syndromes will often require more invasive techniques, such as spinal opioids, nerve block, or neurostimulation.

Adjuvant Therapies

Antidepressants

The analgesic effect of tricyclic antidepressants appears to be related to inhibition of norepinephrine and serotonin reuptake, making these neurotransmitters more available within central nervous system pain inhibitory pathways.

Anticonvulsants

The older anticonvulsants, such as carbamazepine and clonazepam, relieve pain by blocking sodium channels. These compounds are very useful in the treatment of neuropathic pain, especially pain with episodic, lancinating qualities. Gabapentin seems to have several different mechanisms of action, although calcium ion channel blockade is thought to be its main pain-inhibiting mechanism. The analgesic doses of gabapentin reported to relieve pain in non-end-of-life pain conditions ranged from 900 mg/day to 3600 mg/day in divided doses. A common reason for inadequate relief is failure to titrate upward after prescribing the usual starting dose of 100 mg by mouth 3 times daily.

Corticosteroids

Corticosteroids are particularly useful for neuropathic, visceral, and bone pain syndromes. Dexamethasone produces the least amount of mineralocorticoid effect, making it the least toxic choice. Dexamethasone is available in oral, intravenous, subcutaneous, and epidural formulations. The standard dose is 16-24 mg/day and can be administered once daily due to the long half-life of this drug, but divided doses are usually used to mitigate high-dose toxic effects, such as psychosis and severe blood sugar abnormalities in diabetic patients. Doses as high as 100 mg may be given with severe pain crises, similar to the doses used in acute neurologic emergencies. Intravenous bolus doses should be administered over several minutes to reduce untoward reactions, such as burning sensations.

Local Anesthetics

Local anesthetics are useful for relieving neuropathic pain. Local anesthetic gels and patches have been used to prevent the pain that is associated with needlestick and other minor procedures.

Calcitonin

Subcutaneous calcitonin may be effective in the relief of neuropathic or bone pain. The nasal form of this drug may be more acceptable in end-of-life care when other therapies are ineffective. Usual doses are 100-200 IU/day subcutaneously or nasally.

Chemotherapy and Radiation Therapy

Palliative chemotherapy is the use of antitumor therapy to relieve the symptoms that are associated with malignancy. Examples of symptoms that may improve with chemotherapy include relief of chest wall pain from reduced tumor ulceration through the use of hormonal therapy in breast cancer. Similarly, newer agents, such as docetaxel, reduce pain and improve quality of life in hormone-refractory prostate cancer, and topotecan and epidermal growth factor receptor inhibitors accomplish similar results for patients with lung cancers. Radiation therapy is also a highly useful adjunct to control pain from bone metastasis and pressure-inducing and ulcerative malignancies.

Baclofen, a skeletal muscle relaxant, is also useful for the relief of spasm-associated pain, and it may be helpful in the treatment of intractable hiccups, which can be painful and cause sleep disturbance. Doses begin at 10 mg/day, increasing every few days. Feelings of weakness and confusion or hallucinations often occur with doses above 60 mg/day. Slow downward titration is necessary to prevent withdrawal-related seizures.

Calcium channel blockers are believed to provide pain relief in certain pain syndromes as well. For instance, nifedipine 10 mg orally may be useful to relieve ischemic or neuropathic pain syndromes.

Managing Adverse Effects

There are a variety of adverse effects that drugs for pain can cause patients in palliative care. The normal side effects associated with pain relief medications are often exacerbated by changes in metabolism caused by end-stage disease, polypharmacy associated with old age, and other factors. Patients in palliative care frequently experience constipation, in part due to opioid therapy. Avoid bulking agents, such as psyllium, because these tend to increase desiccation time in the large bowel, and debilitated patients can rarely take in sufficient fluid to facilitate the action of bulking agents. Instead use cost-effective and palatable products, such as senna tea and fruit.

Excessive sedation may occur with the initial doses of opioids. If sedation persists after 24-48 hours and other correctable causes have been identified and treated, the use of psychostimulants may be beneficial. These include dextroamphetamine 2.5-5 mg by mouth every morning and midday or methylphenidate 5-10 mg by mouth every morning and 2.5-5 mg mid-day. Adjust both the dose and timing to prevent nocturnal insomnia, and monitor for undesirable psychotomimetic effects (such as agitation, hallucinations, and irritability). Nausea is common and vomiting is an occasional adverse effect associated with opioids due to activation of the chemoreceptor trigger zone in the medulla, vestibular sensitivity, and delayed gastric emptying, but habituation occurs in most cases within several days. Myoclonic jerking can occur with high-dose opioid therapy. Clonazepam 0.5-1 mg by mouth every 6-8 hours, to be increased as needed and tolerated, may be useful in treating myoclonus inpatients who are still alert, able to communicate, and take oral preparations. Lorazepam can be given sublingually if the patient is unable to swallow. Otherwise, parenteral administration of diazepam is indicated if symptoms are distressing. Grand mal seizures associated with high-dose parenteral opioid infusions have been reported and may be due to preservatives in the solution.

Pruritus can occur with most opioids, although it appears to be most common with morphine. Fentanyl and oxymorphone may be less likely to cause histamine release. Most antipruritus therapies cause sedation, so the patient must see this as an acceptable trade-off. Antihistamines (such as diphenhydramine) are the most common first-line approach to this opioid-induced symptom when treatment is indicated. Ondansetron and paroxetine have been reported to be effective in relieving opioid-induced pruritus, but no randomized, controlled studies.

The ultimate hour

Clinical competence, willingness to educate, and calm and empathic reassurance are critical to helping patients and families in the last hours of living. Clinical issues that commonly arise in the last hours of living include the management of feeding and hydration, changes in consciousness, delirium, pain, breathlessness, and secretions. Management principles are the same at home or in a health care institution. However, death in an institution requires accommodations to assure privacy, cultural observances, and communication that may not be customary. In anticipation of the event, inform the family and other professionals about what to do and what to expect. Care does not end until the family has been supported with their grief reactions and those with complicated grief have been helped to get care.

Preparing for the Last Hours of Life

During the last hours of their lives, most patients require continuous skilled care. This can be provided in any setting as long as the professional, family, and volunteer caregivers are appropriately prepared and supported throughout the process. The environment must allow family and friends access to their loved one around the clock without disturbing others and should be conducive to privacy and intimacy. Medications, equipment, and supplies need to be available in anticipation of problems, whether the patient is at home or in a health care institution. As the patient's condition and the family's ability to cope can change frequently, both must be reassessed regularly and the plan of care modified as needed. Changes in the patient's condition can occur suddenly and unexpectedly, so caregivers must be able to respond quickly. This is particularly important when the patient is at home, if unnecessary readmission is to be avoided.

If the last hours of a person's life are to be as positive as possible, advance preparation and education of professional, family, and volunteer caregivers are essential, whether the patient is at home, in an acute care or skilled nursing facility, a hospice or palliative care unit, prison, or other setting. Everyone who participates must be aware of the patient's health status, his or her goals for care (and the parents' goals if the patient is a child), advance directives, and proxy for decision-making. They should also be knowledgeable about the potential time course, signs, and symptoms of the dying process, and their potential management.

Help families to understand that what they see may be very different from the patient's experience. If family members and caregivers feel confident, the experience can be a time of final gift giving. For example, when parents feel confident about providing for the needs of their dying child, their sense that they are practicing good parenting skills is reinforced. If they are left unprepared and unsupported, they may spend excessive energy worrying about how to handle the next event. If things do not go as hoped for, family members may live with frustration, worry, fear, or guilt that they did something wrong or caused the patient's death.

Establish in advance whether potential caregivers, including professionals who work in institutions, are skilled in caring for patients in the last hours of life. Do not assume that anyone, even a professional, knows how to perform basic tasks. Those who are inexperienced in this particular area will need specific training in areas such as body fluid precautions. Written materials can provide additional support to caregivers when experts are not present. Although we often sense that death will either come quickly over minutes or be protracted over days to weeks, it is not possible to predict when death will occur with precision. Some patients may appear to wait for someone to visit, or for an important event such as a birthday or a special holiday, and then die soon afterward. Others experience unexplained improvements and live longer than expected. A few seem to decide to die and do so very quickly, sometimes within minutes. While it is possible to give families or professional caregivers a general idea of how long the patient might live, always advise them about the inherent unpredictability of the moment of death.

Physiologic Changes and Symptom Management

There are a variety of physiologic changes that occur in the last hours and days of life, and when the patient is actually dying. Each can be alarming if it is not understood.

Fatigue and weakness

Weakness and fatigue usually increase as the patient approaches the time of death. It is likely that the patient will not be able to move around in the bed or raise his or her head. Joints may become uncomfortable if they are not moved. Continuous pressure on the same area of skin, particularly over bony prominences, will increase the risk of skin ischemia and pain. As the patient approaches death, providing adequate cushioning on the bed will lessen the need for uncomfortable turning.

Cutaneous ischemia

At the end of life, fatigue need not be resisted and most treatment to alleviate it can be discontinued. Patients who are too fatigued to move and have joint position fatigue may require passive movement of their joints every 1 to 2 hours. To minimize the risk of pressure ulcer formation, turn the patient from side to side every 1 to 1.5 hours and protect areas of bony prominence with hydrocolloid dressings and special supports. Do not use "donut-shaped" pillows or cushions, as they paradoxically worsen areas of breakdown by compressing blood flow circumferentially around the compromised area.

A draw sheet can assist caregivers to turn the patient and minimize pain and shearing forces to the skin. If turning is painful, consider a pressure-reducing surface (eg, air mattress or airbed). As the patient approaches death, the need for turning lessens as the risk of skin breakdown becomes less important. Intermittent massage before and after turning, particularly to areas of contact, can both be comforting and reduce the risk of skin breakdown by improving circulation and shifting edema. Avoid massaging areas of non-blanching erythema or actual skin breakdown.

Decreasing appetite and food intake

Most dying patients lose their appetite. Unfortunately, families and professional caregivers may interpret cessation of eating as "giving in" or "starving to death." Yet, studies demonstrate that parenteral or enteral feeding of patients near death neither improves symptom control nor lengthens life. Anorexia may be helpful as the resulting ketosis can lead to a sense of well-being and diminish discomfort.

Clinicians can help families understand that loss of appetite is normal at this stage. Remind them that the patient is not hungry, that food either is not appealing or may be nauseating, that the patient would likely eat if he or she could, that the patient's body is unable to absorb and use nutrients, and that clenching of teeth may be the only way for the patient to express his/her desire not to eat.

Whatever the degree of acceptance of these facts, it is important for professionals to help families and caregivers realize that food pushed upon the unwilling patient may cause problems such as aspiration and increased tension. Above all, help them to find alternative ways to nurture the patient so that they can continue to participate and feel valued during the dying process.

Decreasing fluid intake and dehydration

Most dying patients stop drinking. This may heighten onlookers' distress as they worry that the dehydrated patient will suffer, particularly if he or she becomes thirsty. Most experts feel that dehydration in the last hours of living does not cause distress and may stimulate endorphin release that promotes the patient's sense of well-being. Low blood pressure or weak pulse is part of the dying process and not an indication of dehydration. Patients who are not able to be upright do not get light-headed or dizzy. Patients with peripheral edema or ascites have excess body water and salt and are not dehydrated.

Parenteral fluids, given either intravenously or subcutaneously using hypodermoclysis, are sometimes considered, particularly when the goal is to reverse delirium. However, parenteral fluids may have adverse effects that are not commonly considered. Intravenous lines can be cumbersome and difficult to maintain. Changing the site of the angiocatheter can be painful, particularly when the patient is cachectic or has no discernible veins. Excess parenteral fluids can lead to fluid overload with consequent peripheral or pulmonary edema, worsened breathlessness, cough, and orotracheobronchial secretions, particularly if there is significant hypoalbuminemia.

Mucosal and conjunctival care

To maintain patient comfort and minimize the sense of thirst, even in the face of dehydration, maintain moisture on mucosal membrane surfaces with meticulous oral, nasal, and conjunctival hygiene.[16] Moisten and clean oral mucosa every 15 to 30 minutes with either baking soda mouthwash (1 teaspoon salt, 1 teaspoon baking soda, 1 quart tepid water) or an artificial saliva preparation to minimize the sense of thirst and avoid bad odors or tastes and painful cracking. Treat oral candidiasis with topical nystatin or systemic fluconazole if the patient is able to swallow. Coat the lips and anterior nasal mucosa hourly with a thin layer of petroleum jelly to reduce evaporation. If the patient is using oxygen, use an alternative nonpetroleum-based lubricant. Avoid perfumed lip balms and swabs containing lemon and glycerin, as these can be both desiccating and irritating, particularly on open sores. If eyelids are not closed, moisten conjunctiva with an ophthalmic lubricating gel every 3 to 4 hours or artificial tears or physiologic saline solution every 15 to 30 minutes to avoid painful dry eyes.

Cardiac dysfunction and renal failure

As cardiac output and intravascular volume decrease at the end of life, there will be evidence of diminished peripheral blood perfusion. Tachycardia, hypotension, peripheral cooling, peripheral and central cyanosis, and mottling of the skin (livedo reticularis) are normal. Venous blood may pool along dependent skin surfaces. Urine output falls as perfusion of the kidneys diminishes. Oliguria or anuria is normal. Parenteral fluids will not reverse this circulatory shut down.

Decreasing level of consciousness

The majority of patients traverse the "usual road to death." They experience increasing drowsiness, sleep most if not all of the time, and eventually become unarousable. Absence of eyelash reflexes on physical examination indicates a profound level of coma equivalent to full anesthesia.

Communication with the unconscious patient

Families will frequently find that their decreasing ability to communicate is distressing. The last hours of life are the time when they most want to communicate with their loved one. As many clinicians have observed, the degree of family distress seems to be inversely related to the extent to which advance planning and preparation occurred. The time spent preparing families is likely to be very worthwhile.

While we do not know what unconscious patients can actually hear, extrapolation from data from the operating room and "near death" experiences suggests that at times their awareness may be greater than their ability to respond. Given our inability to assess a dying patient's comprehension and the distress that talking "over" the patient may cause, it is prudent to presume that the unconscious patient hears everything. Advise families and professional caregivers to talk to the patient as if he or she were conscious.

Encourage families to create an environment that is familiar and pleasant. Surround the patient with the people, children, pets, objects, music, and sounds that he or she would like. Include the patient in everyday conversations. Encourage family members to say the things they need to say. At times, it may seem that a patient may be waiting for permission to die. If this is the case, encourage family members to give the patient permission to "let go" and die in a manner that feels most comfortable. The physician, nurse, social worker, chaplain, or other caregivers might suggest to family members other words like:

- "I know that you are dying; please do so when you are ready."
- "I love you. I will miss you. I will never forget you. Please do what you need to do when you are ready."
- "Mommy and Daddy love you. We will miss you, but we will be okay."

As touch can heighten communication, encourage family members to show affection in ways they are used to. Let them know that it is okay to lie beside the patient in privacy to maintain as much intimacy as they feel comfortable with.

Terminal delirium

An agitated delirium may be the first sign to herald the "difficult road to death." It frequently presents as confusion, restlessness, and/or agitation, with or without day-night reversal. To the family and professional caregivers who do not understand it, agitated terminal delirium can be very distressing. Although previous care may have been excellent, if the delirium goes misdiagnosed or unmanaged, family members will likely remember a horrible death, "in terrible pain," and cognitively impaired "because of the drugs," and they may worry that their own death will be the same.

In anticipation of the possibility of terminal delirium, educate and support family and professional caregivers to understand its causes, the finality and irreversibility of the situation, and approaches to its management. It is particularly important that all onlookers understand that what the patient experiences may be very different from what they see.

If the patient is not assessed to be imminently dying, it may be appropriate to evaluate and try to reverse treatable contributing factors. However, if the patient is in the last hours of his or her life, the condition is by definition irreversible. Focus on the management of the symptoms associated with the terminal delirium in order to settle the patient and the family.

When moaning, groaning, and grimacing accompany the agitation and restlessness, these symptoms are frequently misinterpreted as physical pain. However, it is a myth that uncontrollable pain suddenly develops during the last hours of life when it has not previously been a problem. If the trial of increased opioids does not relieve the agitation or makes the delirium worse by increasing agitation or precipitating myoclonic jerks or seizures (rare), then pursue alternative therapies directed at suppressing the symptoms associated with delirium.

Benzodiazepines are used widely to treat terminal delirium as they are anxiolytics, amnestics, skeletal muscle relaxants, and antiepileptics. Common starting doses are:

- Lorazepam, 1-2 mg as an elixir, or a tablet predissolved in 0.5-1.0 mL of water and administered against the buccal mucosa every hour as needed will settle most patients with 2-10 mg/24 hours. It can then be given in divided doses, every 3-4 hours, to keep the patient settled. For a few extremely agitated patients, high doses of lorazepam, 20-50+ mg/24 hours, may be required.
- Midazolam 1-5 mg/hour subcutaneously or intravenously by continuous infusion, preceded by repeated loading boluses of 0.5 mg every 15 minutes to effect, may be a rapidly effective alternative.

Benzodiazepines may paradoxically excite some patients. These patients require neuroleptic medications to control their delirium.

- Haloperidol 0.5-2.0 mg intravenously, subcutaneously, or rectally every hour (titrated to effect, then nightly to every 6 hours to maintain) may be effective.
- Chlorpromazine 10-25 mg orally, rectally, or intramuscularly nightly to every 6 hours and titrated to effect intravenously or rectally is a more sedating alternative.

Barbiturates or propofol have been suggested as alternatives. Seizures may be managed with high doses of benzodiazepines. Other antiepileptics such as intravenous phenytoin, subcutaneous fosphenytoin, or phenobarbital 60-120 mg rectally, intravenously, or intramuscularly every 10-20 minutes as needed may become necessary until control is established. Alternatively, carbamazepine 200 mg rectally 3-4 times per day can be used.

Respiratory dysfunction

Changes in a dying patient's breathing pattern may be indicative of significant neurologic compromise. Breaths may become very shallow and frequent with a diminishing tidal volume. Periods of apnea and/or Cheyne-Stokes pattern respirations may develop. (Cheyne-Stokes is a disorder characterized by recurrent central apneas during sleep, alternating with a crescendo-decrescendo pattern of tidal volume. Accessory respiratory muscle use may also become prominent. A few (or many) last reflex breaths may signal death.

Families and professional caregivers frequently find changes in breathing patterns to be one of the most distressing signs of impending death. Many fear that the comatose patient will experience a sense of suffocation. Knowledge that the unresponsive patient may not be experiencing breathlessness or "suffocating," and may not benefit from oxygen (which may actually prolong the dying process) can be very comforting. Low doses of opioids or benzodiazepines are appropriate to manage any perception of breathlessness.

Some clinicians express concern that the use of opioids or benzodiazepines for symptom control near the end of life will hasten death. Consequently, they feel they must invoke the ethical principle of "double effect" to justify treatment. The principle of double effect applies in situations where there is a difference in the effects of an intended action (alleviating suffering) and the unintended possible consequences of the same action (hastening death). To be acceptable, the action must comply with the following requirements:

- The treatment proposed must be beneficial or at least neutral (relief of intolerable symptoms);
- The clinician must intend only the good effect (relieving pain or symptoms), although some untoward effects might be foreseen (hastening death or loss of consciousness);
- The untoward effect must not be a means (not necessary) to bring about the good effect; and
- The good result (relief of suffering) must outweigh the untoward outcome (hastening death).

Loss of ability to swallow

Weakness and decreased neurologic function frequently combine to impair the patient's ability to swallow. The gag reflex and reflexive clearing of the oropharynx decline and secretions from the tracheobronchial tree accumulate. These conditions may become more prominent as the patient loses consciousness. Buildup of saliva and oropharyngeal secretions may lead to gurgling, crackling, or rattling sounds with each breath. Some have called this the "death rattle" (a term that should be avoided, as it is frequently disconcerting to families and caregivers).

Once the patient is unable to swallow, cease oral intake. Warn families and professional caregivers of the risk of aspiration. Scopolamine or glycopyrrolate will effectively reduce the production of saliva and other secretions. Common starting doses of these medications are:

- Scopolamine, 0.2-0.4 mg subcutaneously every 4 hours, or Scopolamine, 1-3 transdermal patches every 72 hours, or Scopolamine, 0.1-1.0 mg/hr by continuous intravenous or subcutaneous infusion.
- Glycopyrrolate, 0.2 mg subcutaneously every 4-6 hours, or Glycopyrrolate, 0.4-1.2 mg daily by continuous intravenous or subcutaneous infusion.

These drugs will minimize or eliminate the gurgling and crackling sounds and may be used prophylactically in the unconscious dying patient. Anecdotal evidence suggests that the earlier treatment is initiated, the better it works, as larger amounts of secretions in the upper aerodigestive tract are more difficult to eliminate. However, premature use in the patient who is still alert may lead to unacceptable drying of oral and pharyngeal mucosa. While atropine may be equally effective, it has an increased risk of producing undesired cardiac and/or central nervous system excitation.

If excessive fluid accumulates in the back of the throat and upper airways, it may need to be cleared by repositioning of the patient or postural drainage. Turning the patient onto one side or into a semiprone position may reduce gurgling. Lowering the head of the bed and raising the foot of the bed while the patient is in a semiprone position may cause fluids to move into the oropharynx, from which they can be easily removed. Do not maintain this position for more than a few minutes at a time, as stomach contents may also move unexpectedly.

Oropharyngeal suctioning is not recommended. Suctioning is frequently ineffective, as fluids are beyond the reach of the catheter, and may only stimulate an otherwise peaceful patient and distress family members who are watching.

Loss of sphincter control. Fatigue and loss of sphincter control in the last hours of life may lead to incontinence of urine and/or stool. Both can be very distressing to patients and family members, particularly if they are not warned in advance that these problems may arise. If they occur, attention needs to be paid to cleaning and skin care. A urinary catheter may minimize the need for frequent changing and cleaning, prevent skin breakdown, and reduce the demand on caregivers. However, it is not always necessary if urine flow is minimal and can be managed with absorbent pads or surfaces. If diarrhea is considerable and relentless, a rectal tube may be similarly effective.

Pain

While many people fear that pain will suddenly increase as the patient dies, there is no evidence to suggest that this occurs. Though difficult to assess, continuous pain in the semiconscious or obtunded patient may be associated with grimacing and continuous facial tension, particularly across the forehead and between the eyebrows. The possibility of pain must also be considered when physiologic signs occur, such as transitory tachycardia that may signal distress. However, do not overdiagnose pain when fleeting forehead tension comes and goes with movement or mental activity (e.g. dreams or hallucinations). Do not confuse pain with the restlessness, agitation, moaning, and groaning that accompany terminal delirium. If the diagnosis is unclear, a trial of a higher dose of opioid may be necessary to judge whether pain is driving the observed behaviors.

Knowledge of opioid pharmacology becomes critical during the last hours of life. The liver conjugates codeine, morphine, oxycodone, and hydromorphone into glucuronides. Some of their metabolites remain active as analgesics until they are renally cleared, particularly morphine. As dying patients experience diminished hepatic function and renal perfusion, and usually become oliguric or anuric, routine dosing or continuous infusions of morphine may lead to increased serum concentrations of active metabolites, toxicity, and an increased risk of terminal delirium. To minimize this risk, discontinue routine dosing or continuous infusions of morphine when urine output and renal clearance stop. Titrate morphine breakthrough (rescue) doses to manage expressions suggestive of continuous pain. Consider the use of alternative opioids with inactive metabolites such as fentanyl or hydromorphone.

Loss of ability to close eyes

Eyes that remain open can be distressing to onlookers unless the condition is understood. Advanced wasting leads to loss of the retro-orbital fat pad, and the orbit falls posteriorly within the orbital socket. As eyelids are of insufficient length to both extend the additional distance backward and cover the conjunctiva, they may not be able to fully appose. This may leave some conjunctiva exposed even when the patient is sleeping. If conjunctiva remains exposed, maintain moisture by using ophthalmic lubricants, artificial tears, or physiologic saline.

Medications

As patients approach death, reassess the need for each medication and minimize the number of drugs that the patient is taking. Continue only those medications needed to manage symptoms such as pain, breathlessness, excess secretions, and terminal delirium and to reduce the risk of seizures. Choose the least invasive route of administration: the buccal mucosa or oral routes first, the subcutaneous or intravenous routes only if necessary, and the intramuscular route almost never. Rectal administration can also be considered, especially if the oral route is not possible.

When death is imminent, it is appropriate that patients remain with caregivers they know rather than be transferred to another facility. Institutions can help by making the environment as home-like as possible. It is appropriate for the physician, nurse practitioner, or physician assistant to order a private room where family can be present continuously and be undisturbed with the patient if they so choose. The clinician will want to talk with the professional staff and encourage continuity of care plans across nursing shifts and changes in house staff.

When Death Occurs

No matter how well families and professional caregivers are prepared, they may find the time of death to be challenging. Families, including children, and caregivers may have specific questions for health professionals.

Signs of Death

- The heart stops beating
- Breathing stops
- Pupils become fixed and dilated
- Body color becomes pale and waxen as blood settles
- Body temperature drops
- Muscles and sphincters relax (muscles stiffen 4-6 hours after death as rigor mortis sets in)
- Urine and stool may be released
- Eyes may remain open
- The jaw can fall open
- Observers may hear the trickling of fluids internally, even after death

When an expected death occurs, the focus of care should shift from the patient to the family and those who provided care. Even though the loss has been anticipated for some time, no one will know what it feels like until it actually occurs, and indeed it may take hours to days to weeks or even months for each person to realize the full effect.

Many experts assert that the time spent with the body immediately after death will help people deal with acute grief. Those present, including caregivers, may need the clinician's permission to spend the time to come to terms with the event and say their good-byes. There is no need to rush, even in the hospital or other care facility. Encourage those who need to touch, hold, and even kiss the person's body as they feel most comfortable (while maintaining universal body fluid precautions).

Notifying Others of the Death

Spiritual advisors or other interdisciplinary team members may be instrumental in orchestrating events to facilitate the experience of those present. Those who have not been present for the death may benefit from listening to a recounting of how things went leading up to the death and afterward. Grief reactions beyond cultural norms suggest a risk of significant ongoing or delayed grief reactions.

Once family members have had the time they need to deal with their acute grief reactions and observe their customs and traditions, then preparations for burial or cremation and a funeral can begin. Some family members may find it therapeutic to help bathe and prepare the person's body for transfer to the funeral home or the hospital morgue. For many, such rituals will be their final act of direct caring.

All will require a completed death certificate to proceed with any body preparation and registration of the death. To avoid delaying the process, ensure that the clinician who will complete the certificate has ample warning that one will be required.

Immediately after the death, those who survive will need time to recover. A bereavement card from the physician, nurse, or health care professional and attendance at the patient's funeral may be appropriate. Many members of the professional team consider it a part of their professional duty of care to encourage follow-up visits from bereaved family members in order to assess the severity of their grief reactions and the effectiveness of their coping strategies, and to provide emotional support.

Most clinicians have little or no formal training in managing the dying process or death. Many have neither watched someone die nor provided direct care during the last hours of life. Families usually have even less experience or knowledge about death and dying. Based on media dramatization and vivid imaginations, most people have developed an exaggerated sense of what dying and death are like. However, with appropriate management, it is possible to provide smooth passage and comfort for the patient and all those who watch.

Euthanasia

'Can the benefit of a 'smooth ride' be extended to countless people who are languishing in hospitals with terminal ailments, burdening the already stretched health care system or dumped in a corner of the house in a state of total neglect, with a lot of physical and mental pain to bear. Can anybody offer the end on demand of the sufferer when the possibility of cure has 'extinguished'?

Neither law nor medical ethics requires that 'every possible damn thing be done' to keep a person alive, when the medical procedures and aids only add to his torture. It would also be cruel and inhumane to prolong his misery and cause a financial ruin of the family. Some proponents share the view that modern medicine keeps human beings alive for much longer than their natural longevity would permit. There comes a time when continued attempts to cure are not compassionate, wise, or medically sound. There is no point forcing people to stay alive 'hooked up' to machines, artificial feeding and hydration through a nasogastric tube and excretionary functions regulated by a catheter and by enemas, since the existence is vegetative. We see many elderly patients with debilitating chronic illnesses such as terminal chronic heart failure (CHF), chronic obstructive pulmonary disorder (COPD), malignancies and dementias. Many such patients need 24-hour care for several months, with no prospects of cure. When the undisputed consensus of eminent medical opinion is that there is no prospect whatsoever that patient would ever make recovery from his present condition, but that there is every likelihood that he will maintain his present state of vegetative existence for a long time, provided that painful interventions, which he is now receiving were continued, what could be the objectives at that stage? Proponents of euthanasia emphasize that when a person faces unbearable pain or disability, and the dignity in his/her life is lost; it is only noble that the state grants him/her the right to choose to have death hastened.

It is debatable 'whether ethics would dictate that the death be brought about quickly (by administering a lethal drug), rather than a prolonged torture of stopping artificial feeding and other treatment. Recently many persons in this category have written to the President asking his permission to end their lives. Legalized euthanasia raises the potential for a situation in which families and the society could find themselves better off financially if a seriously ill or disabled person 'chooses' to die rather than receive long-term care. In India's context where the health services are scarce and expensive, old age social security is non existent, the love and care to the ageing and ailing is missing the end of the older family member seems to bring a sense of great relief to all concerned.

Many people feel guilty for not choosing death, when it is inevitable. Financial considerations, added to the concern about 'being a burden'. However, doctors treating terminal cases are frequently too obsessed with the control of symptoms of disease and have little concern for the patient as a person. Doctors need to start talking to patients and their family about the futility of treatments that only prolong death. Until this major block is overcome, we will not be able to proceed to the next step-putting the wishes of the patient in writing in such a manner that they are legally binding on the medical profession.

Euthanasia has, so far been legalized in Northern Australia in 1995, the US state of Oregon in 1998, Netherlands in 2001 and Belgium in 2002. Once legalized, euthanasia becomes nearly impossible to control and leads inevitably to patients being killed out of greed of his property or revenge, without consent. Euthanasia, they say, erodes patient autonomy and creates an atmosphere in which it is considered 'easier to kill a patient than to treat'. The safeguard on this account have to be foolproof. It does not mean stopping all decisions of voluntary dying in every circumstance viz. A soldier throws himself on a grenade to save his fellow-beings, pedestrian leaps into the path of a truck to save a child; fire-fighters remain in a collapsing building rather than abandon trapped victims. These, too, are decisions to embrace death, yet we leave them to the conscience of the persons concerned. Then why tar all reasons for physician-assisted suicide with a common brush? Given that we do not have the power to ameliorate every disease and never will, why withhold from individuals the power to lessen the duration of their own pain and also financial and emotional burdens that dying process imposes on their loved ones? The dying are persons—not always in need of one more investigation or operation, but a kind word, an affectionate squeeze, a warm pep talk; in short, love. The stage of acceptance of end', is a time when the patient comes to terms with the prospect of death, and makes peace with it. Should not all of us, even in health, weave this thread of the acceptance of death into the very fabric of our life?

The fairest deaths are those that are voluntary; 'Death never takes the wise man by surprise; He is always ready to go.' Can Indian society offer the romance of smooth ride to many of its members who need and demand the same in public interest?

What is euthanasia?

It is widely defined as 'the intentional killing by act or omission of a dependent human being for his or her alleged benefit'. Voluntary euthanasia refers to a situation where the person who is killed has requested to be killed. Involuntary Euthanasia refers to a situation where the person who is killed made an expressed wish to the contrary. Non-voluntary euthanasia refers to a situation where the person who is killed made no request and gave no consent. Assisted suicide refers to a situation where someone provides an individual with the information, guidance, and means to take his or her own life with the intention that they will be used for this purpose. When it is a doctor who helps another person, to kill themselves it is called 'physician assisted suicide' Euthanasia By Action refers to a situation of intentionally causing a person's death by performing an action such as by giving a lethal injection. Euthanasia is usually suggested as a measure of relief for 'terminally ill' persons, who are bound to face death in a short span of time. The measure is meant to alleviate suffering, by hastening the inevitable death. The argument that is usually raised is that in medicine, one cannot ever say for certain what a person's life expectancy will be like, even if their medical condition is really hopeless. Increasingly, however, euthanasia activists have dropped references to terminal illness, replacing them with such phrases as 'hopelessly ill', 'desperately ill', 'incurably ill', 'hopeless condition', and 'meaningless life.'

Euthanasia has, so far been legalized in Northern Australia in 1995, the US state of Oregon in 1998, Netherlands in 2001 and Belgium in 2002. The Netherlands and Belgium have legalized euthanasia as well as assisted suicide, whereas Oregon has legalized assisted suicide. Both euthanasia and assisted suicide have been widely practiced in the Netherlands since 1973 although they were against the law until 2002.

Euthanasia has not been specifically covered in any Indian statute. The closest the issue has come to be addressed, is in section 309 of the Indian Penal Code,1860, which states that an attempt to suicide is a criminal offence. While it is considered as an offence under the same section, any person assisting an attempt to commit euthanasia, can be accused u/s 306 of IPC for abetment to suicide. A bench comprising Justice Y.K. Sabharwal and Mr. Justice P P Naolekar issued notice to the Centre on the PIL by NGO Common Cause which argued that right to life under Article 21 of the Constitution included right to live with human dignity. Every individual should have a right to execute a 'Living Will' expressing his or her desire to have or not to have an extraordinary life prolonging measures when his or her recovery from any terminal illness is not possible. The petition argued that a person should be allowed to execute a Living Will before getting into a state of permanent vegetative state, the petition said, adding that he should have a right to refuse treatments like feeding through hydration tubes, being kept on ventilators or other life supporting machines.

References

AGS Panel on Persistent Pain in Older Persons. Clinical guideline for assessment and management of persistent pain in older persons. *J Am Geriatr Soc.* 2000;50:S205-S224.

Ahronheim JC, Gasner MR. The sloganism of starvation. Lancet. 1990;335:278-279. Abstract

American College of Physicians. Parenteral nutrition inpatients receiving cancer chemotherapy. *Ann Intern Med.* 1989;110:734-735. Abstract 526

American Pain Society. Principles of Analgesic Use in the Treatment of Acute Pain and Cancer Pain. 5th ed. Glenview, Ill: American Pain Society; 2003.

Andersen G, Jensen NH, Christrup L, Hansen SH, Sjogren P. Pain, sedation and morphine metabolism in cancer patients during long-term treatment with sustained-release morphine. *Palliat Med.* 2002;16:107-114.

Aspen Reference Group. Palliative Care Patient and Family Counseling Manual. Gaithersburg, Md: Aspen Publishers Inc; 1996.

Backonja M, Beydoun A, Edwards KR, *et al.* Gabapentin for the symptomatic treatment of painful neuropathy inpatients with diabetes mellitus: a randomized controlled trial. *JAMA.* 1998;280:1831-1836.

Barbano RL, Herrmann DN, Hart-Gouleau S, Pennella-Vaughan J, Lodewick PA, Dworkin RH. Effectiveness, tolerability, and impact on quality of life of the 5% lidocaine patch in diabetic polyneuropathy. *Arch Neurol.* 2004;61:914-918.

Barrueto F Jr, Green J, Howland MA, Hoffman RS, Nelson LS. Gabapentin withdrawal presenting as status epilepticus. *J Toxicol Clin Toxicol.* 2002;40:925-928.

Bernabei R, Gambassi G, Lapane K, *et al.* Management of pain in elderly patients with cancer. SAGE Study Group. Systematic assessment of geriatric drug use via epidemiology. *JAMA.* 1998;279:1877-1882.

Berry PE, Ward SE. Barriers to pain management in hospice: a study of family caregivers. *Hosp J.* 1995;10:19-33.

Billings JA. Comfort measures for the terminally ill: is dehydration painful? J Am Geriatr Soc. 1985;33:808-810.

Brescia FJ, Portenoy RK, Ryan M, Krasnoff L, Gray G. Pain, opioid use, and survival in hospitalized patients with advanced cancer. *J Clin Oncol.* 1992;10:149-155.

Bruera E, Fainsinger RL. Clinical management of cachexia and anorexia. In: Doyle D, Hanks GWC, MacDonald N, eds. Oxford Textbook of Palliative Medicine. 2nd ed. Oxford, England: Oxford University Press; 1998:548.

Bruera E, Legris MA, Kuehn N, Miller MJ. Hypodermoclysis for the administration of fluids and narcotic analgesics inpatients with advanced cancer. *J Pain Symptom Manage.* 1990;5:218-220. Abstract

Bruera E, Neumann CM, Mazzocato C, Stiefel F, Sala R. Abstract attitudes and beliefs of palliative care physicians regarding communication with terminally ill cancer patients. *Palliat Med.* 2000;14:287-298.

Bruera E, Palmer JL, Bosnjak S, *et al.* Methadone versus morphine as a first-line strong opioid for cancer pain: a randomized, double-blind study. *J Clin Oncol.* 2004;22:185-192.

Caraceni A, Weinstein SM. Classification of cancer pain syndromes. Oncology (Williston Park). 2001;15:1627-1640, 1642; *Discussion* 1642-1623, 1646-1627.

Cassel CK. ICD-9 code for palliative or terminal care. *N Engl J Med* 1996;335:1232-4. 2. Sullivan AD, Hedberg K, Hopkins D. Legalized physician-assisted suicide in Oregon, 1998-2000. *N Engl J Med* 2001;344:605-7.

Cassileth, Vickers, Magill. (2003). Music therapy for mood disturbance during hospitalization for autologous stem cell transplantation: a randomized controlled trial (abstract). PubMed, NCBI. Retrieved on March 07, 2006.

Census of India 2001: Provisional Population Totals.Registrar General and Census Commissioner GOI.

Center to Advance Palliative Care, www.capc.org

Central Bureau of Health Intelligence.Directorate General of Health Services, Ministry of Health and Family Welfare. Health Information of India 2000 and 2001.

Chang H-M. Pain and its management inpatients with cancer. *Cancer Invest.* 2004;22;799-809.

Chang VT, Hwang SS, Feuerman M, Kasimis BS. Symptom and quality of life survey of medical oncology patients at a veterans affairs medical center: a role for symptom assessment. *Cancer.* 2000;88:1175-1183.

Cleeland CS, Gonin R, Baez L, Loehrer P, Pandya KJ. Pain and treatment of pain in minority patients with cancer. The Eastern Cooperative Oncology Group Minority Outpatient Pain Study. *Ann Intern Med.* 1997;127:813-816.

Cleeland CS, Gonin R, Hatfield AK, *et al.* Pain and its treatment in outpatients with metastatic cancer. *N Engl J Med.* 1994;330:592-596.

CLIP: Current Learning in Palliative Care. Online tutorials. Help the Hospices. Retrieved on March 07, 2006.

Cohen LM, Germain M, Poppel DM, Woods A, Kjellstrand CM. Dialysis discontinuation and palliative care. *Am J Kidney Dis.* 2000;36:140-144.

Cole BE. The psychiatric management of end-of-life pain and associated psychiatric comorbidity. *Curr Pain Headache Rep.* 2003;7:89-97.

Coleman RE. Bisphosphonates: clinical experience. *The Oncologist.* 2004;9 (supp l4):14-27.

Coluzzi PH, Schwartzberg L, Conroy JD, *et al.* Breakthrough cancer pain: a randomized trial comparing oral transmucosal fentanyl citrate (OTFC) and morphine sulfate immediate release (MSIR). *Pain.* 2001;91:123-130.

Coluzzi PH. Sublingual morphine: efficacy reviewed. *J Pain Symptom Manage.* 1998;16:184-192.

Coyle N, Adelhardt J, Foley KM, Portenoy RK. Character of terminal illness in the advanced cancer patient: pain and other symptoms during the last four weeks of life. [comment]. *J Pain Symptom Manage.* 1990;5:83-93.

David Alimi *et al.* (2003). Analgesic Effect of Auricular Acupuncture for Cancer Pain: A Randomized, Blinded, Controlled Trial. Journal of Clinical Oncology. Retrieved on March 07, 2006.

Davis MP, Varga J, Dickerson D, Walsh D, LeGrand SB, Lagman R. Normal-release and controlled-release oxycodone: pharmacokinetics, pharmacodynamics, and controversy. *Support Care Cancer.* 2003;11:84-92.

Davis MP, Walsh D. Methadone for relief of cancer pain: a review of pharmacokinetics, pharmacodynamics, drug interactions and protocols of administration. [see comment]. *Support Care Cancer.* 2001;9:73-83.

Deer TR, Caraway DL, Kim CK, Dempsey CD, Stewart CD, McNeil KF. Clinical experience with intrathecal bupivacaine in combination with opioid for the treatment of chronic pain related to failed back surgery syndrome and metastatic cancer pain of the spine. *Spine J.* 2002;2:274-278.

Deer TR. Current and future trends in spinal cord stimulation for chronic pain. *Curr Pain Headache Rep.* 2001;5:503-509.

Degner LF, Kristjanson LJ, Bowman D, *et al.* Abstract Information needs and decisional preferences in women with breast cancer. *JAMA.* 1997;277:1485-1492.

Degner LF, Sloan JA, Venkatesh P. The Control Preferences Scale. Can J Nurs Res. 1997;29:21-43.

Degner LF, Sloan JA. Abstract decision-making during serious illness: what role do patients really want to play? *J Clin Epidemiol.* 1992;45:941-950.

Doverty M, Somogyi AA, White JM, *et al.* Methadone maintenance patients are cross-tolerant to the antinociceptive effects of morphine. *Pain.* 2001;93:155-163.

Doyle D, Hanks G, Cherny NI, Calman K, eds. Oxford Textbook of Palliative Medicine. 3rd ed. Oxford, United Kingdom: Oxford University Press; 2003.

Doyle D. Domiciliary palliative care. In: Doyle D, Hanks GWC, MacDonald N, eds. Oxford Textbook of Palliative Medicine. 2nd ed. Oxford, England: Oxford University Press; 1998:957-973.

Du X, Skopp G, Aderjan R. The influence of the route of administration: a comparative study at steady state of oral sustained release morphine and morphine sulfate suppositories. *Ther Drug Monit.* 1999;21:208-214.

Duggal,Ravi. Operationalizing Right to Health Care in India. Right to Health Care, Moving from Idea to Reality. CEHAT Mumbai, 2003.

Dworkin RH, Backonja M, Rowbotham MC, *et al.* Advances in neuropathic pain: diagnosis, mechanisms, and treatment recommendations. [see comment]. *Arch Neurol.* 2003;60:1524-1534.

Eisele JH Jr, Grigsby EJ, Dea G. Clonazepam treatment of myoclonic contractions associated with high-dose opioids: case report. [see comment]. *Pain.* 1992;49:231-232.

Ellershaw J, Ward C. Care of the dying patient: the last hours or days of life. *BMJ.* 2003;326:30-34.

Ellershaw JE, Sutcliffe JM, Saunders CM. Dehydration and the dying patient. *J Pain Symptom Manage.* 1995;10:192-197. Abstract Musgrave CF, Bartal N, Opstad J. The sensation of thirst in dying patients receiving IV hydration. *J Palliat Care.* 1995;11:17-21.

Fainsinger R, Schoeller T, Boiskin M, Bruera E. Palliative care round: cognitive failure and coma after renal failure in a patient receiving captopril and hydromorphone. *J Palliat Care.* 1993;9:53-55.

Fainsinger RL, Tapper M, Bruera E. A perspective on the management of delirium in terminally ill patients on a palliative care unit. *J Palliat Care.* 1993;9:4-8. Abstract

Farrar JT, Portenoy RK. Neuropathic cancer pain: the role of adjuvant analgesics. Oncology (Huntingt). 2001;15:1435-1442, 1445; *Discussion* 1445, 1450-1433.

Feldman MD. Paradoxical effects of benzodiazepines. NC Med J. 1986;47:311-312.

Ferris FD, Flannery JS, McNeal HB, Morissette MR, Cameron R, Bally GA, eds. Module 4: Palliative care. In: A Comprehensive Guide for the Care of Persons with HIV Disease. Toronto, Ontario: Mount Sinai Hospital and Casey House Hospice, Inc.; 1995.

Ferris FD, von Gunten CF, Emanuel LL. Competency in end of life care: The last hours of living. *J Palliat Med.* 2003;6:605-613. Abstract

Ferris TG, Hallward JA, Ronan L, Billings JA. When the patient dies: a survey of medical housestaff about care after death. *J Palliat Med.* 1998;1:231-239. Abstract

Field MJ, Cassel CK, eds. Approaching Death: Improving Care at the End of Life. Washington, DC: National Academy Press; 1997:28-30.

Fine PG, Miaskowski C, Paice JA. Meeting the challenges in cancer pain management. *J Support Oncol.* 2004;2(suppl4):5-22.

Fine PG, Portenoy RK. A Clinical Guide to Opioid Analgesia. Minneapolis, Minn: McGraw-Hill Health Care Information; 2004.

Fine PG. Analgesia issues in palliative care: bone pain, controlled release opioids, managing opioid-induced constipation and nifedipine as an analgesic. *J Pain Palliat Care Pharmacother.* 2002;16:93-97.

Fine PG. Opioid analgesic drugs in older people. Clin Geriatr Med. 2001;17:479-487.

Fine PG. Opioid insights: opioid-induced hyperalgesia and opioid rotation. *J Pain Palliat Care Pharmacother.* 2004;18:75-59.

Fine PG. The ethical imperative to relieve pain at life's end. *J Pain Symptom Manage.* 2002;23: 273-277.

Fine PG. The evolving and important role of anesthesiology in palliative care. *Anesth Analg.* 2005; 100:183-188.

Finucane TE, Christmas C, Travis K. Tube feeding inpatients with advanced dementia: a review of the evidence. *JAMA.* 1999;282:1365-1370. Abstract

Freemon FR. Delirium and organic psychosis. In: Organic Mental Disease. Jamaica, NY: SP Medical and Scientific Books; 1981:81-94.

Fulton CL, Else R. Physiotherapy. In: Doyle D, Hanks GWC, MacDonald N, eds. Oxford Textbook of Palliative Medicine. 2nd ed. Oxford, England: Oxford University Press; 1998:821-822.

Ganzini L, Goy ER, Miller LL, Harvath TA, Jackson A, Delrot MA. Nurses' experiences with hospice patients who refuse food and fluids to hasten death. *N Engl J Med* 2003;349:359-65.

Garnett M. Sustaining the cocoon: the emotional inoculation produced by complementary therapies in palliative care. *Eur J Cancer Care* (Engl). 2003;12:129-136.

Gazelle G, Fine PG. Methadone for the treatment of pain. *J Palliat Med.* 2003;6:621-622.

George S, Pulimood S, Jacob M, Chandi SM. Pain in multiple leiomyomas alleviated by nifedipine. *Pain.* 1997;73:101-102.

Goudas LC, Bloch R, Gialeli-Goudas M, Lau J, Carr DB. The epidemiology of cancer pain. *Cancer Invest.* 2005;23:182-190.

Gralla RJ. Quality-of-life considerations inpatients with advanced lung cancer. Effect of topotecan on symptom palliation and quality of life. *Oncologist.* 2004;9(suppl6):14-24.

Gray H. Anatomy of the Human Body, 29th ed. Philadelphia, *Pa: Lea and Febiger;* 1985:1303-1313.

Grealish L, Lomasney A, Whiteman B. (2000). Foot massage. A nursing intervention to modify the distressing symptoms of pain and nausea inpatients hospitalized with cancer (abstract). PubMed, NCBI. Retrieved on March 07, 2006.

Hagen N, Swanson R. Strychnine-like multifocal myoclonus and seizures in extremely high-dose opioid administration: treatment strategies. [see comment]. *J Pain Symptom Manage.* 1997;14:51-58.

Hahn K, Arendt G, Braun JS, *et al*; German Neuro-AIDS Working Group. A placebo-controlled trial of gabapentin for painful HIV-associated sensory neuropathies. *J Neurol.* 2004;251:1260-1266.

Hall EJ, Sykes NP. Analgesia for patients with advanced disease: part 1. *Postgrad Med J.* 2004;80:148-154.

Hammack JE, Michalak JC, Loprinzi CL, *et al.* Phase III evaluation of nortriptyline for alleviation of symptoms of cis-platinum-induced peripheral neuropathy. *Pain.* 2002;98:195-203.

Hartsell WF, Scott CB, Bruner DW, *et al.* Randomized trial of short- versus long-course radiotherapy for palliation of painful bone metastases. *J Natl Cancer Inst.* 2005;97:798-804.

Health Survey and Development Committee, GOI 1946 (Bhore Report) Mahal A. www.worldbank.org

Hoppmann RA, Peden JG, Ober SK. Central nervous system side effects of nonsteroidal anti-inflammatory drugs. Aseptic meningitis, psychosis, and cognitive dysfunction. *Arch Intern Med.* 1991;151:1309-1313.

Hughes AC, Wilcock A, Corcoran R. Management of "death rattle." *J Pain Symptom Manage.* 1996;12:271-272.

Ingham J, Breitbart W. Epidemiology and clinical features of delirium. In: Portenoy RK, Bruera E, eds. Topics in Palliative Care, vol. 1. New York: Oxford University Press; 1997:7-19.

Integration of behavioral and relaxation approaches into the treatment of chronic pain and insomnia.. NIH Technology Assessment Panel on Integration of Behavioral and Relaxation Approaches into the Treatment of Chronic Pain and Insomnia. The Journal of the American Medical Association (archives) (1996). Retrieved on March 07, 2006.

International Institute for Population Sciences and ORC Macro. National Family Health Survey (NFHS-II) 1998-99. India.

International Institute for Population Sciences. Facility Survey.1999.

International Institute for Population Sciences. RCH-RHS India 1998-1999. National Crime Records Bureau. Ministry of Home Affairs. Accidental Deaths and Suicides In India 2000.

Inturrisi CE. Pharmacology of analgesia: basic principles. In: Bruera E, Portenoy RK, eds. Cancer Pain: Assessment and Management. Cambridge, United Kingdom: Cambridge University Press; 2003.

Irvine P. The attending at the funeral. *N Engl J Med.* 1985;312:1704-1705. Abstract

Iserson KV. The gravest words: notifying survivors about sudden unexpected deaths. Resident Staff Physician. 2001;47:66-72.

Iserson KV. The gravest words: sudden death notification and emergency care. *Ann Emerg Med.* 2000;36:75-77. Abstract

Jenkins V, Fallowfield L, Saul J. Abstract Information needs of patients with cancer: results from a large study in UK cancer centres. *Br J Cancer.* 2001;84:48-51.

Joanne Lynn (2004). Sick to death and not going to take it anymore!: reforming health care for the last years of life. Berkeley: University of California Press, 72. ISBN 0-520-24300-5.

Keefe FJ, Ahles TA, Porter LS, *et al.* The self-efficacy of family caregivers for helping cancer patients manage pain at end-of-life. *Pain.* 2003;103:157-162.

Kellar N, Martinez J, Finis N, Bolger A, von Gunten CF. Characterization of an acute inpatient hospice palliative care unit in a US teaching hospital. *J Nurs Admin.* 1996;26:16-20.

Konski A, Feigenberg S, Chow E. Palliative radiation therapy. *Semin Oncol.* 2005;32:156-164.

Langer CJ. Emerging role of epidermal growth factor receptor inhibition in therapy for advanced malignancy. Focus on NSCLC. *Int J Radiat Oncol Biol Phys.* 2004;58:991-1002.

Larijani GE, Goldberg ME, Rogers KH. Treatment of opioid-induced pruritus with ondansetron: report of four patients. *Pharmacotherapy.* 1996;16:958-960.

Larue F, Brasseur L, Musseault P, *et al.* Pain and symptoms during HIV disease. A French national study. *J Palliat Care.* 1994:10;95.

Lasch K, Greenhill A, Wilkes G, Carr D, Lee M, Blanchard R. Why study pain? A qualitative analysis of medical and nursing faculty and students' knowledge of and attitudes to cancer pain management. *J Palliat Med.* 2002;5:57-71.

Lauretti GR, Oliveira GM, Pereira NL. Comparison of sustained-release morphine with sustained-release oxycodone in advanced cancer patients. *Br J Cancer.* 2003;89:2027-2030.

Lee MA, Leng ME, Tiernan EJ. Retrospective study of the use of hydromorphone in palliative care patients with normal and abnormal urea and creatinine. *Palliat Med.* 2001;15:26-34.

Lethen W. Mouth and skin problems. In: Saunders C, Sykes N. The Management of Terminal Malignant Disease, 3rd ed. Boston: Edward Arnold; 1993:139-142.

Lichter I, Hunt E. The last 48 hours of life. J Palliat Care. 1990;6:7-15.

Liu MC, Caraceni AT, Ingham JM. Altered mental status inpatients with cancer: a delirium update. Principles and Practice of Supportive Oncology Updates. Philadelphia, Pa: JB Lippincott Co; 1999:2.

Lucas LK, Lipman AG. Recent advances in pharmacotherapy for cancer pain management. *Cancer Pract.* 2002;10 (suppl1):S14-20.

Lutz S, Spence C, Chow E, *et al.* Survey on use of palliative radiotherapy in hospice care. *J Clin Oncol.* 2004;22:3581-3586.

MacDonald N, ed. Palliative Medicine, a Case-Based Manual. Oxford, NY: Oxford University Press; 1998:263.

Maddocks I, Somogyi A, Abbott F, Hayball P, Parker D. Attenuation of morphine-induced delirium in palliative care by substitution with infusion of oxycodone. *J Pain Symptom Manage.* 1996;12:182-189. Abstract

Magrane BP, Gilliland MG, King DE. Certification of death by family physicians. *Am Fam Physician.* 1997;56:1433-1438. Abstract

Maizels M, McCarberg B. Antidepressants and antiepileptic drugs for chronic non-cancer pain. *Am Fam Physician.* 2005;71:483-490.

Mao J, Chen LL. Systemic lidocaine for neuropathic pain relief. Pain. 2000;87:7-17.

Marchand LR, Kushner KP. Death pronouncement: survival tips for residents. *Am Fam Physician.* 1998;58:284-285. Abstract

Martinez J, Wagner S. Hospice care. In: Groenwald SL, Frogge M, Goodman M, Yarbro M, Jones CH, eds. Cancer Nursing: Principles and Practices. 4th ed. Boston, Mass: Bartlett Publishers; 1997.

Martinez MJ, Roque M, Alonso-Coello P, Catala E, Garcia JL, Ferrandiz M. Calcitonin for metastatic bone pain. *Cochrane Database Syst Rev.* 2003:CD003223.

Matching Services to needs. Copenhagen, WHO Regional Office for Europe, 2002 (document EUR/RC50/10)

McCaffery M, Martin L, Ferrell BR. Analgesic administration via rectum or stoma. *J ET Nurs.* 1992;19:114-121.

McCann RM, Hall WJ, Groth-Juncker A. Comfort care for terminally ill patients: the appropriate use of nutrition and hydration. *JAMA.* 1994;272:1263-1266. Abstract

McIver B, Walsh D, Nelson K. The use of chlorpromazine for symptom control in dying cancer patients. *J Pain Symptom Manage.* 1994;9:341-345. Abstract

Menten J, Desmedt M, Lossignol D, Mullie A. Longitudinal follow-up of TTS-fentanyl use inpatients with cancer-related pain: results of a compassionate-use study with special focus on elderly patients. *Curr Med Res Opin.* 2002;18:488-498.

Mercadante S, Fulfaro F, Casuccio A. A randomised controlled study on the use of anti-inflammatory drugs inpatients with cancer pain on morphine therapy: effects on dose-escalation and a pharmacoeconomic analysis. *Eur J Cancer.* 2002;38:1358-1363.

Mercadante S, Fulfaro F, Casuccio A. The use of corticosteroids in home palliative care. *Support Care Cancer.* 2001;9:386-389.

Mercadante S. The use of anti-inflammatory drugs in cancer pain. *Cancer Treat Rev.* 2001;27:51-61.

Meuser T, Pietruck C, Radbruch L, Stute P, Lehmann KA, Grond S. Symptoms during cancer pain treatment following WHO-guidelines: a longitudinal follow-up study of symptom prevalence, severity and etiology. *Pain.* 2001;93:247-257.

Miaskowski C, Cleary J, Burney R, *et al.* Guideline for the Management of Cancer Pain in Adults and Children, APS Clinical Practice Guidelines Series, No. 3. Glenview, Ill: American Pain Society; 2005. Available at: http://www.ampainsoc.org/pub/cancer.htm#panel Accessed September 14, 2005.

Miller KE, Miller MM, Jolley MR. Challenges in pain management at the end of life. *Am Fam Physician.* 2001;64:1227-1234.

Misra, Chatterjee, Rao. India Health Report.Oxford University Press, New Delhi, 2003

Montagnini M, Lodhi M, Born W. The utilization of physical therapy in a palliative care unit. *J Palliat Med.* 2003;6:11-17.

Morbidity and Treatment of Ailments. NSS Fifty second round. Government of India. 1998. Changing the Indian Health System—Draft Report, ICRIER, 2001.

Morley JS, Bridson J, Nash TP, Miles JB, White S, Makin MK. Low-dose methadone has an analgesic effect in neuropathic pain: a double-blind randomized controlled crossover trial. Palliat *Med.* 2003;17:576-587.

Mount BM. Care of dying patients and their families. In: Bennett JC, Plum F. Cecil Textbook of Medicine. 20th ed. Philadelphia, Pa: WB Saunders Company; 1996:6-9.

Moyle J. The use of propofol in palliative medicine. *J Pain Symptom Manage.* 1995;10:643-646. Abstract

Muijsers RB, Wagstaff AJ. Transdermal fentanyl: an updated review of its pharmacological properties and therapeutic efficacy in chronic cancer pain control. *Drugs.* 2001;61:2289-2307.

Musgrave CF. Terminal dehydration: to give or not to give intravenous fluids? Cancer Nurs. 1990;13:62-66. Abstract.

Myskja A. Therapeutic use of music in nursing homes. Tidsskr Nor Laegeforen. 2005;125:1497-1499. Kemper KJ, Danhauer SC. Music as therapy. *South Med J.* 2005;98:282-288.

National Coordination Committee for the Jana Swasthya Sabha. Health for All NOW. 2004.

National Institutes of Health Consensus Development Statement. Acupuncture. November 3-5, 1997. Revised draft 11/5/97. Available at: http://www.healthy.net/LIBRARY/Articles/NIH/Report.htm Accessed August 12, 2005.

National Sample Survey Organization. Department of Statistics. GOI. 42nd and 52nd Round.

Naughton MT. Pathophysiology and treatment of Cheyne-Stokes respiration. *Thorax.* 1998;53:514-518. Abstract

Nelson KA, Glare PA, Walsh D, Groh ES. A prospective, within-patient, crossover study of continuous intravenous and subcutaneous morphine for chronic cancer pain. *J Pain Symptom Manage.* 1997;13:262-267.

Ng K, von Gunten CF. Symptoms and attitudes of 100 consecutive patients admitted to an acute hospice/palliative care unit. *J Pain Symptom Manage.* 1998;16:307-316.

Nuland S. How We Die. New York: Vintage Books; 1995.

Nurmikko TJ, Haanpaa M. Treatment of postherpetic neuralgia. *Curr Pain Headache Rep.* 2005;9:161-167.

O'Brien T, Mortimer PG, McDonald CJ, Miller AJ. A randomized crossover study comparing the efficacy and tolerability of a novel once-daily morphine preparation (MXL capsules) with MST Continus tablets in cancer patients with severe pain. *Palliat Med.* 1997;11:475-482.

O'Gorman SM. Death and dying in contemporary society. J Adv Nurs. 1998;27:1127-1135. Abstract

Osias RR, Pomerantz DH, Brensilver JM. Fast Facts and Concepts #76 and 77: Telephone Notification of Death. Milwaukee, Wi: End of Life Physician Education Resource Center. Available at: http://www.eperc.mcw.edu/ff_index.htm. Accessed August 1, 2006.

Osler W. Canada Lancet. 1909;42:899-912.

Otis JA, Fudin J. Use of long-acting opioids for the management of chronic pain. US Pharmacist. Available at: http://www.uspharmacist.com/index.asp?page'ce/10163/default.htm Accessed September 12, 2005.

Ottawa Charter for Health Promotion (http://www.who/int/hpr/NPH/docs/ottawa_charter_hp.pdf). Ottawa, WHO, 1986 (accessed 4 March 2004).

Page GG. The immune-suppressive effects of pain. *Adv Exp Med Biol.* 2003;521:117-125.

Pai M *et al.* A high rate of Cesaerean sections in affluent section of Chennai, is it a cause for concern? *Nat Med J India,* 1999,12:156-158.

Paice J, Fine PG. Pain management at end of life. In: Ferrell B, Coyle N, eds. Oxford Textbook of Pálliative Nursing. 2nd ed. New York: Oxford University Press. In press.

Paice JA, Fine PG. Pain at the end of life. In: Ferrell BR, Coyle N, eds. Oxford Textbook of Palliative Nursing. 2nd ed. New York: Oxford University Press; 2001.

Paice JA, Toy C, Shott S. Barriers to cancer pain relief: fear of tolerance and addiction. *J Pain Symptom Manage.* 1998;16:1-9.

Paqueta C, Kergoata M-J, Dube L. The role of everyday emotion regulation on pain in hospitalized elderly: insights from a prospective within-day assessment. *Pain.* 2005;115:355-363.

Phadke A. Drug Supply and Use. Towards a Rational Policy in India. Sage Publications New Delhi. Ministry of Chemicals and Fertilizers.

Planning Commission, Government of India. Tenth Five Year Plan 2002-2007. Volume II.

Potter VT, Wiseman CE, Dunn SM, Boyle FM. Patient barriers to optimal cancer pain control. *Psychooncology.* 2003;12:153-160.

Quill TE, Lo B, Brock DW. Palliative options of last resort: a comparison of voluntarily stopping eating and drinking, terminal sedation, physician-assisted suicide, and voluntary active euthanasia. *JAMA* 1997;278:2099-104.

Rabow MW, Petersen J, Schanche K, Dibble SL, McPhee SJ. The comprehensive care team: a description of a controlled trial of care at the beginning of the end of life. *J Palliat Med.* 2003;6:489-499.

Radbruch L, Sabatowski R, Petzke F, Brunsch-Radbruch A, Grond S, Lehmann KA. Transdermal fentanyl for the management of cancer pain: a survey of 1005 patients. *Palliat Med.* 2001;15:309-321.

Ripamonti C. Pharmacology of opioid analgesia: clinical principles. In: Bruera E, Portenoy RK, eds. Cancer Pain: Assessment and Management. Cambridge, United Kingdom: Cambridge University Press; 2003:124-149.

Rosen LS, Gordon D, Kaminski M, *et al.* Long-term efficacy and safety of zoledronic acid compared with pamidronate disodium in the treatment of skeletal complications inpatients with advanced multiple myeloma or breast cancer: a randomized, double-blind, multicenter, comparative trial. *Cancer.* 2003;98:1735-1744.

Rosen LS, Gordon D, Tchekmedyian NS, *et al.* Long-term efficacy and safety of zoledronic acid in the treatment of skeletal metastases inpatients with nonsmall cell lung carcinoma and other solid tumors: a randomized, phase III, double-blind, placebo-controlled trial. *Cancer.* 2004;100:2613-2621.

Rosen LS, Gordon DH, Dugan W Jr, *et al.* Zoledronic acid is superior to pamidronate for the treatment of bone metastases in breast cancer patients with at least one osteolytic lesion. *Cancer.* 2004;100:36-43.

Rowbotham MC, Twilling L, Davies PS, Reisner L, Taylor K, Mohr D. Oral opioid therapy for chronic peripheral and central neuropathic pain. [comment]. *N Engl J Med.* 2003;348:1223-1232.

Saad F, Gleason D, Murray R, *et al.* Zoledronic acid is well tolerated for up to 24 months and significantly reduces skeletal complications inpatients with advanced prostate cancer metastatic to bone. *J Urol.* 2003;169(suppl):394.

Schiodt FV, Rochling FA, Casey DL, Lee WM. Acetaminophen toxicity in an urban county hospital. *N Engl J Med.* 1997;337:1112-1117.

See Existential pain—an entity, a provocation, or a challenge? in Journal of Pain Symptom and Management, Volume 27, Issue 3, Pages 241-250 (March 2004)

Seymour, J. E; D. Clark, M. Winslow (2004). "Morphine use in cancer pain: from 'last resort' to 'gold standard'. Poster presentation at the Third research Forum of the European Association of Palliative Care.". *Palliative Medicine* 18 (4): 378.

Shaiova L, Sperber KT, Hord ED. Methadone for refractory cancer pain. *J Pain Symptom Manage.* 2002;23:178-180.

Shariff Abusaleh. India Human Development Report.Oxford University Press New Delhi.

Sheldon F. Communication. In: Saunders C, Sykes N, eds. The Management of Terminal Malignant Disease. Boston, Mass: Edward Arnold: 1993:29-31.

Shuster JL. Delirium, confusion, and agitation at the end of life. *J Palliat Med.* 1998;1:177-186. Abstract

Sloan P, Basta M, Storey P, von Gunten C. Mexiletine as an adjuvant analgesic for the management of neuropathic cancer pain. *Anesth Analg.* 1999;89:760-761.

Smeltzer SC, Bare BG, eds. Brunner and Suddarth's Textbook of Medical Surgical Nursing. 7th ed. Philadelphia, Pa: JB Lippincott Company; 1992:1657-1602.

Smith MT. Neuroexcitatory effects of morphine and hydromorphone: evidence implicating the 3-glucuronide metabolites. *Clin Exp Pharmacol Physiol.* 2000;27:524-528.

Smith TJ, Staats PS, Deer T, *et al.* Randomized clinical trial of an implantable drug delivery system compared with comprehensive medical management for refractory cancer pain: impact on pain, drug-related toxicity, and survival. [see comment]. *J Clin Oncol.* 2002;20:4040-4049.

Soden K, Vincent K, Craske S, Lucas C, Ashley S. A randomized controlled trial of aromatherapy massage in a hospice setting. *Palliat Med.* 2004;18:87-92.

SRS Bulletin. Government of India.1998.

Storey P. Symptom control in dying. In: Berger A, Portenoy RK, Weissman D, eds. Principles and Practice of Supportive Oncology Updates. Philadelphia, Pa: Lippincott-Raven Publishers; 1998:741-748.

Swica Y, Breitbart W. Treating pain inpatients with AIDS and a history of substance use. *West J Med.* 2002;176:33-39.

Sykes N, Thorns A. Sedative use in the last week of life and the implications for end-of-life decision-making. *Arch Intern Med.* 2003;163:341-344.

Sykes N, Thorns A. Sedative use in the last week of life and the implications for end-of-life decision-making. *Arch Intern Med.* 2003;163:341-344. Abstract

Sykes N, Thorns A. The use of opioids and sedatives at the end of life. *Lancet Oncol.* 2003;4:312-318.

Tanaka E, Yamazaki K, Misawa S. Update: the clinical importance of acetaminophen hepatotoxicity in non-alcoholic and alcoholic subjects. *J Clin Pharm Ther.* 2000;25:325-332.

TB India 2003. RNTCP Stats Report.Central TB Division.DDHS GOI.

Teno JM, Weitzen S, Wetle T, Mor V. Persistent pain in nursing home residents. *JAMA.* 2001;285:2081.

The Hospice Institute of the Florida Suncoast, Hospice Training Program. Care at the Time of Death. Largo, Fl: The Hospice Institute of the Florida Suncoast; 1996.

The International Society for Quality in Health Care. Alpha and accreditation (http://www.isqua.org.au/isquaPages/Alpha.html). Victoria, Isqua, 2003 (accessed 4 March 2004).

Tilden VP, Drach LL, Tolle SW. Complementary and alternative therapy use at end-of-life in community settings. *J Altern Complement Med.* 2004;10:811-817.

Truog RD, Berde CB, Mitchell C, Grier HE. Barbiturates in the care of the terminally ill. *N Engl J Med.* 1992;337:1678-1682.

Twycross R, Lichter I. The terminal phase. In: Doyle D, Hanks GWC, MacDonald N, eds. Oxford Textbook of Palliative Medicine. 2nd ed. Oxford, England: Oxford University Press; 1998:977-992.

Twycross R, Lichter I. The terminal phase. In: Doyle D, Hanks GWC, MacDonald N, eds. Oxford Textbook of Palliative Medicine. 2nd ed. Oxford, England: Oxford University Press; 1998:987-988.

Twycross R, Lichter I. The terminal phase. In: Doyle D, Hanks GWC, MacDonald N, eds. Oxford Textbook of Palliative Medicine. 2nd ed. Oxford, England: Oxford University Press; 1998:985-6.

Twycross RB, Lack SA. Therapeutics in Terminal Cancer. 2nd ed. London, England: *Churchill Livingstone*; 1990:134-136.

US Food and Drug Administration, Department of Health and Human Services. Center for Drug Evaluation and Research. Questions and answers: FDA regulatory actions for the COX-2 selective and non-selective non-steroidal anti-inflammatory drugs (NSAIDs). Created April 7, 2005. Available at: http://www.fda.gov/cder/drug/infopage/COX2/COX2qa.htm Accessed September 12, 2005.

US Food and Drug Administration, Department of Health and Human Services. MedWatch, The FDA Safety Information and Adverse Event Reporting Program. 2005 safety alerts for drugs, biologics, medical devices, and dietary supplements. Posted July 15, 2005. Available at: http://www.fda.gov/MedWatch/SAFETY/2005/safety05.htm#Fentanyl Accessed September 12, 2005.

Van Poppel H. Recent docetaxel studies establish a new standard of care in hormone refractory prostate cancer. *Can J Urol.* 2005;12(suppl):81-85.

Vienna Recommendations for Health Promoting Hospitals (http:/Iwww.euro.who.int/document/IHB/hphviennarecom.pdf) (accessed 4 March 2004).

Vogl D, Rosenfeld B, Breitbart W, *et al.* Symptom prevalence, characteristics, and distress in AIDS outpatients. *J Pain Symptom Manage.* 1999;18:253-262.

Voltz R, Borasio GD. Palliative therapy in the terminal stage of neurological disease. J Neurol. 1997;244(suppl 4):S2-S10. Abstract

Walker P, Watanabe S, Bruera E. Baclofen, a treatment for chronic hiccup. *J Pain Symptom Manage.* 1998;16:125-132.

Walker P. The pathophysiology and management of pressure ulcers. In: Portenoy RK, Bruera E, eds. Topics in Palliative Care, Voi. 3. New York: Oxford University Press; 1998:253-270.

Walker, Walker *et al.* (1999). Psychological, clinical and pathological effects of relaxation training and guided imagery during primary chemotherapy (abstract). PubMed, National Center for Biotechnology Information (NCBI). Retrieved on March 07, 2006.

Wallace MS, Magnuson S, Ridgeway B. Efficacy of oral mexiletine for neuropathic pain with allodynia: a double-blind, placebo-controlled, crossover study. *Reg Anesth Pain Med.* 2000;25:459-467.

Walsh D, Gombeski W, Goldstein P, Hayes D, Armour M (1994). "Managing a palliative oncology program: the role of a business plan". *J Pain Symptom Manage* 9 (2): 109. PMID 7517428.

Walsh D, Gombeski WR, Goldstein P, Hayes D, Armour M. Managing a palliative oncology program: the role of a business plan. *J Pain Symptom Manage.* 1994;9:109-118. Abstract

Ward SE, Berry PE, Misiewicz H. Concerns about analgesics among patients and family caregivers in a hospice setting. *Res Nurs Health.* 1996;19:205-211.

Watanabe S, Pereira J, Hanson J, Bruera E. Fentanyl by continuous subcutaneous infusion for the management of cancer pain: a retrospective study. *J Pain Symptom Manage.* 1998;16:323-326.

Weber M, Ochsmann R, Huber C. Laying out and viewing the body at home—a forgotten tradition? *J Palliat Care.* 1998;14:34-37.

Webster L, Andrews M, Stoddard G. Modafinil treatment of opioid-induced sedation. *Pain Med.* 2003;4:135-140.

Weiner DK, Ernst E. Complementary and alternative approaches to the treatment of persistent musculoskeletal pain. *Clin J Pain.* 2004;20:244-255.

Weissman DE, Heidenreich CA. Fast Facts and Concepts #4: Death Pronouncement in the Hospital. Milwaukee, Wi: End of Life Physician Education Resource Center. Available at: http://www.eperc.mcw.edu/ff_index.htm. Accessed August 1, 2006.

Wells N. Pain intensity and pain interference in hospitalized patients with cancer. *Oncol Nurs Forum.* 2000;27:985-991.

WHO Definition of Palliative Care. World Health Organization. Retrieved on March 07, 2006.

WHO Regional Office for Europe. Health Promoting Hospital, (http://www.euro.who.int/healthpromohosp). Copenhagen, WHO Regional Office for Europe, 2002 (accessed 4 March 2004).

WHO Standards Working Group. Development of standards for disease prevention and health promotion. WHO, Meeting on standards for disease prevention and health promotion, Bratislava, 14 May 2002.

Wolfe MM, Lichtenstein DR, Singh G. Gastrointestinal toxicity of nonsteroidal antiinflammatory drugs. [comment]. [erratum appears in *N Engl J Med.* 1999;341:548]. *N Engl J Med.* 1999;340:1888-1899.

Wooldridge JE, Anderson CM, Perry MC. Corticosteroids in advanced cancer. Oncology (Huntingt). 2001;15:225-234; *Discussion* 234-226.

World Health Organization. The World Health Report 2003.

Wright AW, Mather LE, Smith MT. Hydromorphone-3-glucuronide: a more potent neuro-excitant than its structural analogue, morphine-3-glucuronide. *Life Sci.* 2001;69:409-420.

Zaw-tun N, Bruera E. Active metabolites of morphine. *J Palliat Care.* 1992;8:48-50. Abstract

Zerzan, J.; S. Stearns, L. Hanson (2000). "Access to palliative care and hospice in nursing homes". Journal of the American Medical Association 284: 2489 - 2494.

Zylicz Z, Smits C, Krajnik M. Paroxetine for pruritus in advanced cancer. *J Pain Symptom Manage.* 1998;16:121-124.

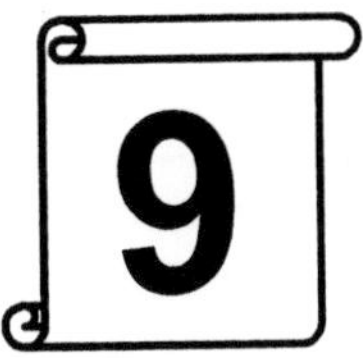

Chronically Ill Patients with Bedsores: Challenge to Hospital's Management

A horse riding accident transformed Christopher Reed from an actor identified with SUPERMAN into a quadriplegic, who later died from complications of a bedsore. Each year, about one million people in the U.S. develop bedsores also called decubitus ulcers, simply from prolonged pressure on the skin, generally, resulting and ranging from mild inflammation to deep wounds. In India the number would be much higher, given the dismal state of nursing care available in the hospitals, Nursing homes or even own homes. Bedsores (bedsores), more properly known as pressure ulcers or decubitus ulcers, are lesions caused by unrelieved pressure to any part of the body, especially portions over bony or cartilaginous areas. Although completely treatable if found early, without medical attention, bedsores can become life-threatening. In its most basic description, a bedsore is an open sore. Bedsores progress in four stages, as classified by the National Pressure Ulcer Advisory Panel (NPUAP) in the United States. Bedsores are marked by a breakdown of the tissue in ulcerated area, high risk of infection, and a LONG healing time.

RISK FACTORS

Pressure sores are more likely to develop persons who are at higher risk due to one or more risk factors. A number of risk factors have been identified which put individuals at higher risk. Once a person is identified as being at increased risk for pressure sores, measures should be undertaken to reduce or eliminate those risks. Thus, health care providers must be aware of these risk factors when caring for patients in order to prevent the unnecessary development of pressure sores. While risk factors may vary depending upon the particular circumstances, the following represents a list of the most common:

1. Confinement to bed, chair, or wheelchair. Persons confined to beds, chairs, or wheelchairs who are unable to move themselves, can develop pressure-induced injuries in as little as 1-2 hours if the pressure is not relieved;
2. Inability to change positions without help. (e.g., an individual in a coma, who is paralyzed, or recovering from a hip fracture or other mobility limitation.)
3. Loss of bowel or bladder control. Sources of moisture on the skin from urine, stool, or perspiration can irritate the skin.
4. Poor nutrition and/or dehydration. Bedsores are more likely to form when the skin is not properly nourished.
5. Decreased mental awareness. An individual with decreased mental awareness may not have the level of sensory perception or ability to act to prevent the development of pressure-induced injury. The lack of mental awareness may arise from medications.

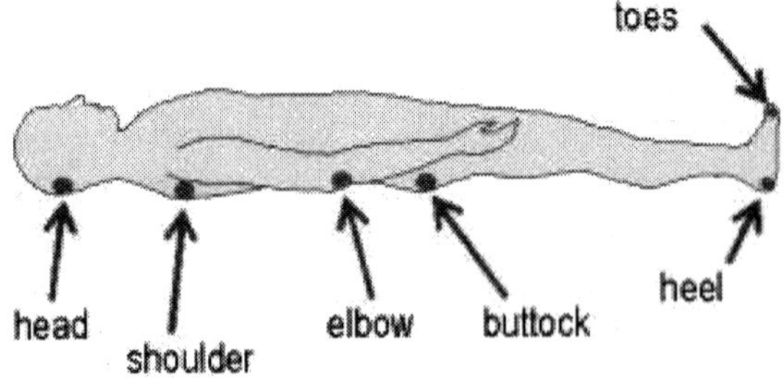

The following merit attention:

- Pressure ulcers or bedsores are a frequent complication in bedridden patients.
- Pressure sores develop quickly, progress rapidly, and are often difficult to heal if allowed to progress, but can usually be cured with proper care.
- Key preventive measures can also encourage healing.
- Patients transferred from a hospital to a nursing home are particularly vulnerable, with 10% to 35% having sores at the time they are admitted to the nursing home.
- Studies show that 50% of patients with pressure ulcers are over the age of 70 and among these elderly; bedsores means a four-fold increase in the rate of death.
- About 60,000 deaths a year are attributed to complications caused by bedsores. Incidence of bedsores varies among nursing homes anywhere between 12-26% in the U.S.A.
- Among those who are ulcer free at admission 13% develop stage 2 through 4 ulcers by one year and an alarming 21% by two years.

- Organs affected: buttocks, shoulder blades, elbows, heels, ankles, knees, lower back, spine, and hip.
- Bedsores can lead to other severe medical complications, infections, arthritis, and scar carcinoma.
- $2.57 million is spent on preventable decubitus ulcers yearly in the U.S. (2000-2).

What is bedsore?

Bedsores range from mild inflammation to ulceration (breakdown of tissue) and deep wounds that involve muscle and bone. This painful condition usually starts with shiny red skin that quickly blisters and deteriorates into open sores. These sores become a target for bacterial contamination and will often harbor life-threatening infection. Bedsores are not contagious or cancerous, although the most serious complication of chronic bedsores is the development of malignant degeneration, which is a type of cancer.

Bedsores develop as a result of pressure that cuts off the flow of blood and oxygen to tissue. Constant pressure pinches off capillaries, the tiny blood vessels that deliver oxygen and nutrients to the skin. If the skin is deprived of essential oxygen and nutrients (a condition known as ischemia) for even as little as an hour, tissue cells can die (anoxia) and bedsores can form. Even the slightest rubbing, called shear, or friction between a hard surface and skin stretched over bones, can cause minor pressure ulcers. They can also develop when a patient stretches or bends blood vessels by slipping into a different position in a bed or chair.

Since urine, feces, or other moisture increases the risk of skin infection, people who suffer from incontinence, as well as immobility, have a greater than average risk of developing bedsores.

Unfortunately, people who have been successfully treated for bedsores have a 90% chance of developing them again. While the pressure sores themselves can usually be cured, about 60,000 deaths per year are attributed to complications caused by bedsores. They can be slow to heal, particularly when the patient's overall status may be weakened. Without proper treatment, bedsores can lead to:

- gangrene (tissue death),
- osteomyelitis (infection of the bone beneath the bedsore),
- sepsis (a poisoning of tissue or the whole body from bacterial infection), and
- other localized or systemic infections that slow the healing process, increase the cost of treatment, lengthen hospital or nursing home stays, or cause death.

Bedsores are most apt to develop on bony parts of the body, including:

- ankles
- back of the head
- heels
- hips
- knees
- lower back
- shoulder blades
- spine

Although impaired mobility is a leading factor in the development of pressure sores, the risk is also increased by illnesses and conditions that weaken muscle and soft tissue, or that affect blood circulation and the delivery of oxygen to body tissue, leaving skin thinner and more vulnerable to breakdown and subsequent infection. These conditions include:

- atherosclerosis (hardening of arteries) that restricts blood flow
- diabetes
- diminished sensation or lack of feeling, unable to feel pain
- heart problems
- incontinence (inability to control bladder or bowel movements)
- malnutrition
- obesity
- paralysis
- poor circulation
- infection
- prolonged bed rest, especially in unsanitary conditions or with wet or wrinkled sheets
- spinal cord injury

Classification of bedsores

It is described in four stages of ulceration, based primarily on the depth of a sore at the time of examination. This helps standardize the language and encourages effective communication of medical personnel caring for patients with bedsores. Not all bedsores follow the stages directly from I to IV. The four most widely accepted stages are described as:

Stage 1 Bedsore

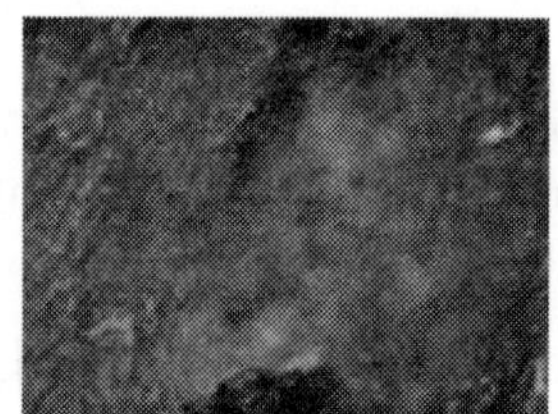

Stage 2 Bedsore

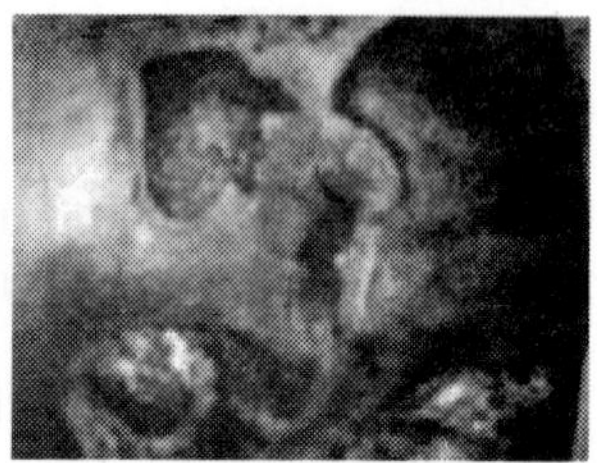

Stage 3-4 Bedsore

- Stage I: intact skin with redness (erythema) and sometimes with warmth.
- Stage II: partial-thickness loss of skin, an abrasion, swelling, and possible blistering or peeling of skin.
- Stage III: full-thickness loss of skin, open wound (crater), and possible exposed under layer.
- Stage IV: full-thickness loss of skin and underlying tissue extends into muscle, bone, tendon, or joint. Possible bone destruction, dislocations, or pathologic fractures (not caused by injury).

In addition to observing the depth of the wound, the presence or absence of wound drainage and foul odors, or any debris in the wound, such as pieces of dead skin tissue or other material, should also be noted. Any condition that could likely contaminate the wound and cause infection, such as the presence of urine or feces from incontinence, should be noted as well.

How the sore develops

An area of skin breakdown that occurs when sustained pressure cuts off blood circulation—usually inpatients confined to their beds in hospitals and nursing homes—a bedsore can result in a wound so deep and painful that some patients require narcotics. If a bedsore becomes infected, the complications can be fatal.

"They are not just little sores," said Susan Horn, senior scientist at the Institute for Clinical Outcomes Research in Salt Lake City. "If you've ever seen a very bad one, frankly, it would make you sick. You see a very reddened outer area, then you see, depending on how deep it is, just this hole in the skin, and it goes right down to the bone."

Experts estimate that two million Americans suffer from pressure ulcers each year, usually through some combination of immobility, poor nutrition, dehydration and incontinence. The Centers for Disease Control and Prevention does not keep statistics on fatalities, but one prominent victim was the actor Christopher Reeve, who died of a bedsore infection in 2004 in the middle of a heroic battle against paralysis.

New research is suggesting that the battle against bedsores requires a team approach, enlisting everyone from nurses and nursing assistants to laundry workers, nutritionists, maintenance workers and even in-house beauticians.

Causes

Although pressure on the skin is the main cause of bedsores, other factors often contribute to the problem. These include:

- *Shearing and friction*

Shearing and friction causes skin to stretch and blood vessels to kink, which can impair blood circulation in the skin. In a person confined to bed, shearing and friction can occur when the person is dragged or slid across the bed sheets. This can also occur when the head of the bed is raised more than 30 degrees. This increases shearing forces over the lower back and tailbone.

- *Moisture*

Wetness from perspiration, urine or feces can make the skin too soft and more likely to be injured by pressure. For this reason, people who can't control their bladders or bowels (people who are incontinent) are at high risk of developing bedsores.

- *Decreased movement*

Bedsores are common in people who can't move because they are paralyzed, recuperating from surgery for a prolonged time, being treated in intensive care for a long time, or are incapacitated by severe arthritis, *stroke* or a neurological problem such as *multiple sclerosis.* (People who can move without assistance have a lower risk of bedsores because they can shift their weight periodically.)

- *Decreased sensation*

Bedsores are common in people who have spinal cord injuries or other neurological problems that decrease their ability to feel pain or discomfort. Without these feelings, the person cannot feel the effects of prolonged pressure on the skin.

- *Circulatory problems*

People with atherosclerosis, circulatory problems from long-term diabetes or localized swelling (edema) may be more likely to develop bedsores. This is because the blood flow in their skin is weak even before pressure is applied to the skin. People with anemia are also at risk because their blood cannot carry enough oxygen to skin cells, even though circulation may be normal.

- *Poor nutrition*

Studies show that bedsores are more likely to develop in people who don't get enough protein, vitamin C, vitamin E, calcium or zinc.

- *Age*

Elderly people, especially those over 85, are more likely to develop bedsores because skin usually becomes thinner with age. Also, as we age, fat tends to shift away from the body surface, where it acts as a cushion, to deeper areas of the body.

Prevention

It is usually possible to prevent bedsores from developing or worsening. In 1989, the NPUAP set a goal that pressure sores be reduced by 50% by 2000. Because of the varying ways in which the number of cases were recorded during this timeframe, the NPUAP is finding it difficult to analyze accurate incident accounts. However even with the diversity of recording methods and the difficulties in comparing data, small group data indicates that progress has been made with the standardization of guidelines and care.

Bedsores can still form even if a patient is receiving excellent medical care or household care they are not necessarily a sign of neglected needs. Still, health care experts believe that at least 50% of bedsores can be prevented by using simple measures to relieve pressure and decrease the skin's vulnerability to injury. To help prevent bedsores in a person who is confined to a bed or chair, a plan of care may include these strategies:

- *Relieve pressure on vulnerable areas*

Change the person's position every two hours when in bed and every hour when sitting in a chair. Use pillows to raise the person's arms, legs, buttocks and hips. Relieve pressure on the back with an egg-crate foam mattress, a water mattress or a sheepskin. Two types of beds air-fluidized beds and low-air-loss beds have been shown to reduce the likelihood that a pressure ulcer will form.

- *Reduce shear and friction*

Avoid dragging the person across the bed sheets. Either lift the person or have the person use an overhead trapeze to briefly raise his or her body. Keep the bed free from crumbs and other particles that can rub and irritate the skin. Do not raise the head of the bed more than 30 degrees, unless your doctor tells you otherwise. Use sheepskin boots and elbow pads to reduce friction on heels and elbows. Wash the person gently. Avoid rubbing or scrubbing the skin.

- *Inspect the person's skin at least once each day*

Early detection can prevent stage I redness from becoming worse.

- *Minimize irritation from chemicals*

Avoid irritating antiseptics, hydrogen peroxide, povidone iodine solution or other harsh chemicals to clean or disinfect the skin.

- *Encourage the person to eat well*

The diet should include enough calories, protein, calcium, and zinc and vitamins C and E. If the person cannot eat enough food, ask your doctor about nutritional supplements.

- *Encourage daily exercise*

Exercise increases blood flow and speeds healing. In many cases, even bedridden people can do stretches and simple exercises.

- *Keep the skin clean and dry*

Clean the skin with saline (a non-irritating salt solution) rather than harsh soaps. Use absorbent pads to draw moisture away from vulnerable areas. If the person is incontinent, ask your doctor about ways to control or limit the leakage of urine or feces.

All patients recovering from illness or surgery or confined to a bed or wheelchair long-term should be inspected regularly; they should be bathed or should shower every day using warm water and mild soap; and patients should avoid cold or dry air. Bedridden patients, who are either mentally unaware or physically unable to turn themselves, must be repositioned regularly by caregivers at least once every two hours while awake. People who use a wheelchair should be encouraged to shift their weight every 10 or 15 minutes, or be repositioned by caregivers at least once an hour. It is important to lift, rather than to drag, a person being repositioned. Bony parts of the body should not be massaged. Even slight friction can remove the weakened top layer of skin and damage blood vessels beneath it.

If the patient is bedridden, sensitive body parts can be protected by:

- sheepskin pads
- special cushions placed on top of a mattress
- a water-filled mattress
- a variable-pressure mattress with individually inflatable sections to redistribute pressure

Pillows or foam wedges can prevent a bedridden patient's ankles from irritating each other, and pillows placed under the legs from mid-calf to ankle can raise the heels off the bed. Raising the head of the bed slightly and briefly can provide relief, but raising the head of the bed more than 30 degrees can cause the patient to slide, thereby causing damage to skin and tiny blood vessels.

A person who uses a wheelchair should be encouraged to sit up as straight as possible. Pillows behind the head and between the legs can help prevent bedsores, as can a special cushion placed on the chair seat. Donut shaped cushions should not be used because they restrict blood flow and cause tissues to swell.

Special support surfaces are manufactured and readily available for care in medical facilities or at home, including: air-filled mattresses and cushions, low-air loss beds, and air-fluidized beds. These devices give adequate support while reducing pressure on vulnerable skin. They have been shown to exert less pressure on the skin of compromised patients than do regular mattresses. Patients using these devices and beds must still be repositioned every two hours.

A doctor should be notified whenever a person:

- will be bedridden or immobilized for an extended time period
- is very weak or unable to move
- develops redness (inflammation) and warmth or peeling on any area of skin

Immediate medical attention is required whenever:

- skin turns black or becomes inflamed, tender, swollen, or warm to the touch
- the patient develops a fever during treatment
- a bedsore contains pus or has a foul-smelling discharge

Prompt medical attention can prevent surface pressure sores from deepening into more serious infections. The first step is always to reduce or eliminate the pressure that is causing bedsores. For minor bedsores, stages I and II, treatment involves relieving pressure, keeping the wound clean and moist, and keeping the area around the ulcer clean and dry. This is often accomplished with saline washes and the use of sterile medicated gauze dressings that both absorb the wound drainage and fight infection-causing bacteria. Antiseptics, soaps, and other skin cleansers can damage new tissue and should be avoided. Only saline solution should be used to cleanse bedsores whenever fresh non-stick dressings are applied. The patient's doctor may prescribe infection-fighting antibiotics, special dressings or drying agents, and/or lotions or ointments to be applied to the wound in a thin film three or four times a day. Warm whirlpool treatments are sometimes recommended for sores on the arm, hand, foot, or leg. Zinc and vitamins A, C, E, and B complex provide necessary nutrients for the skin and help it to repair injuries and stay healthy. Large doses of vitamins or minerals should not be used without a doctor's approval.

A poultice made of equal parts of powdered slippery elm (Ulmus fulva), marsh mallow (Althaea officinalis), and echinacea blended with a small amount of hot water can relieve minor inflammation. An infection-fighting rinse of two drops of essential tea tree oil (Melaleuca) to every 8 oz (0.23 g) of water can also be administered. An herbal tea made from calendula (Calendula officinalis) is also an effective antiseptic and wound healing agent. Calendula cream can also be used.

Contrasting hot and cold compresses applied to the bedsore site can increase circulation to the area and help flush out waste products, speeding the healing process. The temperatures should be extreme (very hot and ice cold), yet tolerable to the skin. Hot compresses should be applied for three minutes, followed by 30 seconds of cold compress application, repeating the cycle three times. The cycle should always end with a cold compress.

Other treatment options are described later in this chapter.

Symptoms

- *Stage I (earliest signs of skin damage)*

  White people or people with pale skin develop a lasting patch of red skin that does not turn white when you press it with your finger. In people with darker skin, the patch may be red, purple or blue and may be more difficult to detect. The skin may be tender or itchy, and may feel warm or cold and firm.

- *Stage II*

  The injured skin blisters or develops an open sore or abrasion that does not extend through the full thickness of the skin. There may be a surrounding area of red or purple discoloration, mild swelling and some oozing.

- *Stage III*

  The ulcer becomes a crater and that goes below the skin surface.

- *Stage IV*

  The crater deepens and reaches into a muscle, bone, tendon or joint.

Because broken skin can allow bacteria to enter, bedsores are extremely vulnerable to infection. This is especially true if the sore is contaminated by urine or feces. Signs of infection in a bedsore can include:

- Pus draining from the sore
- A foul smelling odor
- Tenderness, heat and increased redness in the surrounding skin
- Fever

A doctor or nurse can diagnose a bedsore by examining the skin. Testing is usually unnecessary unless there are symptoms of infection. If a person with bedsores develops an infection, a doctor may order tests to find out if the infection has moved into the soft tissues, into bones, into the bloodstream or to another site. Tests may include blood tests, a laboratory examination of tissue or secretions from the bedsore, and an x-ray, a magnetic resonance imaging scan (MRI scan) or a bone scan to look for evidence of a bone infection called osteomyelitis. If you care for a family member who is in a bed or wheelchair, your doctor or home care nurse can teach you how to identify the earliest signs of bedsores. You'll learn which areas of skin are particularly vulnerable and what to look for. When you find signs of skin damage, you can take steps to prevent areas of redness from becoming full-blown ulcers.

Many factors influence how long a bedsore lasts, including the severity of the sore and the type of treatment, as well as the person's age, overall health, nutrition and ability to move. For example, there is a good chance that a Stage II bedsore will heal within one to six weeks in a relatively healthy older person who eats well and is able to move. Stage II and stage IV ulcers may take six weeks to three months to heal. Often, they can last longer. Thirty percent of stage II ulcers, 50% of stage III ulcers, and 70% of stage IV ulcers take longer than six months to heal.

Bedsores can be an ongoing problem in chronically ill people who have multiple risk factors, such as incontinence, the inability to move and circulatory problems.

Treatment

First, areas of unbroken skin near the bedsore are covered with a protective film or a lubricant to protect them from injury. Next, special dressings are applied to the injured area to promote healing or to help remove small areas of dead tissue. If necessary, larger areas of dead tissue may be trimmed away surgically or dissolved with a special medication. Deep craters may need skin grafting and other forms of reconstructive surgery.

If the person's skin does not begin to heal within a few days after treatment starts, the doctor may prescribe antibiotics, which may be applied as an ointment, taken as a pill or given intravenously (into a vein). Antibiotics also are used to treat bedsores that show obvious signs of infection. The Electron-Active™ Silver Oxide compound brings Silver and Oxygen together in a single molecule, which has been estimated to be up to 40 times more potent than simple silver or oxygen alone. So Terrasil can kill the underlying causes of infection faster (and safer) than anything else on the market.

How to Use Terrasil Cream for Bedsores

- Clean the bed sore well. Repeat at least once daily, removing dead tissue if possible.
- Apply a moderate amount directly into the affected area. If the ulcer is in an early stage and not deep, rub Terrasil in until it disappears. It is generally quite safe to use Terrasil in open bedsores. Continue three or more times daily until the bed sore is completely healed.
- Use as much of the cream as needed. For deep or large bedsores several jars of Terrasil may be needed.
- After applying the cream, cover with a sterile gauze or bandage.
- Goes on smooth and begins to work right away.
- Safe and non-irritating.
- Can be used on all skin types, for all ages and at any stage of bed sore.

Debridement

The removal of *necrotic* tissue is an absolute must in the treatment of pressure sores. Because dead tissue is an ideal area for bacterial growth, it has the ability to greatly compromise wound healing. There are at least seven ways to excise necrotic tissue.

1. Autolytic debridement is the use of moist dressings to promote autolysis with the body's own enzymes. It is a slow process, but mostly painless.
2. Biological debridement, or *maggot debridement therapy,* is the use of medical maggots to feed on necrotic tissue and therefore clean the wound of excess bacteria. Although this fell out of favour for many years, in January 2004, the FDA approved maggots as a live medical device.
3. Chemical debridement, or enzymatic debridement, is the use of prescribed enzymes that promote the removal of necrotic tissue.
4. Mechanical debridement is the use of outside force to remove dead tissue. A quite painful method, this involves the packing of a wound with wet dressings that are allowed to dry and then are removed. This is also unpopular because it has the ability to remove healthy tissue in addition to dead tissue. Lastly, with Stage IV ulcers, there is the chance that overdrying of the dressings can lead to bone fractures and ligament snaps.
5. Sharp debridement is the removal of necrotic tissue with a scalpel or similar instrument.
6. Surgical debridement is the most popular method, as it allows a surgeon to quickly remove dead tissue with little pain to the patient.
7. Ultrasound-assisted wound therapy is the use of ultrasound waves to separate necrotic and healthy tissue.

Infection control

Infection has one of the greatest effects on the healing of a wound. Purulent discharge provides a breeding ground for excess bacteria, a problem especially in the immunocompromised patient. Symptoms of systemic infection include fever, pain, erythema, oedema, and warmth of the area, not to mention purulent discharge. Additionally, infected wounds may have a gangrenous smell, be discoloured, and may eventually exude even more pus.

In order to eliminate this bioburden, it is imperative to apply antiseptics and antimicrobials at once. It is not recommended to use hydrogen peroxide for this task as it is difficult to balance the toxicity of the wound with this. New dressings have been developed that have cadexomer iodine and silver in them, and they are used to treat bad infections. Duoderm can be used on smaller wounds to both provide comfort and protect them from outside air and infections.It is not recommended to use systemic antibiotics to treat infection of a bedsore, as it can lead to bacterial resistance.

Nutritional support

Upon admission, the patient should have a consultation with a dietitian to determine the best diet to support healing, as a malnourished person does not have the ability to synthesize enough protein to repair tissue. The dietitian should conduct a nutritional assessment that includes a battery of questions and a physical examination. If malnourishment is suspected, lab tests should be run to check serum albumin and lymphocyte counts. Additionally, a bioelectrical impedance analysis should be considered.

If the patient is found to be at risk for malnutrition, it is imperative to begin nutritional intervention with dietary supplements and nutrients including, but not limited to, arginine, glutamine, vitamin A, vitamin B complex, vitamin E, vitamin C, magnesium, manganese, selenium and zinc. It is very important that intake of these vitamins and minerals be overseen by a physician, as many of them can be detrimental in incorrect dosages.

Proper care

The most important care for a patient with bedsores is the relief of pressure. Once a bedsore is found, pressure should immediately be lifted from the area and the patient turned at least every two hours to avoid aggravating the wound. Nursing homes and hospitals usually set programs to avoid the development of bedsores in bedridden patients such as using a standing frame to reduce pressure and ensuring dry sheets by using catheters or impermeable dressings. For individuals with paralysis, pressure shifting on a regular basis and using a cushion featuring pressure relief components can help prevent pressure wounds.

Pressure-distributive mattresses are used to reduce high values of pressure on prominent or bony areas of the body. However, methods to evaluate the efficacy of these products have only been developed in recent years.

Educating the caregiver

In the case that the patient will be returning to home care, it is very important to educate the family about how to treat their loved one's pressure ulcers. The cross-specialization wound team should train the caregiver in the proper way to turn the patient, how to properly dress the wound, how to properly nourish the patient, and how to deal with crisis, among other things.

As this is a very difficult undertaking, the caregiver may feel overburdened and depressed, so it may be best to bring in a psychological consult.

Wound intervention

Once the patient has reached the point that intervention is possible, there are many different options. For patients with Stages I and II ulcers, the wound care team should use guidelines established by the American

Medical Directors Association (AMDA) for the treatment of these low-grade sores.

For those with Stage III or IV ulcers, most interventions will likely include surgery such as a tissue flap, skin graft or other closure methods. A more recent intervention is Negative Pressure Wound Therapy, which is the application of topical negative pressure to the wound. This technique, developed by scientists at Wake Forest University, uses foam placed into the wound cavity which is then covered in a film which creates an airtight seal. Once this seal is established, the technician is able to remove exudate and other infectious materials in addition to aiding the body produce granulation tissue, the best bed for the creation of new skin.

Surgical options are often considered for non-healing wounds. When deep wounds are not responding well to standard medical procedures, consultation with a plastic surgeon may be needed to determine if reconstructive surgery is the best possible treatment. In a procedure called debriding, a scalpel may be used to remove dead tissue or other debris from Stage III and IV wounds. A surgical procedure called urinary (or fecal) diversion may also be used with incontinent patients to divert the flow of urinary or fecal material—this keeps the wound clean and encourages wound healing. Reconstruction involves the complete removal of the ulcerated area and surrounding damaged tissue (excision), debriding the bone, and reducing the amount of bacteria in the area with vigorous flushing (lavage) with saline solution. The surgical wound is then drained for a period of days until it is clear that no infection is present and that healing has begun. Plastic surgery may follow to close the wound with a flap (skin from another part of the body), providing a new tissue surface over the bone. For surgery to succeed, infection must not be present. Complications can occur after reconstructive surgery; these include bleeding under the skin (hematoma), wound infection, and the recurrence of pressure sores. Infection in deep wounds can progress to life-threatening systemic infection. Amputation may be required when a wound will not heal or when reconstructive surgery is not an option for a particular patient.

There are, unfortunately, contraindications to the use of negative pressure therapy. Most deal with the unprepared patient, one who has not gone through the previous steps toward recovery, but there are also wound characteristics that bar a patient from participating: a wound with inadequate circulation, a raw debridled wound, a wound with necrotised tissue and eschar, and a fibrotic wound. After Negative Pressure Wound Therapy, the patient should be reevaluated every two weeks to determine future therapy.

Complications

Pressure sores can trigger other ailments, cause patients considerable suffering, and be expensive to treat. Some complications include autonomic dysreflexia, bladder distension, osteomyelitis, pyarthroses, sepsis, amyloidosis, anemia, urethral fistula, gangrene and very rarely malignant transformation. Sores often recur because patients do not follow recommended treatment or develop seromas, hematomas, infections, or dehiscence. Paralytic patients are the most likely people to have pressure sores recur. In some cases, complications from pressure sores can be life-threatening. The most common causes of fatality stem from renal failure and amyloidosis.

Abuse and neglect by Nursing Homes

It is becoming one of the fastest growing industries in the legal system today secondary to the large increase in the elderly population." Some sources call abused seniors and dependant adults, the "silent victims." Experts estimate that at least 4% of all elders age 65 and over in the U.S. are abused. Bedsores are at the top of the list of elder abuse cited by the legal system, followed by falls, fixtures, malnutrition and dehydration. In India the aged embers of the family, who suffer from chronic ailments are dumped in the garage of the house or in a charitable hospital, waiting for his/her death.

Most pressure sores can be prevented, and those which have formed need not necessarily get worse. Each patient's individual circumstances must be taken into consideration by the caregiver in order to develop a plan of care which will best assure the patient will not unnecessarily suffer from a pressure sore. The following generally represent some of the precautions which health care providers should, but too often fail to undertake:

1. An appropriate and thorough and systematic assessment must be made of the patient's risk for developing a pressure sore;
2. Appropriate periodic reassessment should be made of the patient's risk;
3. The patient should be bathed appropriately;
4. The patient's incontinence should be assessed and treated to assure that moisture on the skin does not contribute to the development of a pressure sore;
5. Appropriate nutrition and hydration must be maintained;
6. Repositioning of the patient should occur with a frequency to assure that the pressure is adequately relieved;
7. Use of appropriate support devices should be maintained to relieve pressure from troublesome areas;
8. Postural alignment, distribution of weight, balance and stability, and pressure relief should be considered when positioning persons in chairs or wheelchairs;
9. Appropriate lifting devices and techniques should be used to assure that shear and friction related injuries are avoided;
10. Education should be given to the patient, family, and caregivers on measures to be taken to avoid pressure sores, and appropriate documentation of such measures.

It is essential to remember that every individual is different, and has different risk factors, thus requiring a customized plan of care and diligence in carrying out the plan of care.

Prognosis

Firstly, aggressive, intensive treatment and wound management intervention by our fully licensed, experienced surgeons of Coast to Coast Wound Care is essential in assessing and caring for any signs of an ulceration in its earliest stages. Bedsores that are advanced and will not readily heal can require incision, drainage, skin flaps, skin grafts, and bone resection. Our surgeons can also provide conservative sharp bedside debridement of wounds, but wounds that are exceedingly progressed or unresponsive, may require plastic surgery. In later stages, also, deep craters may need skin grafting and other forms of reconstructive surgery.

Stages II, III, IV—In many cases, however, with skilled care, the prognosis for bedsores is good. Expertise bedside treatment can heal most Stage II bedsores within a few weeks or longer. If conservative methods fail to heal a Stage III or Stage IV bedsore, reconstructive surgery often can repair the damaged area. Without proper treatment, however, they can lead to: gangrene, osteomyelitis, fractures, sepsis, and other localized or systemic infections, increased cost of treatment, lengthen nursing home stays, or even cause death.

In spite of this, forecast issues, or overall 'prognosis' of bedsores, by their nature are still unpredictable, because of the many and diverse outcome possibilities; duration, health, complication, recovery prospects, survival rates, death rates, and other issues.

A clinical study on bedsores

In a study of a collaborative program involving 52 nursing homes around the country, The Journal of the American Geriatrics Society reported last August that team efforts had reduced the number of severe pressure ulcers acquired in-house by 69 percent. "Preventing pressure ulcers is a 24/7/365 kind of job," said Jeff West, a clinical reviewer at Qualis Health in Seattle, who helped to set-up the collaborative in 2003. "It's not as if one person can get it all done. And if it fails just a little bit, just during the weekends, for instance, you're not going to get the results. It takes tremendous consistency." At the Lutheran Home in Fort Wayne, Indiana, for instance, "the laundry workers helped us see that some clothes weren't fitting the residents properly and were restricting their skin," said Jeanie Langschied, a registered nurse there. The kitchen staff began putting protein powders in cookies to boost nutrition. They added buffet dining, so residents would not remain in one position for so long, compressing fragile skin.

Even the beauty shop "realized that wait times needed to decrease," Langschied said, and residents should be repositioned while getting their hair done. "It was all departments looking at everything, and it was just amazing the information that flowed through."

Lutheran Home was one of the 52 facilities that took part in the collaborative, sponsored by the Centers for Medicare and Medicaid Services. Dr. Joanne Lynn, who helped begin the project when she was a senior natural scientist with the RAND Corporation (she has since joined the Medicare centers), said the goal was to educate nursing home workers in bedsore prevention and to encourage them to come up with creative, low-tech solutions of their own. "It was a combination of education, cheerleading and something like systems engineering," Lynn recalled.

The number of superficial bedsores did not decrease to a statistically significant degree, for reasons that are unclear.

At David Place, a nursing home in David City, Nebraska, staff members say they focused on assessing each resident's risk for bedsores, and noted this risk on the assignment sheets used by nursing assistants.

"The residents at highest risk," said Dan Smith, director of nursing, "would be the last up for meals and the first down after meals so they would not be in their wheelchairs for long periods of time putting pressure on their bottoms." Residents at risk from weight loss were given yellow plates, so that staff members would remember to encourage them to eat more.

David Place also bought new mattresses made of high-density foam to reduce pressure in key areas. Staff members say they redoubled efforts to keep feet elevated with pillows so that bedsores would not develop on the heels. And they began to use new moisture barrier creams with residents who were incontinent, since lingering moisture can speed the development of sores.

Staff members at Palatka Health Care Center in Palatka, Florida, initiated a similar blend of measures. They created a "skin-watch action team," or SWAT, to identify vulnerable residents and to make sure that their heels were floated, that they were given pressure-reducing cushions and that they were repositioned frequently, said Carol Jones, a risk manager at the center. "We got the grass-roots level, the certified nursing assistants, much more involved, and they were held accountable," Jones said. If a bedsore began to develop, she said, "we'd ask them, how did this happen?"

Initially, as the collaborative collected data from participating facilities, the incidence of pressure ulcers did not appear to change, Lynn said. It was only when researchers focused on data for the most severe bedsores that they saw an improvement.

Clinicians document four stages of pressure ulcers, in which Stages 1 and 2 are superficial sores and Stages 3 and 4 are deep wounds that result from death of the skin and underlying tissues.

"In good care, almost all new stage 3 or 4 pressure ulcers show up fully formed," Lynn said, meaning that they do not begin as superficial bruises that then go deeper. The injury, she said, "appears to be in the deep tissues from the start, though it can take a few days for the extent of dead tissue to become apparent."

The deeper sores may have different underlying causes than the superficial ones, she said. But it is unclear why the less severe ones did not respond as well to the practices instituted by the collaborative.

Horn, of the Institute for Clinical Outcomes Research, praised the collaborative as "the first major national effort driven by Medicare to reduce pressure ulcers." But she said that better outcomes could be achieved if more nursing homes improved their documentation, so that all of the information on a given resident, including details on eating, urinary and bowel function, appeared on a single sheet, with key reminders to nursing assistants and other staff members about best practices.

Institutional change and work-flow redesign are critical, she added, given the high rates of turnover in nursing home staff across the country.

The changes need to become hard-wired in an organization, said West, of Qualis. "A lot of places do well when they have a lot of support," he said. "But it's hard to keep that momentum going. That's the real challenge."

Statewide efforts to reduce pressure ulcers are also under way in California, New Jersey, New York and elsewhere.

Bedsores are "a major quality-of-life issue, and a self-esteem issue," said Joanie Jones, a nurse at David Place in Nebraska. "No one wants to have sores on their bottom. I don't care how old you are. You still want your skin intact."

References

510(k)s Final Decisions Rendered for January 2004: DEVICE: MEDICAL MAGGOTS". FDA. http://www.fda.gov/cdrh/510k/sumjan04.html.

Alexander's Care of the Patient in Surgery by Jane C Rothrock, Thirteenth Edition, 2007. Mosby.

Bain DS, Ferguson-Pell M (2002). "Remote monitoring of sitting behavior of people with spinal cord injury". *J Rehabil Res Dev* 39(4): 513–20. PMID 17638148.

Brem H, Kirsner RS, Falanga V (2004). "Protocol for the successful treatment of venous ulcers". *Am. J. Surg.* 188 (1A Suppl): 1–8. doi:10.1016/S0002-9610(03)00284-8. PMID 15223495.

Jiricka MK, Ryan P, Carvalho MA, Bukvich J (1995). "Pressure ulcer risk factors in an ICU population". *Am. J. Crit. Care* 4(5): 361–7. PMID 7489039.

Niezgoda JA, Mendez-Eastman S (2006). "*The effective management of pressure ulcers*". *Adv Skin Wound Care* 19 Suppl 1: 3–15. PMID 16565615. http://meta.wkhealth.com/pt/pt-core/template-journal/lwwgateway/media/landingpage.htm?an=00129334-200601001-00001.

Pressure ulcers in America: prevalence, incidence, and implications for the future. An executive summary of the National Pressure Ulcer Advisory Panel monograph". *Adv Skin Wound Care* 14(4): 208–15. 2001. *PMID 11902346.* http://meta.wkhealth.com/pt/pt-core/template-journal/lwwgateway/media/landingpage.htm?issn=1527-7941&volume=14&issue=4&spage=208.

Thomas DR, Diebold MR, Eggemeyer LM (2005). "A controlled, randomized, comparative study of a radiant heat bandage on the healing of stage 3-4 pressure ulcers: a pilot study". *J Am Med Dir Assoc* 6(1): 46–9. doi:10.1016/j.jamda.2004.12.007. PMID 15871870.

APPENDIX

HOSPITAL PROJECT REDUCES 'BEDSORES' TO AN INDUSTRY LOW

By : *Senaida (Cindy) Garza, Veronica Okere, Jackson Igbinoba, Kristi Novosad and Carolyn Pexton*

Lying in a hospital bed, patients can receive the best that medical knowledge, compassion and technology have to offer. But they also can be at risk. A lack of mobility—especially for a prolonged period of time—can increase the chance of developing bedsores, or pressure ulcers as they are most often referred to among practitioners. Pressure ulcers are lesions caused by unrelieved pressure, which leads to damage in underlying tissue.

This condition is a major concern for both patients and caregivers. Along with the obvious cost in terms of human suffering, hospitals spend at least $2.2 billion every year treating pressure ulcers.

Safety and quality are top priorities at Memorial Hermann Southwest Hospital in Houston, Texas, USA, and methods such as Lean Six Sigma and Work-Out are among the hospital's strategies to help improve the patient care environment. When the hospital found it had a 12 percent incidence of pressure ulcers in 2004—exceeding the 7 percent national average—it put a team in place and launched a project to reduce the incidence of hospital-acquired pressure ulcers by half within a nine-month period.

They outlined several anticipated benefits from the project:

- Raise customer satisfaction through better skin and wound care.
- Avoid the risk of lawsuits.
- Avoid fines from regulatory agency (Centers for Medicare and Medicaid Services).
- Reduce specialty bed rental cost by $125,000.
- Reduce length of stay associated with Stage 3, Stage 4 and "unable-to-stage" pressure ulcers.
- Increase International Classification of Diseases coding for pressure ulcers.
- Reduce supply costs.

Beginning the Team Effort

The team included three nurses—a Black Belt guiding the process and two Green Belts. Eventually skin and wound Champions were included to enact specific changes. The team also received input from a physician and a certified wound-ostomy-continence nurse.

The project targeted any area where pressure ulcer prevention and reduction should be a main concern, and excluded the normal newborn nursery unit, emergency department (at least in the beginning) and labor and delivery. A defect was defined as a patient with one or more pressure ulcers acquired while in the hospital.

Various stakeholders in the organization were consulted to collect the voice of the customer. This provided valuable information on incidence rates, process steps and potential factors that may lead to pressure ulcers. The team also examined data from other hospitals to compare performance and identify best practices.

Team members also made sure that the process they were using for data collection would be accurate. Tools such as gage R&R addressed inconsistencies, and provided all the required information. The skin and wound Champions used this process to gather data from each room. They also used the Braden Scale to score a patient's risk for developing pressure ulcers. The scale is comprised of six subscales that measure functional capabilities—sensory perception, moisture, activity, mobility, nutrition, and friction and shear. A lower Braden Scale score indicates lower levels of functioning.

Keys: Communication and Focus

Before the team could move ahead with analysis, it had to be sure the skin and wound Champions could accurately identify a wound, beyond the normal assessment capabilities. Expertise and oversight from a newly hired wound-ostomy-continence nurse proved valuable in this regard.

Communication also was a key element in the team's success, as it sought to build awareness and acceptance for the initiative. The team developed an elevator speech as a brief, consistent description of the project and used change acceleration process tools to foster better understanding and participation.

A fishbone diagram captured any underlying factors such as personnel, materials and environment, and helped the team narrow its focus on the most critical elements. Interestingly, nurses surfaced as a more pivotal group than physicians in terms of critical Xs.

During the Analyze phase, the team also effectively used failure mode and effects analysis (FMEA) to determine how a patient might acquire a pressure ulcer. Through FMEA, the team was able to review and improve existing safeguards to catch opportunities for failure. Tools such as FMEA and regression analysis revealed important information and helped to set the right priorities and direction for the project.

Solutions: Piloting New Procedures

The nurses had been empowered to begin planning and implementing three pilots during the Improve phase. The team conducted a Work-Out session to get everyone involved in creating workable solutions.

Pilot A involved weekly skin documentation audits using a tool based on chart review. Skin and wound Champions would note whether a skin assessment and Braden Scale score had been done both upon admission and then on a daily basis. Additional elements were added later. After a successful two-week pilot, the process moved to other units of the hospital.

Pilot B involved nurse-to-nurse communication to increase reporting on the patient's skin status, Braden Scale score and interventions. Some areas audio tape reports from shift to shift, so skin and wound Champions would ask nurses not to erase reports before an audit could be performed. The intensive care unit implemented "daily interdisciplinary rounds" which involves pharmacists, infection control and a case manager coming together to discuss a patient. This provided the opportunity to talk about the Braden Scale score or skin status and treatment. Pilot B also was monitored for two weeks before taking it hospital-wide.

Nurse-to-physician communication was identified as the third pilot, but a decision was made to postpone this phase until nurses completed their process changes. They would then work with physician Champions to develop new skin and wound management protocols.

Figure 9.1: Pressure Ulcers Acquired in Memorial Hermann

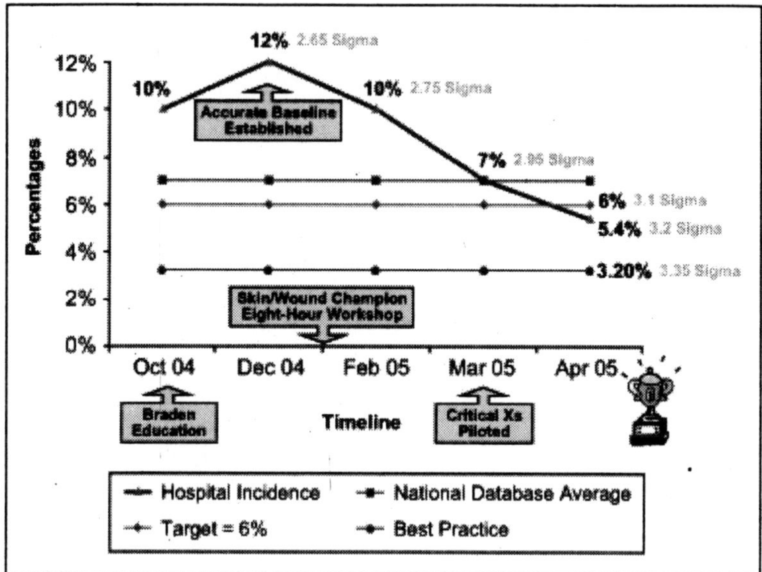

Results an Industry Best

When new procedures were in place and functioning, the hospital saw excellent results. In the Control phase, the team surpassed its goal of 6 percent (a 50-percent reduction), and actually achieved a rate of just 5.4 percent. This subsequently improved to 2.7 percent, considered the best practice in the industry. Memorial Hermann Southwest Hospital was able to reduce hospital-acquired pressure ulcers by 78 percent. Along with safety and quality improvement, the financial benefits from the project include a $1.2 million cost savings within the first six months and a projected $2.4 million annualized cost savings.

Skin audits and monitoring continues to make sure the results are maintained. The team found that one of the most positive outcomes of the project was development of a strong network among the nurses. Better collaboration and communication should translate to providing better care for patients.

TABLE 9.1

Implement Process Control: Risk Assessment Plan

Risk Element	*Probability*	*Impact*	*Total*	*Abatement Plan*
Skin Assessment Documentation (Admission/Daily) Not Performed Documentation	3	5	15	> Weekly Skin Assessment Audits with Reports to Directors > Daily Pressure Ulcer Reporting (Charge Nurse) > Nurse-to-Nurse Shift Report
Braden Pressure Ulcer Risk Score (Admission/Daily) Not Performed	3	5	15	> Weekly Skin Assessment Documentation Audits with Reports to Directors > Nurse-to-Nurse Shift Report
Pressure Ulcers Not Managed	3	5	15	> Daily Pressure Ulcer Reporting (Charge Nurse) > Wound Documentation Form > Wound Management Protocol > Stage 1 and 2 Pressure Ulcers are Reported to Skin/Wound Champions > Stage 3 and 4 Pressure Ulcers are Reported to Certified Wound-Ostomy
Continence Nurse Skin/Wound Team Commitment Declines	1	5	5	> Project Champions Identified to Lead Team > Team Members to Oversee Initiatives Specialty Bed Rentals Fall
Out of Protocol	1	3	3	> Sign-on Provided

APPENDIX I

TOTAL QUALITY MANAGEMENT

A. Chakravarti (JAHA, Vol. 15, No. 1, 5-6)

The last decade has witnessed a revolutionary array in health care dimensions. Terms like "Total Quality Management", 'ISO-9000', 'Continuous Quality Management', 'Re-engineering', Benchmarking and Accreditation have embraced and got incorporated in the delivery of health care services. Globalization, economic liberalization, privatization of health services, patient's enhanced awareness and expectations from providers of health care have made 'Quality' an inseparable part of the health care delivery system.

To achieve quality is thus an essential ingredient and to formulate, evaluate standards as per predetermined objectives is a requisite which has become universally applicable to all health care institutions.

Total Quality Management (TQM) and Accreditation are two main strategic essentials which have to be initiated, evolved and sustained in all health care institutions. These are imperative managerial tools to successfully function a complex, matrix and a multidisciplinary institution, i.e. the modern hospital.

Quality is not the end; it is a means to an end. Quality is not an absolute standard but must be worked at and consciously achieved. Quality in health care institutions is different from other organizations since the product, i.e. health care is a multifaceted and multidimensional product and it delivered personally to the customer. Interaction between the provider and consumer significantly affects perception of quality.

TQM is a philosophy as well as a set of guiding principles and practices that represent the foundations of a continuously improving organization. It integrates fundamental management techniques, existing improvement efforts, futuristic quality plans, innovations and their successful implementation.

In the management of any type of system, success can most readily be attained if appropriate goals are first established. The development of appropriate hospital standards provides these goals. Hospital administrators may then focus an attaining levels of care, that although challenging are achievable. With the availability of standards, managers are less likely to become solely occupied by day-to-day problems and more likely to place some effort in a proactive search for institutional improvement.

A successful accreditation programme is educational in nature rather than punitive. The standards that are developed should facilitate improvement in quality of care, must be realistic and achievable within the available resources.

The standards used in accreditation programmes previously focused on structural evaluation but now attention is being given also to outcome evaluation. Accreditation programmes are operated to ensure that good quality services are provided by health institutions, their evaluation standards contain all the components of quality care. Modern accreditation programmes contain all aspects of the three components of quality care, i.e. structure, process and outcome. A modern hospital is a matrix organization, an amalgam of human resources, architecture wonders and technological advancement. Traditional Quality Assurance efforts are focused on retrospective review of documented patient care mainly in form of conventional medical audits. Outcome in the form of patient review are not included in these audits. TQM focuses on all the facets of effectiveness and efficiency in an organization. In traditional Quality Assurance, effort is to be achieve local or national standards, however in TQM attempts are also made.

Operation Room Utilization

- There is marked difference in utilization of operation theatres between the perception of surgical consultants and reality.
- Non-availability of anesthetic service after 14.30 hrs., improper utilization of time between two surgeries and late starting of OTs are important areas needing attention of Hospital Administrators to improve utilization.
- There is an imperative need to expand OT timings, especially in view of long waiting lists.

A study was carried out at a tertiary care hospital with objective of assessment of utilization of OTs and identification of bottlenecks, if any for optimum utilization. The study revealed that the utilization though satisfactory could be further maximized by increasing the operational timing of OT, functioning two shifts of 08 hours each and performing minor procedures in minor OTs of the OPD. The study identified the main bottlenecks as the non-availability of the Operating Room Manual and non-adherence to OT timings.

The surgical suite typically consumes 9-10% of the hospital budget. Surgical suites once needed only 20% utilization to produce a positive bottom line. However, economics of the OR environment have changed dramatically in the past 25 years. Technological advances like minimally invasive surgery which need costly equipment, payments based on diagnosis related groups, captivated payment and discounted fee—for service have all significantly reduced margins in the surgical business. It is therefore, not surprising that this area is earmarked by many hospitals as a place to reduce expenses. All of us who work in the OR must be cost efficient and must maximize productivity for long-term success. Achieving these goals requires reliable data to help various stakeholders, chief executive officer, chief financial officer, nurses, surgeons and anesthetists—all have to align what sometimes appear as disparate goals. We need to examine traditional OR management practices. Traditional utilization measurements that look only at the time patients are in the OR reward surgeons for occupying ORs but do not addresses cost efficiency or productivity. One measure of how well an OR function: is the "utilization".

OR utilization is defined by Donham and colleagues as the quotient of hours of OR time actually used during elective resource hours and the total number of elective resource hours available for use Optimum utilization of the OT time has always been a priority area for Hospital Administrators. Baker had opined that accurate records, weekly analysis of recorded data, establishment of operating room rules and regulations and strict adherence to and enforcement of approved policies and procedures are essential ingredients for an efficient operating of an operating room. Thus it is clear that study of operating room records can provide means of assessment of the degree of utilization of operation theatres.

Analysis of the data collected from various O.Ts. with regard to O.T. utilization revealed that by and large all the O.T.s are adequately utilized as per the current working schedule. The overall O.T. Utilization % of M.O.T. Complex was 90.4%. The average O.T. case start time was 8.45 a.m., case end time was 3.55 p.m. and theatre closure time was 6.30 p.m. (Table 4)

Resource hours—total number of hours scheduled to be available for performance of procedures (i.e. the sum of all available block time and open time). Taking 5½ days a week and 8 hours a day as theatre resource time, it was found that in O.T.-2, 3, 4, 5, 6, 9 and 10 resource hours were fully utilized. (7, 12 to 7.47 hours). O.T.-7 was under utilized with utilization of 6.20 hours of resource time. O.T.-8, 8A and 11 were running beyond resource hours and are over utilized (utilization hours: 8.12 to 8.18 hours).

Room Clean up time—time from patient out of room to room clean-up finished and next case taken. The clean up time ranged from 5 minutes (when O.T. was not cleaned and next case was taken up immediately) as in O.T.-8A (ENT minor cases) and O.T.-11 (Ped. Surgery) to 26.6 minutes as in O.T.-2 where lengthy, HCV and HbsAg positive and complicated cases were usually taken up. O.T.-4, 5 (General Surgery) and O.T.-7 (Urology) had clean up time of less than 10 minutes. The average clean up time of all OTs ranged between 10 to 15 minutes which is within the acceptable range Thus, it can be seen that not much time is wasted for cleaning the operation theatres.

Due to unrealistic scheduling and shortage of OT time it has been seen that nearly 26% of total cases posted in all the OTs are cancelled. Inaccurate prediction of the duration of surgical operations resulted in over utilization, under utilization and frustration for those involved in caring for patients coming to the OR. It was observed that each surgical service has a different use pattern for OR resources. Some surgical services work largely in allocated scheduled time and use very little out of scheduled time. Other surgical services regularly push in to after hours time starts; still others are in consistent in their pattern of utilization.

Medical Errors reflect on the quality

Health Care institutions of today are complex matrix organizations. Errors are bound to occur in any complex human endeavor, and health care is no exception. Medical errors are ubiquitous and the costs (human and financial) are substantial. Many practice systems have developed by evolution rather than design. The inherent faults that lead to errors are a result of the organizational pathologies—the "Vulnerable System Syndrome". Approaches to patient safety should focus on the latent errors, which represent the failure of system design and processes. The top priority must be to redesign systems geared to prevent, detect and minimize effects of undesirable combinations of design, performance, and circumstance. Safety improvement through system monitoring and feedback, and system and process redesign from aviation and nuclear power industries hold many lessons for health care. Health Care institutions with patient safety as high priority should have a blame-free, non-punitive system for reporting errors in medical care to peer-review protected committees that are empowered to institute changes for system-wide improvements to prevent future errors.

Newspaper and television stories of catastrophic injuries occurring at the hands of clinicians spotlight the problem of medical error but provide little insight into its nature or magnitude. These horrific cases that make the headlines are just the tip of the iceberg.

A report from the Institute of Medicine, USA, states that around 100 000 patients a year die from preventable errors in hospitals in America. The annual toll exceeds the combined number of deaths and injuries from motor and air crashes, suicides, falls, poisonings, and drowning. Medical error is the third most frequent cause of death in Britain after cancer and heart disease.........kills four times more people than die from all other types of accidents. Around 850,000 medical errors occur per year resulting in up to 40,000 unintended patient deaths plus other harm in UK.

Medical errors are ubiquitous and the costs (human and financial) are substantial. Patients injured as a result of a medical error spend longer in hospital and have higher hospital costs. The length of stay increased by 1.9 to 2.2 days as a result of adverse drug events in Utah and Harvard studies. The annual costs of 'loss' is estimated to be around 20% of budget to NHS organizations, UK. The total expenditure on health care in India is expected to be more than double by the year 2012 to around Rs. 2,00,000 crore, according to the CII-Mckinsey study in 2002. It will be a huge amount lost due to medical errors, even if we go by the western standards of health care.

Brennan *et al* reviewed the medical charts of 30121 patients admitted to 51 acute care hospitals and found that 69% of injuries were caused by errors. The Harvard study of medical practice and a study of the quality of Australian health care, have found that medical errors occur in 4-17 percent of admissions and 30-51 percent of these adverse events were considered to be preventable and represent suboptimal care. In contrast, non-preventable adverse events suggest, that anticipated and unavoidable "complications" were present. Donchin *et al* have reported that 1.7 errors per patient per bed occurred in a medical-surgical intensive care unit, by an observational study at university hospital in Israel. All physicians, after all, have had the unwelcome experience of becoming what Wu calls "the second victim," being involved in an error or patient injury and feeling the attendant sense of guilt or remorse as responsible professionals. Familiar too, are Helmreich's findings that doctors, like pilots, tend to overestimate their ability to function flawlessly under adverse conditions, such as under the pressures of time, fatigue, or high anxiety.

VULNERABLE SYSTEM SYNDROME

Health Care institutions complexity derives from several factors, but perhaps the most significant is the presence of many defenses, barriers, safeguards, and administrative controls designed to protect potential victims from the local hazards. As in all well defended systems, a mishap requires some assistance from chance in order to bring about such a low probability event. The greater the complexity of the system, the more likely it is that these tactics can be deployed to support any of the three strategic components of error prevention, detection, and mitigation and most importantly, review.

Risk Management Process

An effective risk-management programme will be based on the following core elements:

- identifying each risk
- measuring the identified risk in terms of magnitude and frequency of occurrence
- prioritizing and controlling the risk
- constantly monitoring the effectiveness of control measures

STEPS IN THE RISK MANAGEMENT OF ERRORS

Based on the concepts of active and latent errors described above, accident analysis is generally broken down into the following steps:

Data collection: establishment of what happened through structured interviews, document review and/or field observation. These data are used to generate a sequence or timeline of events preceding and following the event. Data analysis: an iterative process to examine the sequence of events generated above with the goals of determining the common underlying factors—

- Establishment of how the event happened, by identification of active failures in the sequence.
- Establishment of why the event happened, through identification of latent failures in the sequence, which are generalisable.

Health Care practitioners themselves are best placed to identify where weak system's links may lie. So, practitioners must be encouraged to carry out self-assessment of risks and the effectiveness of the measures in place for managing those risks.18 Steps proposed are—

Step I : Identifying risks

Practitioners examine the processes within their work and identify the key operational risks, e.g., systems for repeat prescriptions, handling of test results18, checking instruments before and after surgery, receipt of telephone messages, and so on.

Step 2 : Determining the cause

Practitioners then identify the sort of situations that could cause a breakdown in care. For example, the absence of a system ensuring that the test results are seen.

Appendix 2

PARKWAY HEALTH GROUP OF HOSPITALS

It is one of Asia's leading health care providers. With an extensive network of hospitals and integrated health care facilities, the Group is committed to maintain a high standard of patient-centered quality health care.

PARKWAY'S THREE ACUTE CARE HOSPITALS IN SINGAPORE

MOUNT ELIZABETH, GLENEAGLES AND EAST SHORE

Offer the services of experienced and renowned specialists, quality nursing care from dedicated nursing staff and state of the art technology to keep it's services abreast with advanced medical care of international standard.

If you or your loved ones require advanced medical treatment in Singapore, we can be of assistance to help you identify the right medical institute and medical specialist. Seeking treatment abroad can be very expensive and we can help you with financial estimates and also help you book your hotels and apartment rooms.

SOME ADVANCED TREATMENTS

- Liver and renal transplants of Acute liver and renal failure cases.
- Specialized oncology procedures and bone marrow transplants and stem cell transplants.
- Position Emission Tomography (PET) functional assessment of growths and malignancies.
- The use of Stereoactic Radiosurgery for Neurological Tumours and Cerebral Aneurysms.
- Surgical Management of Epilepsy and Parkinson's disease.
- Advanced In-Vitro Fertilization (IVF) techniques for childless couples.
- Special CT scan procedures such as Virtual Colonoscopy and CT angiograms.
- Arthroscopic techniques for knee and shoulder injuries.
- Open Heart Surgery and specialized Angioplasty procedures including Cypher Stent Insertion.
- Electrophysiology studies and high radiofrequency catheter ablation for Arrhythmia problems.

- Lasik procedures for vision correction.
- Emergency Air Evacuation.

MEDICAL SPECIALISTS AND SERVICES AVAILABLE

- Cancer treatment
- Obstetrics
- Cardiology
- Ophthalmology
- Cardical Surgery
- Orthopaedic Surgery
- Clinical Medicine
- Paediatric Surgery
- Dental Surgery
- Paediatrics
- Dermatology
- Plastic Surgery
- E.N.T.
- Psychiatry
- Endocrinology
- Radiology
- Gastroenterology
- Renal Medicine
- General Surgery
- Respiratory Medicine
- Gynaecology
- Rheumatology
- Haematology
- Sleep Disorders
- Lasik
- Thoracic Surgery
- Neurology
- Vascular Surgery
- Neurosurgery
- Urology

INTERNATIONAL REACH

ParkwayHealth is constantly seeking new frontiers and establishing new business opportunities in existing and overseas markets to extend our network of services worldwide.

Embarking upon international growth, we strive to engage our expertise across the globe and deliver the finest quality in medical excellence that ParkwayHealth is widely recognized for.

Our current overseas ventures include:

- The Gleneagles JPMC Cardiac Centre (Brunei), and Cancer Centre in 2008

- The Shanghai Gleneagles International Medical and Surgical Centre (China)
- The Apollo Gleneagles Hospital (India)
- Pantai Irama Ventures Sdn Bhd-a partnership with Khazanah Nasional Berhad (Malaysia)
- Parkway Shenton International Clinic (Vietnam)

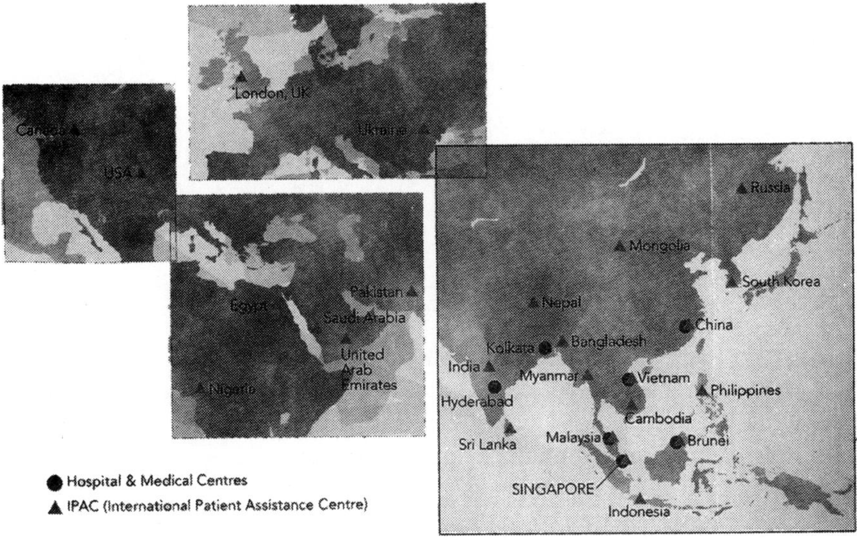

Our extended reach is further attributed to ParkwayHealth's growing network of International Patient Assistance Centres (IPAC) worldwide, Spanning the globe, our IPACs are poised to aid various localities including Egypt, India, Nigeria, United Kingdom, Russia and Saudi Arabia.

These successful facilities reflect ParkwayHealth's aim and efforts to become an international health care provider of choice.

ENTERPRISE STRATEGY MAP 2008-2010

Mission

To make a difference in people's lives through excellent patient care.

Vision

To be the global leader in value-based integrated health care.

Brand Essence

Community, Innovation, Excellence, Confidence, Global Leadership.

Values

People, Excellence, Results.

PEOPLE
Attract, Develop, Retain Engaged Employees
Create Competitive Compensation & Benefit Plans
Enhance Leadership Development & Succession Plans
Develop Competent Staff
Enhance Safety Culture
Build "Parkway Pride"& Employee Engagement Programmes
QUALITY
Achieve The Finest Clinical Outcomes
Meet Or Exceed Globally Recognized Clinical Outcomes & Benchmarks
Build Strong Relationships With Doctors & Other Partners
Build A Reputation For Clinical Excellence
Create Climate of Open Communication
SERVICE
Attain Highest Levels of Service Excellence
"Journey To Excellence"
Create Patient-focused Environment
Continuous Process Improvement
FINANCE
Meet And Exceed Our Financial Goals
Exceed International Benchmarks For Operational Efficiency
Increase Bargaining Power
Optimise Use of Facilities
Minimise Financial Risk
Improve Profitability Through Bundling
Improve Marketability of Programmes
GROWTH
Grow The System Per Our Strategic Plans
Singapore Operations
International Operations
Grow The Reit
Develop Good Networks In Target Markets

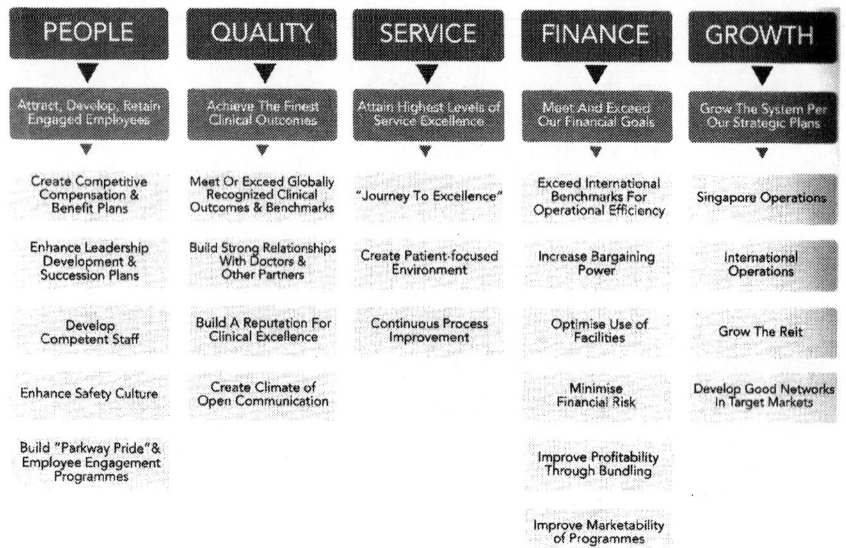

QUALITY TEAM AND FRAMEWORK

ParkwayHealth has developed a comprehensive and robust quality framework. Currently, the Quality Division is organized into five teams that look after each critical domain of quality system:

- Medical Affairs
- Quality Management
- Clinical Safety and Risk Management
- Infection Control
- Strategic Clinical Projects

These teams work closely with clinical departments. They oversee, administer and support the following quality programmes and initiatives:

- The Hospital Occurrence System
- Clinical Review Programme
- Clinical Quality Scorecard
- Clinical Practice Improvement Projects
- Environmental and Occupational Safety
- Clinical Safety and Risk Management Programme
- Infection Control Programme
- Monitoring of Clinical Outcomes for the 8 Clinical Programmes

In addition the Quality Division is also responsible for Accreditation and Licensing of our Hospitals. Parkway Hospitals in Singapore have the rare distinction of being the only private hospital group fully accredited by Joint Commission International (JCI).

STEM CELL TRANSPLANT

Previously incurable or possibly fatal blood disorders such as multiple myeloma, chronic lymphatic leukemia and Thalassaemia Major cannot be cured using conventional therapy, such as chemotherapy and radiotherapy.

However, in recent years, there have been dramatic breakthroughs in the field of hematology and stem cell transplant that offer new therapies help patients live longer and lead better quality lives.

With allogeneic stem cell transplant, cure rates for some of these previously "incurable" disorders are as high as 90%. Besides increasing survival rates, quality of life is also enhanced. Stem cell transplantation allows for much higher doses of chemotherapy than usual to achieve significantly higher cure rates.

The Haematology and Stem Cell Transplant (HSCT) Centre at Mount Elizabeth Hospital, Singapore was established to provide a full range of facilities and services to diagnose and treat blood disorders and blood cancers, including various types of anaemias, marrow aplasias, coagulation disorders, acute and chronic leukaemias, myelomas, lymphomas and lymphoproliferative disorders.

The Centre is spearheaded by Dr. Patrick Tan, a world renowned specialist who has achieved numerous medical milestones and pioneered revolutionary procedures. Amongst other milestones, Dr. Tan was the first in the world to successfully cure a Thalassaemia Major Sufferer with allogeneic stem cell transplant using matched unrelated donors. He was also the first in the world to successfully perform stem cell transplant without the need for high-dose chemotherapy or radiotherapy. Furthermore, he has also expanded the use of this technique for patients with solid tumours.

The Centre aims to help patients beat insurmountable odds to overcome their illness and give them a renewed chance in life.

What are haematopoietic stem cells?

Stem cells are blood cells at the earliest stage of development in the bone marrows. Within the bone marrow, stem cells develop into the different blood cells (red blood cells, white blood cells and platelets).

When cells fully mature, they are released into the bloodstream. Normally, most of the stem cells in the body are in the bone marrow and there are only very small numbers in the bloodstream.

However, it is possible to stimulate the stem cells to move into the bloodstream using injections of a special protein known as growth factor. Blood stem cells can be collected from the bone marrow or bloodstream. They are progenitors or "Mother of All Blood Cells" and have the ability to produce specialized cells and reproduce themselves.

Source of haematopoietic stem cells

- Compatible family member or an unrelated donor (allogeneic transplant)
- An identical twin (syngeniec transplant)
- Patient's own cells previously collected and suitably stored (autologous transplant)

Applications of Stem Cell Transplant

- Replacement therapy as applied to severe aplastic anaemai (marrow failure), and congenital immunodeficiency disorders.
- Gene therapy for Thalassaemia Major and Sickle Cell Anaemia.
- Cell and immunotherapy for the treatment of leukaemias, other haematological malignancies and malignant solid tumours.
- Stem cell rescue therapy, used mainly for certain tumours like lymphomas and myelomas.
- Tolerance induction when stem cell transplant is used to allow development of tolerance to a transplanted organ like the kidney, heart or liver.
- Restoration of deranged immune system as in severe auto-immune disorders.

Future Possibilities

They are currently exploring the use of non-myeloablative allogeneic stem cell as an immunotherapy for elderly patients and for patients with solid cancers, and expanding the use of allogeneic stem cell transplant for severe auto-immune disorders. There is also exploration of the usage of blood stem cell to induce tolerance after organ transplant. In the future, pluripotent stem cells in the marrow or cord blood may be used for organ regeneration. Through continuous research, our Centre is constantly venturing into new uncharted territories to discover new applications and clinical techniques.

Visitor's Guidelines

- Visitors, including family members who are not feeling well, or have fever/flu or other infections are not allowed to visit the patient.
- Restrict the number of visitors in the room.
- Patients and family members are advised not to visit other patients in the ward.
- Patients are encouraged to walk around the ward, but should avoid crowded areas.

Infections Control

- Handwashing is the single most effective way to prevent the spread of infection. Everyone is expected to wash their hands or use handrub before entering and upon leaving the patients room.
- Visitors may be asked to wear face masks when visiting the patient.

Food Guidelines

- Wash hands before eating.
- Eat balanced and nutrition's diet that is freshly prepared for you. Include high protein foods such as eggs, milk/dairy products, meat/poultry, fish, or nutritious supplement such as Ensure, Resource, etc. as much as possible each day.
- All uncooked food may carry risk of bacterial contamination. Do consult doctors or nurses before you eat any fresh fruit, raw food, spices and vegetables. Avoid eating pre-cut raw fruits and vegetables from the restaurant or food court.
- Perishable food (Pasteurized products; juices, milk, cheese, etc.) must be eaten within one hour of visit.
- Drinks are considered perishables. Please bring drinks in single serving sizes. Any opened container should be discarded after four hours.
- Drink amount of fluids as recommended by doctors. Fluids include; beverages (fruit, juice, milk, water, etc.), ice cream porridge and soups, etc.
- Consult doctor before consuming yoghurts or food containing cultured bacteria.

Storage of Food

- Store food at recommended temperature.
- Food kept in refrigerator must be labeled and dated.
- Discard expired food.
- Do not clutter refrigerator with too many items as it will affect the temperature.
- Food such as crackers, cookies and cereal (non-perishables) must be brought into the patient's room unopened.
- Non-perishable items should be stored in resalable containers.
- Use small packages to avoid leftovers.
- Avoid overstocking of food items in the room.

Hygiene Guidelines for Patient

Oral Care

- Rinse mouth frequently, at least four times daily with recommended mothwashes.
- Brush teeth twice a day with a soft bristle toothbrush if it becomes too painful or bleeding occurs, use sponge stick in place of toothbrush.
- Keep lip moist with lip moisturizer that contains paraffin.

Personal Hygiene

- Take shower or bath daily.
- Cover central line before showering to keep water off the dressing.
- Apply skin moisturizer to help skin retain its moisture.
- Avoid alcohol-based products to reduce dryness of skin.
- Avoid exposure to direct sunlight.

Environmental Guidelines

- Fresh or dried flowers and plants are not allowed in the patient's room.
- A family member should regularly wipe and clean patient's personal belonging such as handphone, toys, etc. with a cloth or paper towel dampened with soap and water.
- To help to keep the room as clean as possible, please minimize the number of personal belongings in the room.
- The corridor along the ward and nurses station are not a play area for children. No running, screaming or yelling is allowed. Children are not allowed to play with hospital equipment such as wheelchairs, trolleys and vital sings monitor.

LIVER TRANSPLANT UNIT OF GLENEAGLES, SINGAPORE

The Centre

In recent years, there has been an increase in the number of patients seeking treatment for liver diseases and those needing transplantation. Chronic liver disease as a result of cirrhosis and cancer has become one of the leading causes of death in Singapore. As such, there is a pressing need for a dedicated centre offering a comprehensive range or treatment services to manage these conditions.

Highly specialized and trained health care providers are critical in fulfilling the special needs of these patients.

The Asian Centre For Liver Disease and Transplantation at

Gleneagles Hospital, Singapore, is the first private medical centre in Asia dedicated to the treatment of all types of liver disease. From paediatric to adult patients.

The Centre is unique as it offers highly specialized and diverse medical expertise, with state-of-the-art equipment and facilities. All these are established within a single medical institution, providing comprehensive and seamless care for both children and adults with liver disease.

The Centre also comprises a Liver Intensive Care Unit to complement a highly successful Liver Transplant Programme.

The Asian Centre For Liver Disease and Transplantation features two main facilities—the Liver ICU and the Liver Transplant Programme. Both complement each other to professionally manage the medical and surgical needs of all types of liver disease effectively.

Asian Centre For Liver Disease and Transplantation (ACLDT)

The high medical standards and comprehensive health care facilities, couples with the accumulated experience with the accumulated experience of the ACLDT team in managing all types of liver disease endemic with the Asian region, provide immense benefits towards high quality patient care and better treatment outcomes.

The Centre also offers assistance to overseas patients in facilitating vise applications/extensions and suitable accommodation within walking distance of the hospital.

Among the liver disease treated:

Children

Biliary atresia; Cholecdochal cyst; Inborn error of metabolism; Portal hypertension; Polycytic liver disease; Liver abscess; Liver cancer; Acute Liver failure; Simple Liver Cyst; Budd-Chiari syndrome.

Adults

Viral hepatitis and cirrhosis; Liver cancer; Liver abscess; ile duct and gall bladder cancer; Pancreatic cancer; Acute and chronic pancratitis; Acute liver failure; Alcoholic cirrhosis; Biliary and gallbladder stones; Budd-Chiari syndrome; Portal hypertension.

The services of ACLDT, besides transplantation, range from medical treatment and advice for patients with chronic liver disease to chemotherapy and surgery for liver, gallbladder and pancreatic cancer.

The areas of expertise of this centre includes the following:

- Liver Transplantation
- Liver Surgery
- Pancreatic Surgery
- Gallbladder/Bile Duct Surgery
- Pediatric Liver Surgery and Transplantation

Interventional Radiology and Endoscopy such as:

- Radio-frequency ablation
- Transarterial chemo-embolisation
- Vascular and endoscopic stenting banding/sclero therapy of varices
- TIPSS.

Sophisticated Equipment and Instrument

State-of-the-art technologies and sophisticated equipment are used to facilitate disease treatment and patient recovery. Dedicated operating theaters are a place for liver transplants as well as for other major liver surgical procedures. Advanced radiological equipment is routinely used for liver and biliary diagnostic and interventional therapy.

Hi-tech equipment such as the Molecular Adsorbents Recirculating System (MARS) liver dialysis system support patients with liver failure until such time when a suitable donor organ is available for transplant to be performed. Other patient support systems eoutinely used in the Liver Intensive Care include the intracranial pressure monitoring system, PICO.

Strategic alliance with King's College Hospital Liver Failure Unit in London has been established to provide sophisticated surgical programmes, high level procedure protocols, as well as technology transfer.

Liver Intensive Care Unit

The dedicated Liver Intensive Care Unit, at Gleneagles Hospital, is the first in Asia to have in place a team of multidisiplianry professionals with expertise and extensive experience in the surgery and treatment of liver diseases. It comprises intensive care beds with all necessary specialized equipment dedicated for the treatment of patients with liver disease/failure. The nursing and medical personnel are highly experienced in providing special care needed for these patients.

Patients with liver failure throughout the region can be transported by emergency evacuation to the Liver Intensive care Unit for immediate and highly specialized treatment of this potentially fatal condition.

The Unit is equipped with sophisticated diagnostic tools, monitoring devices, ventilators, advanced kidney dialysis and liver dialysis machines such MARS. For the patients in severe fulminant liver failure, intra-device, PICO are used routinely.

The highly specialized Unit with its state-of-the-are equipment ensures that every patient receives the best possible treatment for their specific liver diseases.

Awards and Accreditation

- People developer Standard
- Asian Hospital Management Award 2004

- Singapore Superbrands 2004/2005
- National Excellent Service Award
- National Model for Work Redesign
- Singapore Quality Circle

GAMMA KNIFE® SURGERY

What is Gamma Knife® surgery?

Gamma Knife® surgery is a well established method to treat targets in the brain. Leksell Gamma Knife® is not a knife in the normal sense of the word. The doctor makes no incisions in the head. Instead, very precisely focused beams of radiation are directed to the treatment area in the brain. The shape an dose of the radiation in optimized to hit only the target, without damaging surrounding healthy tissue. Every year around 30,000 people worldwide undergo Gamma Knife® surgery, the treatment procedure is simple, more or less painless and straightforward.

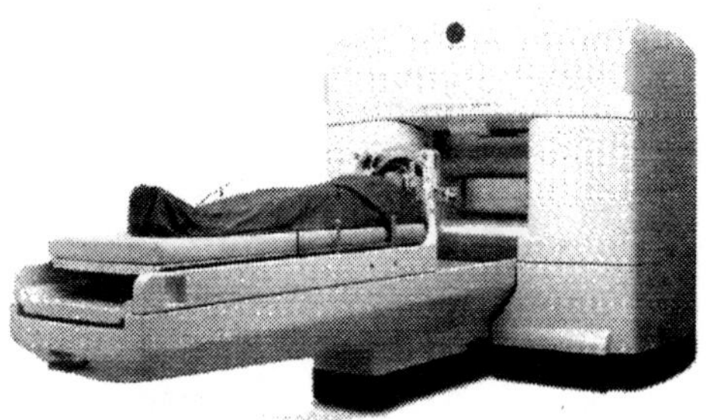

1. The Stereotactic frame

A lightweight metal frame is attached to your head. The frame ensures that the radiation beams can be exactly located and directed with precision to the target. A mild local anaesthetic is applied in the skin in your forehead.

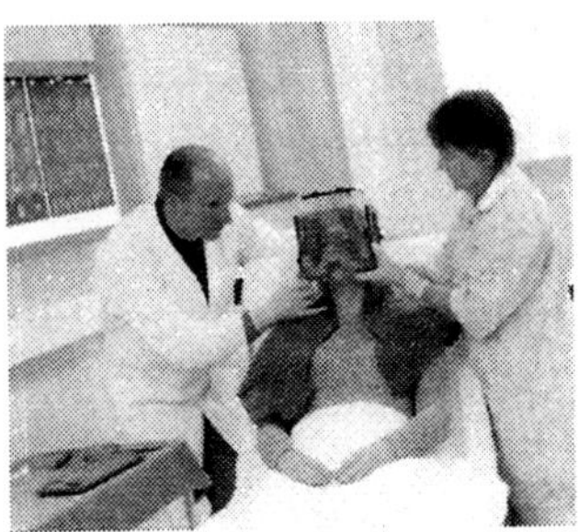

2. Imaging

Magnetic resonance imaging (MRI) computed tomography (CT) or angiography is required to determine the exact size, shape and position of the target in the brain. A coordinate box is placed on the head frame during the procedure.

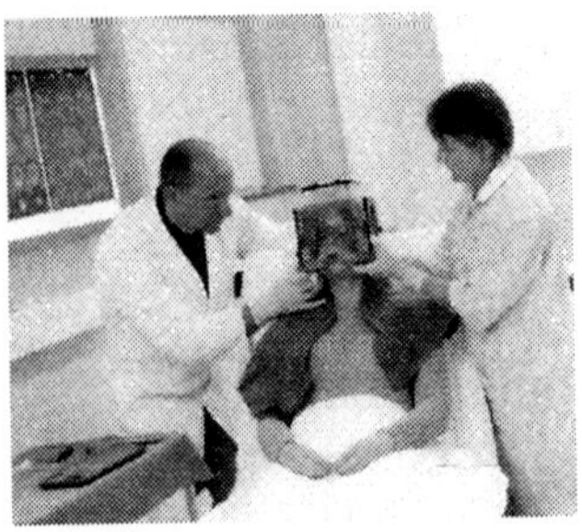

3. Treatment planning

Once your images have been taken, you can rest while your physician develops a treatment plan. The treatment plan is done in a specially designed software and computer and calculates how the treatment should be performed. This usually takes a couple of hours. Meanwhile you can rest.

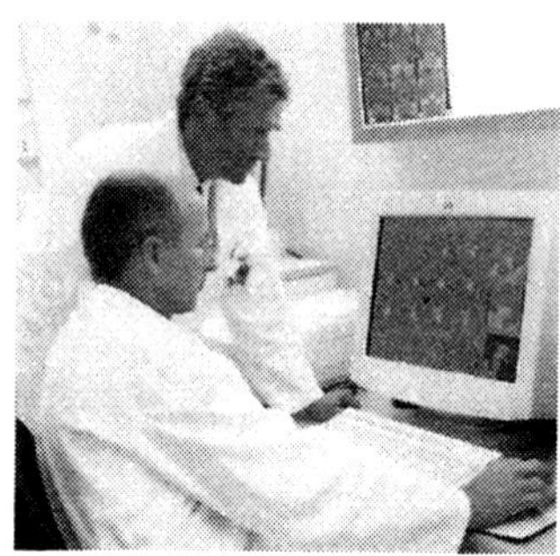

4. Treatment

You are awake during the procedure. When the treatment begins, the couch will move into the dome section of the unit. The treatment is silent and totally painless. It will last a few minutes to more than an hour, depending on your medical condition.

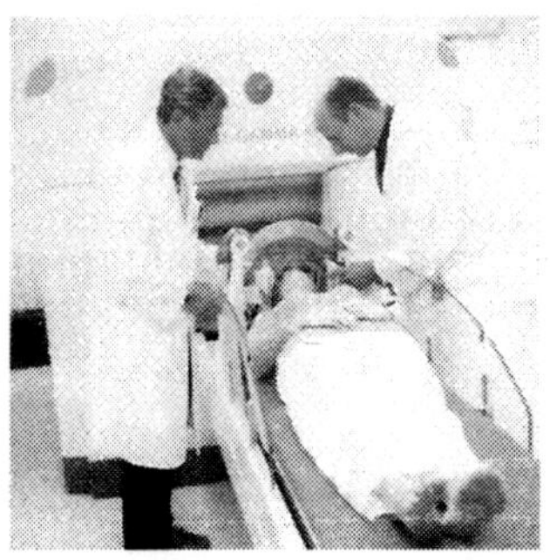

5. After treatment

When the treatment is complete, the head frame will be removed. Some patients might experience a mild ache or minor swelling where the frame was attached, but most report no problems. In a day or so you should be able to return to your normal routines.

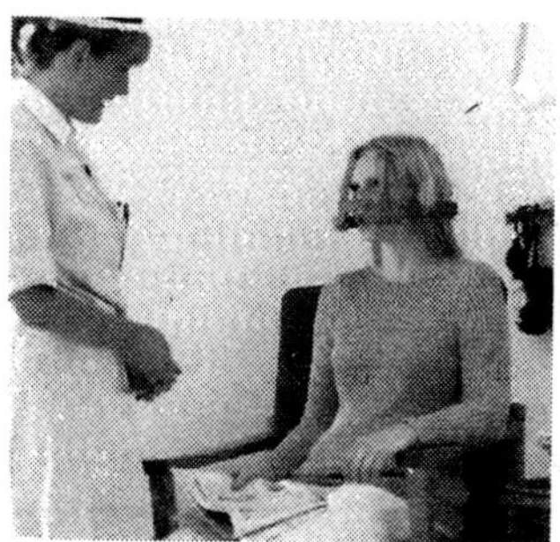

6. Follow-up

The effects of the treatment will occur over time. You doctor will stay in contact with you to assess the progress, which may include follow-up MRI, CT or angiography images. Always consult your doctor if you have any questions.

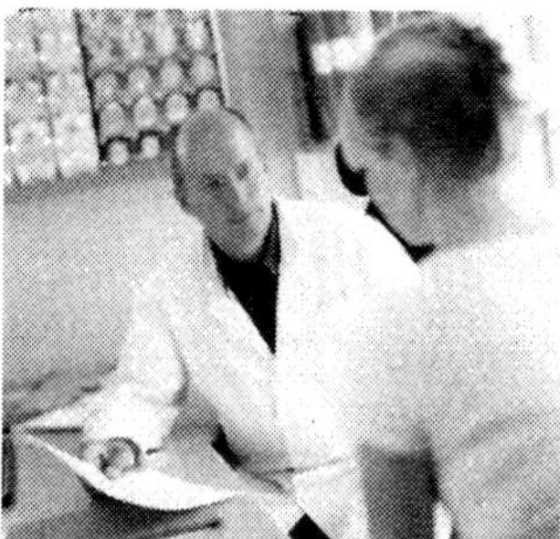

Neuro-Diagnostic Procedures

These include:

- Computerized Tomographic (CT) Scans—Multislice CT scanner
- MRI—Magnetic Resonance Imaging
- EEG—Electroncephlogram
- EMG—Electromyogram
- PET Scan—Positron Emission Tomography
- Digital Substraction Angiography

Stereotactic Radiosurgery/Fractionated Stereotactic Radiotherapy

Our hospitals use modern Linear Accelerator (LINAC) based systems and the Gamma Knife for treating intracranial tumors. Recovery time is shortened as a result as there is, generally, no need for hospitalization for these procedures.

Stereotactic Radiotherapy (SRT) uses one dose, often for small tumors, or a number of fractions of radiation for larger tumours and where the tumor is very closely located to a critical organ, such as the optic nerve. These treatments are non-invasive safe and have been proven to produce good results. Our complete instrument range includes:

- X-knife Stereotactic System (Mount Elizabeth Hospital)
- Tomo Therapy® (Mount Elizabeth Hospital)
- BrainLab Stereotactic Radiosurgery System (Gleneagles Hospital)
- Gamma Knife Radiosurgery (ParwayHealth Day Surgery and Medical Centre)

Key Focus Areas of the ParkwayHealth Neuroscience Clinical Programme

These specially prepared programmes, created to provide our patients assured collective expertise, include the following:

Stroke

Types of stroke include:

— Ischemic Stroke
— Hemorrhagic Stroke

Spine

Treatments include

— Degenerative Diseases of the Spine
— Spinal Tumor
— Spinal Traumas

Neuro-Oncology

Types of treated brain tumors include

— Brain Metastasis
— Glioma
— Low-Grade Glioma
— Astrocytoma
— Glioblastoma
— Oligodendroglioma
— Lymphoma
— Pineal Tumours/Lesions
— Meningioma
— Acoustic Neuroma
— Pituitary Adenoma

Blood Vessel Disorders That Affect The Brain

Type of treated disorders include

— Brain Aneurysm
— Arterio Venous Malformation (AVM)
— Cerebral Haemorrhage
— Cerebral Arteriosclerosis

Others

Treatment for the following are also included:

— Palmar Hyperhydraosis (Seaty Palms)
— Epilepsy
— Parkinson's Disease
— Migraine/Headache

ParkwayHealth Neuro-Rehabilitation Therapy Department provides a comprehensive range of services that includes physiotherapy, occupational therapy and speech therapy under the care and guidance of trained and experienced therapists. The services available for both inpatients and outpatients and it can also be delivered to recuperating patients the comfort of their homes.

The physiotherapist, together with the entire rehab team of doctors, occupational and speech therapists and home care nurses will come up with a treatment regime tailored to the patients need and with the maximum potential for recovery and function.

Who are The Specialists Involved?

- Radiation Therapists/Neurosurgeons
- Interventional Neuroradiologists/Endovascular Neurosurgeons
- Stroke Neurologists
- Neuroradiologists
- Vascular Neurosurgeons

The Radiologic Clinic's equipment at Novena Medical Centre includes:

1. Computerized Tomography

A 64-slice Computed Tomography uses x-rays and special computers to produce cross-sectional images of the body, giving detailed information for diagnosis. The advanced multislice CT equipment produces high resolution scans within a very short scanning time. The data can be reconstructed to produce 3D images with surface rendering, virtual colonoscopy, angiography and cardiac coronary vessels.

2. 1.5T Magnetic Resonance Imaging

Magnetic Resonance Imaging Creates images of the body using a powerful magnetic filed and radio waves only. This versatile, powerful and sensitive tool can generate images of the body from any angle.

3. Cardiac MRI

The Cardiac Magnetic Resonance Imaging (MRI) enables the structure and function of the heart to be studied, creating movie-like images of the beating heart to diagnose a variety of cardiovascular problems, such as viability or location of damaged heart muscles.

4. Ultrasound

Ultrasound imaging uses high-frequency sound waves, which are recorded and displayed as real-time visual images. The transducer, which produces sound waves, is placed on the patient's skin. Special transducers are also used in other openings of the body to take deeper images of the body.

5. Digital Mammography

Digital mammography uses the same technique as film screen mammography but the recorded images are stored directly onto a computer. These digital images can be enlarged or highlighted to allow for better viewing.

6. General Digital X-ray

A new computerized radiography x-ray system is designed for use on the chest, abdomen, pelvis, skull and extremities.

DIGITAL MAMMOGRAPHY

A study published by the *New England Journal of Medicine* revealed that digital mammography was significantly better in screening women in three categories, such as those:

- Under the age of 50;
- Of any age very dense or extremely dense breast;
- Of any age who are pre- or peri-menopausal who are defined as women who have had their final menstrual period within 12 months of their mammograms.

The study's results suggest that for women who fall into these three subgroups, digital mammography may be better than conventional film mammography at detecting breast cancer.

How should I prepare for a Digital Mammogram?

- The best time for a mammogram is one week following your period when you breasts are not tender.

- Wear a comfortable 2-piece outfit.
- Do not use deodorant, perfume, powder or ointment on your underarms or breasts.
- For an accurate diagnosis, you are required to answer a questionnaire before the start of the examination.

How is a Digital Mammogram done?

The Digital Mammogram is performed by a specially trained female radiographer.

- You will stand in front of the special digital x-ray machine.
- The radiographer will lift each breast and place it on a platform that holds the digital imaging detector. Then the breast is gradually pressed against the platform by a specially designed, clear plastic plate.

There might be some slight discomfort but this will only last a few seconds when some pressure is applied to make sure the digital images show as much of the breast as possible. This pressure is not harmful to your breast.

Why is compression of the Breast necessary?

- Even out the breast thickness so that all of the tissue can be visualized.
- Spread out the tissue so that small abnormality wont be obscured by overlying brat tissue.
- Allow the use of a lower x-ray dose since a thinner amount of breast tissue is imaged.
- Hold the breast still in order to eliminate blurring or the image caused by motion.
- Reduce x-ray scatter to increase sharpness of the image.

How often should I have a screening mammogram?

The Health Promotion Board of the Ministry of Health, Singapore, recommends that women aged 40-49 year have regular mammograms every year and women above 50 years of age, every two years.

Women who have a higher risk of developing breast cancer should see a doctor for advice. You may need to go for screening earlier and more frequently.

What are the benefits vs. risks?

Benefits

- Mammograms image the breast to detect small tumours. When

cancers are small, there are more treatment options and a cure is more likely. FFDM is a simple, quick and non-invasive procedure.

- Faster examinations of images as they are acquired in less than a minute.
- With a digital acquisition, it is possible to manipulate the image and reduce the number of extra images required, although the initial set of four images will still be necessary.
- Digital mammography uses relatively lower radiation compared to conventional analog mammogram. The average effective radiation dose from a digital mammogram is about 0.5 5mSv.

Risks

- Women should always inform their doctor or radiographer if there is a possibility that they may be pregnant.
- 5 to 15% of screening mammograms require more testing such as additional mammograms or ultrasound. Most of these tests turn out to be normal.

ROBOTIC SURGERY

What is Da Vinci Surgical System?

Mount Elizabeth Hospital's da Vinci Surgical System is a totally "intuitive" laparoscopic surgical robot that integrates the latest advancements in robotics and computer-enhanced technology with the surgeon's skills.

What are the Benefits of Using the Da Vinci Surgical System Over Traditional Methods of Open Surgery?

Some of the major benefits experienced by surgeons using the da Vinci Surgical System over traditional open methods of surgery include greater surgical precision, increase range of motion, improved dexterity and enhanced 3D visualization.

Benefits that patients have experienced over open surgery include, shorter hospital stay, less pain, less risk of infection, less blood loss and transfusions, less scarring, and faster recovery and return to normal daily activities.

This surgical robot is designed to enable your surgeon to be more precise, to advance his/her technique and to enhance his/her capability to perform complex minimal access surgery. The system replicates your surgeon's movements in real time. It cannot be programmed, nor can it make decisions on its own to move in any way or perform any type of surgical maneuvers without your surgeon's direct control.

What are The Procedures That Can Be Performed With The Da Vinci Surgical System?

Mount Elizabeth Hospital provides a wide spectrum of robotic enhanced surgeries.

Cardiac Procedures

- Endoscopic Single Vessel Beating Heart Bypass, LIMA-LAS Endoscopic Double Vessel Beating Heart Bypass, LIMA-LAD and RIMA-RCA
- IMA Harvesting
- Bilateral IMA Harvesting for Sternotomy Sparing CAGB
- Mitral Valve Repair
- Tricuspid Valve Repair
- Thrombectomy
- Pericardial Window
- Lobectomy
- Mediastinal Tumour Resection
- Pulmonary Wedge Resection
- Transthoracic Esophagectomy
- Thymectomy

General Surgery Procedures

- Nissen Fundoplication
- Cholecystectomy
- Hernia Repair
- Adrenaloectomy
- Esophagogastrectomy
- Gastric Bypass
- Colon Resection
- Pyloroplasty
- Heller Myotomy
- Gastroplaty
- Bowel Resection
- Splenectomy
- Sigmoidectomy
- Hemicolectomy
- Transhital Esophagenctomy

Urology Procedures

- Radical Prostatectomy
- Lymphadenectomy
- Uretero Transplant
- Pyeloplasty

- Ureterolithotomy
- Nephrectomy

Gynaecological Procedures

- Hysterectomy
- Myomectomy
- Radical Hysterectomy
- Tubal Reanastomosis
- Pelvic Floor Reconstruction.

WOCKHARDT GROUP OF HOSPITALS

Among the fastest growing hospital networks in Asia, it operates a chain of super-specialty hospitals in Mumbai, Bangalore, Hyderabad, Nagpur, Kolkata, Surat and Rajkot. Its flagship hospital in Mumbai is dedicated to Cardiac sciences, Neuro sciences, Orthopedics, Ophthalmology and Minimal Access Surgery. As a leading provider of Cardiology/Cardiac Surgery across India, the group operates heart hospitals in Bangalore, Mumbai, Hyderabad and Nagpur. In Kolkata, it runs a super-specialty kidney hospital.

Wockhardt Hospitals Group symbolizes state-of-the-art, high quality care that is comparable to the best in the world. It has an exclusive association in India with Harvard Medical International, the global arm of Harvard Medical School and works towards its mission of "one world, one medicine". Wockhardt Hospitals, Mumbai, recently became the first super-specialty hospital in South Asia to receive the coveted Joint Commission International Accreditation (JCI), which is the global benchmark in health care accreditation. Wockhardt Hospitals is the first hospital group in South Asia to be recognized by the American Blue Cross and Blue Shield association in its worldwide network of participating hospitals. It is recognized by 17 leading insurance providers across the globe, including CIGNA.

In keeping with its mission to expand the reach of quality health care in the country, the Group has launched a Super-Specialty hospital in Bangalore on Bannerghatta Road. This second Wockhardt Hospital in the city has 400 beds and five thrust areas—Cardiac sciences, Neuro sciences, Orthopedics, Women's Health and Minimal Access Surgery. This super-specialty center of medical excellence will provide a boost to critical care in the region and the prominence of Bangalore in the medical map of the world. Wockhardt Hospitals Group has already been a preferred health care destination for patients from Europe, USA, South Asia, South-East Asia, the Middle-East and Africa.

Our association with Harvard Medical International

As an associate hospital of Harvard Medical International (HMI) in India, Wockhardt Hospitals gain from the rich knowledge pool of various Harvard Associated Hospitals in the world and offer patients global standards in medical technology and clinical expertise. Together, "we commit to meet patient expectations through ongoing training, and create a new level of patient care delivery."

This association has helped Wockhardt Hospitals to stay at the forefront of medical technology and techniques, way ahead of the rest.

A self-supporting subsidiary of Harvard Medical School, Harvard Medical International serves as a catalyst in bringing together health care professionals from around the globe towards improving the delivery of health care through education, and implementing its vision that every citizen of the world has access to quality health care in his or her own country. Today, HMI has selective collaboration in 18 countries and 5 continents, working towards its mission, "One world, one medicine".

Patient-friendly

At the heart of Wockhardt lies its patient-friendly approach. Years of elaborate, minute planning have gone into making each feature of this 3-lakh sq ft facility easily accessible, so that a patient can get his or her work done in as little time as possible.

On the ground floor, adjacent to the 13-bed casualty/emergency department, are facilities to carry out all types of diagnosis usually associated with casualty cases so that patients can minimize the use of elevators.

The single-counter-multiple-function facility enables you to complete all registration and billing formalities at the same spot. Here, you can register as an in-patient, pay your bill or enquire about a doctor's availability.

An innovative concept for attendants of ICU patients is the waiting area in the critical care department. Unlike most hospitals, attendants of ICU patients can stay over in the hospital. In twin-sharing cubicles, the attendant gets a cot and a small storage space.

The multi-cuisine dining facility serves a wide variety in meals and snacks. For an occupant of a deluxe room, the elegant interiors and the view of an adjacent terrace garden are designed to make his or her stay not just comfortable but also pleasurable.

Facilities available at the hospital

- 2-hour accident and emergency services, including trauma treatment
- Ambulance services
- Blood bank
- Full service operating threatres including cardiac threatres
- Preventive health check
- Diagnostic and catheterization labotaroy
- Critical and emergency care
- Intensive care/coronary care/neonatal intensive
- Imaging facilities include a 64-slice CT scanner, 1.5 Tesla MRI, a complte Angioplasty (DSA) with CARE package (for Neurovascular Angiography), Fluoroscopy, ultrasound and X-ray.

- Diet Counselling
- Physiotherapy and rehabilitation
- Laboratory and microbiological services
- Stress management and yoga therapist
- 24-hour pharmacy
- Endoscopy unit
- Antenatal classes
- Women's wellness centre
- Labour delivery recovery Post-partum (LDRP) suites.

"Heart is Wockhardt" is how Wockhardt hospitals in Bangalore has come to be known as for the past 17 years. A centre for excellence in Interventional Cardiology and Cardiac Surgeires in the country, it has to its name many path-breaking procedures, such as the first-ever Awake Heart Surgery in India. It has earned the reputation of being a .country-wide leader in this speciality.

Wockhardt Hospitals Cunningham Road has been our first, single-speciality corporate heart hospital. This centre has performed more than 15,000 heart operation and 40,000 interventional cardiology procedures since its inception and has become a renowed tertiary heart care centre. The Institute is now a preferred destination for cardiac patients not only in India but also from neighbouring countries. It is also a teaching centre for clinicians from the sub-continent.

Our cardiac services are driven by an accomplished full-time team of 25 cardiologists and cardiac surgeons. They will continue to Wockhardt legacy of excellence in Heart care across both our facilities in Bangalore, on Bannerghatta Road and Cunnningham Road. A 50 bed ICCU, supported by a highly-trained paramedical and nursing team, is managed and monitored round the clock by our cardiologists to ensure timely care in cardiac emergencies. All these services are supported strongly by the most advanced technology, such as a flat-panel digital cathlab with stent boost software, 64-slice cardiac CT Scan and new generation bedside monitoring system in ICCU and post op SICU.

A dedicated department of pediatric cardiology/cardiac surgery with focused clinical teams provides a new dimension to our highly accomplished adult cardiac program.

Pediatric Cardiology and Cardiac Surgery

- Pediatric Cardiology
- Balloon Atrial Septostomy (BAS)
- Balloon Pulmonary Valvotomy (BPV)
- Balloon Aortic Valvuloplasty (BAV)
- Device Closure of ASD, VSD, PDA
- Embolization ofMAPCA, etc
- Complex Palliative and Collective Intervention

Pediatric Cardiac Surgery

- The entire gamut of cardiac diseases from a newborn to an adolescent
- Dedicated operating rooms and post-operative ICU with state-of-the-art equipment, pediatric cardiac intensivist and experienced staff round-the-clock to provide continuous pediatric care under the supervision of a senior pediatric intensivist and neonatologist.

Procedures performed

- Closed Heart Surgeries like BT Glenn Shunt, PDA Interruption and Coaractation Repair
- Simple Open Heart Surgeries, like ASD Closure and VSD Closure
- Complex Open Heart Surgeries, like Intra-cardiac Repairs, Arterial Switch Operation, Double Switch Operation and Rastelli Operation
- Valve Repairs, Replacements and ROSS Procedures
- ECMO facility

Adult Cardiology and Cardiac Surgery

Interventional Cardiology procedures

- Coronary Angiography, Angioplasty and Stenting
- Angiography and Angioplasty of arteries of neck, leg, arm and kidney
- EP Study Diagnostic and Ablation
- Permanent Pacemaker (Single and Double Chamber)
- Heart Failure Device and AICD Implantation
- Valvuloplasty—Mitral, Aortic, Pulmonary
- Device—ASD, VSD, PDA Closure, Coaractation Replacements
- Endovascular Aneurysm Repair
- Percutaneous Valve Replacements

Cardiothoracic and Vascular Surgery procedures

- Off Pump Bypass Surgeries (since 1992)
- Endoscopic Conduit Harvest for CABG
- Keyhole Bypass Surgery
- Valve Surgeries
  - Valve Repairs and Replacements
  - Maze Procedures for AF
  - ROSS Procedure
- Awake Heart Surgeries (on or off pump cardiac surgeries under

high thoracic epidural anesthesia. Post-operatively managed with patient-controlled, continuous epidural analgesia.

- Surgery for Heart Failure
  - Left Ventricle Remodeling
  - Left Ventricle Support Devices
- The entire gamut of Vascular and Thoracic Surgeries, including VATS (video assisted thoracic surgery)
- Major Aortic Aneurysm Surgeries

Brain and Spine

We believe in investing in the best of technology to enhance our quality of service. In Wockhardt Hospitals Brain and Spine, the advanced microscope with Neuro-nagivation and Endoscopic techniques assist our doctors in attaining precision while conducting complex neurosurgeries.

Wockhardt Hospitals Brain and Spine Care provides 24/7 care for all neurological injuries and emergency neuro-care. The vastly experienced team of Neurosurgeons and Neurologists, backed by the most comprehensive neuro-diagnostic and imaging facilities, positions the hospital among the best in the region. Being part of the comprehensive emergency services, the department caters not only to head an spine injuries but also to all neurological emergencies, poly-trauma and other medical emergencies. Neurological services extend to the very latest in diagnostic equipment such as EEG, ENMG, Video-monitoring 1.5 Telsa MRI and 64-Slice CT Scan.

Wockhardt Hospials Brain and Spine Centre is equipped with two dedicated state-of-the art operation theaters where all complex brain and spine surgeries, from pediatric to geriatric cases, can be performed with precision and complete safety. The operation rooms are equipped with semi-robotic microsopes, the neuro-nagivation facility, cranial and spinal endoscopy, MRI and CT compatible stereotaxy for functional neurosurgery. Minimal invasive techniques, being developed for complex brain and spine surgeons, make the centee among the few to offer such cutting-edge facilities in Inida.

All neurological disorders, including Epilespy, Movement Disorders, Cerebral Strokes and Degenerative Disorders are managed by experienced Neuro-physicians.

Outpatient Services

- Petiatric to Geriatric Neuosurgery Consultations
- Spine Clinic for backache, spondylosis, injury, deformities, tumors, etc.
- Neuro-oncology services
- Neuro-trauma services
- Neuro-rehabilitation and counseling centre
- Elecro-physiological evaluation

- Neuro-psychiatry
- Speech therapy
- Pain management

Inpatient Services

- *Neuro ICU*: For intensive care with complete monitoring facility, ventilator support and trained medical and para-medical staff for post-operative patients.
- *Neuro-HDU (High dependency unit)*: For operative and non-operative, dependent patients of stroke, paralysis, head and spine injury, epilepsy, etc. with intensive nursing care, physiotherapy and basic monitoring facilities.
- *Neuro-rehabilitation—Unit*: Complete with physiatrist, physiotherapists and psychiatrists.
- *Neuro wards*: Dedicated nursing, physiotherapy support in a paralytic-friendly environment.

Brain Surgical Services

- Microsurgery for Brain Tumors
- Endosocpic brain surgery
- Skull base surgery
- Brain trauma surgery
- Congenital cranial deformity
- Stereotaxic Brain Surgery Functional Neurosurgery
- Craniofacial Surgery with FMS (Facio-Maxillary Surgery)
- Brain Surgery for Abnormal Blood vessels
- Brain surgery for Epilepsy
- Brain Surgery for Removal of Blood Clots
- Interventional Neuro-endovascular Therapy for Cerebro-vascular Diseases and Tumors
- Pre-operative Embolization of Brain Lesion.

Surgical Services :

Slipped disc in the neck or lower back

- Microscopic lumbar discecetomy or decompression
- Microscopic anterior cervical discectomy
- Endoscopic discectomy

Lower back spondylosis with pressure on the Nerve/spinal stenosis

- Spinal Decompression with or without fusion
- Endoscopic fusion of the spine

Abnormal Curvature within the spine-scoliosis/kyphosis

- Thoracoscopic Deformity Correction
- Posterior Correction of Scoliosis or Kyphosis with Instrumentation

Degenerative disc diseases

- Minimally-invasive Spinal Fusion and Advanced Instrumentation
- Total Disc Replacement Surgery Spinal Deformity (congenital and acquired) Correction and Stabilization

Osteoporosis of the Spine

- Vertebroplasty
- Kyphoplasty

Slipped Vertebra in Children

- Spondylolisthesis
- Posterior spinal instrumentation

Other Spine surgeries

- TB spine-thoracoscopic spinal surgery with para-spinal abscess drainage
- Spine tumor surgery
- Spine trauma

Bone and Joint

The Bone and joint program at Wockhardt Hospitals makes it a center for excellence in orthopedics with highly-skilled clinical expertise. The hospital provides cutting-edge diagnostic facilities and treatment in orthopedics. It offers excellence in joint replacement surgeries, hip resurfacing and is equipped to treat all types of musculo-skeletal problems for adults, the elderly and children, ranging from minimally-invasive arthroscopic surgeries to complex trauma services.

The most advanced medical equipment emergency care provides the right of full-time orthopedic surgeons, highly experienced in complex and high velocity trauma care. Our computerized navigation and imaging facility ensures the most accurate treatments and joint replacements.

The center has ortho-specialists with micro-specialization in bi-columnar acetabular surgery, failed trauma services, infected joint replacement and neglected trauma fractures. Using the most advanced technology, our surgeons apply the minimal access surgery approach for fractures, which earlier required extensible surgeries.

A comprehensive support of rheumatology and physiotherapy services makes it a complete program.

Centre for Joint Replacements

Total Knee Replacement :

- Unicondylar Knee Replacemnet (which requires only a small incision and assures rapid recovery)
- Hi-flex Knees (where the patient can comfortably move and squat normally, which is not possible in conventional knee replacement)
- Failed or revision join replacement
- Infected Joint Replacement

Total Hip Replacement

- Cementless total Hip replacement (less complicated in terms of fixation of prosthesis)
- Hip Resurfacing/Surface replacements artroplasty
- Cementless bipolar/partial Hip replacements in the elderly with fracture neck femur
- Shoulder Replacement
- Elbow replacement
- Revision Joint Repalcement—for patients whose earlier replacements have failed.

Orthopedic Oncology

- A large experience in custom-made prosthesis
- Extra-Corporeal Irradiation and Re-implantation, followed by Joint Replacement

Complex Trauma Service

- Poly-trauma
- Failed Trauma and Neglected Trauma Services
- Acetabular Fracture Hxation/Pelvic Fractures

Pediatric Orthopedics

- Congenital Deformities—Club Feet, Dislocated Hips, etc.
- Cerebral Palsy with Gate Analysis and Management, Contractures Treatment through Surgery and Botox injection
- Polio (Surgeries, Deformity Correction, Orthotic Acid Prescription

Sports Medicine

- Knee Arthroscopy—ACL reconstructions and Menisectomy
- Shoulder Arthroscopy

Other Services

- Medical or Surgical Management of Rheumatoid Arthritis, Osteoarthritis, Juvenile Arthritis, etc.
- Ligament Repair and Reconstruction
- Arthroscopy and Arthroscopic Treatment
- Physiotherapy and Rehabilitation Program
- Patient Education Program

Women Care

Undoubtedly, the women today faces many challenges because of pressures at the workplace and home. She also needs to take charge of the well-being of her family. To attain this balance, she needs to matianin a healthy lifestyle. We, at Wockhardt understand her requirements. In the homely and caring atmosphere at Wockhardt Hospitals Women Care, she can avail of our extended wellness programs and treatments for healthy living. Specially tained care-givers ensure each women gets the best out of a wellness program or treatment.

A 30,000 sq. ft. area is exclusively dedicated to Woman care with consultation suites, delivery room, operating rooms, with a 112-room neo-natal ICU, a nursery and 13 LDRP (Labour Delivery Recogery Postpartum) rooms. Our women health care programs, besides the operative minimal access gynecological services, also includes preventive clinics (early diagnosis of breast, uterine, ovarian and cervical cancer), infertility clinics and menopausal clinics.

The centre offers exclusive facilities, service, training, preventive and recovery programs required for today's woman. The centre emanates a homely and pleasant atmosphere unlike that of a conventional hospital.

Women's Health Services

Exclusive Clinics for all age groups

- Menopausal clinics
- Post-menopausal Osteoporosis Clinics
- Counselling for Depression and stress

Preventive Clinics for Adolescents

- Early Diagnosis of cancer—uterus, ovaries, cervix, etc.

Infertility clinics

- Women's endocrinology
- Reproductive endocrinology

Minimal Access Gynecological Surgeries

- Laparoscopic hysterectomy
- Laparoscopic tubectomy
- Laparoscopic overectomy

Operative Gynecological Surgeries

- Hysterectomy
- Ovaraian Cysts
- Malignancies
- Surgeries on the Tube
- Removal of fibroids

Training and Counselling

- Breathing Techniques
- Relaxation techniques
- Breast-Feeding Classes

Wockhardt Hospital Woman Care offers 13 private and luxurious LDRP suites where the newborn can stay with the parents after delivery

Inviting every mother-to-be to our exclusive birthing centre.....

If childbirth is one of the most pleasurable moments in life, let the Wockhardt birthing experience enrich the experience for you. With the unqiue 'Birth centre' facility, through the LDRP (Labour Delivery recovery Postpartum) concept, the mother-to-be can minimize the discomforts of childbirth.

The LDRP suite is a concept at Wockhardt Hospital where birthing suits obviate the need of a labour room and help the entire family cherish the once-in-a-lifetime moment. The beds turn into delivery tables when labour progresses. The smart interiors, done in light finish wood and burnt orange add cheer to the place. These luxurious suites have all the necessary medical apparatus required for a safe and hassle-free delivery.

The center allows the women to choose the kind of delivery, the kind of pain relief and various services on offer. She has a choice between the conventional birthing facilities to exclusive birthing suites. We strongly believe that the family has a vital role to play in making the labour process easy. The private suites are designed for the family to experience each phase of birth in a single, luxurious, family-centered setting, making it a memorable experience for all.

Wockhardt is the only hospital in Bangalore to offer 13 private birthing suites with the most modern concepts in obstetric care.

Women Health Services

Our care program promotes normal delivery through various training, counseling and techniques in the process of birthing, one of life's most rewarding experience. Mothers and babies will have to access to all the resourcse of Wockhardt Women Care Centre in a wide range of specialties. We, at Wockhardt Hospitals, offer special neonatal care when extra medical attention is required. The Neonatal Intensive Care Unit is fully equipped to handle babies with severe complications.

Ante-Natal and post-natal classes

- The mother-to-be is taught about safe delivery, exercises, during delivery, ante-natal counseling and labour preparation.
- Lamaze, relaxation and breathing techniques are taught to help in normal delivery.
- Husbands are invited for all counseling classes throughout the pregnancy for diet, exercise and support programes.
- Childbirth education, teen-parenting, grand-parenting and sibling care classes are offered.
- Post-delivery classes and postpartum care—post-delivery exercises, breast-feeding, care of the child, drugs to avoid, diet habits, etc.

Minimal Access Surgery

The field of surgery is undergoing constant evolution. Traditionally, large incisions were a must for successful surgeries, where surgeons had to make wide (>20cm) and deep incision to reach (access) organs for removal or repair. Such large incisions cause pain and are prone to infections/hemia and give a poor cosmetic result. Exposure was the key to a safe and successful operation. Exposure is still essential for a safe and successful operation, except that it can now be provided with minimal skin incision and by using a miniature access approach. For Minimal Access Surgery (MAS), just 2-4 micro incisions of 0.5 cm are done. With the minimal access (endoscopic) approach, surgeons can now achieve the same end results.

Wockhardt Hospitals Minimal Access Surgery is dedicated to performing surgical procedures using minimal access techniques, so that patients enjoy faster recovery and fewer post-surgical complications, and thus minimize surgical trauma, pain and blood loss. The patient's hospital stay is shortened and his or her post-surgery aesthetics improved.

Today, Wockhardt Hosptials has leader in Laparoscopic and Endoscopic surgeries who operate with computer-assisted video-navigational tools. They are assisted by state-of-the-art facilities in endoscopic technology and high-precision hand instruments. Wockhardt undertakes the entire spectrum of minimal access surgeries. It represents the pinnacle for the perfection of surgical skill and dexterity, precision, team work and cutting-edge technology to define new modalities of patient treatment across spcialists.

Minimal Access Surgeries

- Diagnostic Endoscopy
- Upper GI Scopy (Castroscopy)
- Lower GI Scopy (Colonoscopy)
- Endoscopic Retrograde Cholangiopancreatography
- Bronchoscopy
- Therapeutic Endoscopy
- Endoscopic treatment of bleeding in GI Ulcers, Varices Polyps, etc.
- Dilatation of Esophageal strictures
- Removal of CBD stones
- Palliaton of GI and Hepatobilliary Tumors (Stents)
- Laser Therapy
- Laparoscopic Surgery
- Diagnostic Laparoscopy
- Appendectomy
- Cholecystectomy (Removal of Gall Blader)
- Hernia Surgery
- Splenectomy
- Colorectal Surgery
- Rectopexy for prolapse
- Gastric Surgery
- Mytomy for Achalasia Cardia
- Nissen Fundoplication
- Adrenalectomy
- Hepato Biliry Surgery
- Pancreatic Surgery
- Obesity Surgery

Other Minimal Access Surgeries include—

- TURP (Transuretral Resection of Prostrate)
- PCNL (Percutaneous Nephrolithotripys)
- Laparoscopic Urology
- Thoracoscopic Surgery
- Minimal Access Cardiac Surgery

The GI Division of the Minimal Access Centre will also undertake Conventional Gastro-intestinal Surgery with a special focus on Oncology and hepatobiliary Pancreatic Surgery. In due course, Hepatic Transplant will be established.

Wockhardt Hospitals Critical Care

A dedicated team of Intensivists and exclusively trained nursing and paramedical staff are guided by a full-time team of American Board Certified Specialists in Critical Care and Pulmonary Medicine. Besides the entire gamut disciplines associated with the various specialities, Wockhardt Hosptials Critical Care service also offers casualty and emergency health care with high-tech facilities.

The hospital is equipped with over 100 Intensive care beds in Medical, Cardiology, Cardio-Thoracic Surgery, Pediatrics, Neuro-Surgery/ Neurology and Surgical care. Besides these, there are 24 emergency beds.

Each bed is further supported by state-of-art monitors, ventilators, hemo-dynamic monitoring equipment and PACS software. The ICU also offers renal replacement therapy such as dialysis and hemofiltration.

Another endeavor to make the hospital patient-friendly is the facility that we provide for attendants of ICU patients. Unlike other hospitals, here they can stay over in the hospital till such time as the patient is in intensive care.

Wockhardt Hospitals Critical Care

Emergency and Trauma Care

We extend our expertise in critical care to the transportation of critically ill patients by ambulances. Our emergency services are supported by full-time, dedicated ambulances that are connected by Wi-Fi handsets. Timely intervention is crucial in emergency care and special ambulances can provide critical care to the patient in transit. Before the patient reaches hospital, his or her record is exchanged between the doctor in the ambulance and the resident doctor in the hospital, akin to the most advanced EMS system. Needless to say, often this little time saved can be crucial in saving the patient's life or improving his or her post-trauma life.

The casualty and emergency facility has the most advanced equipment to carry out all types of diagnosis associated with such cases, like the 64-Slince CT Scan, 1.5 Tesla MRI and a fully-equipped radiology department that works 24/7.

Wockhardt Hosptials—Wellness Care

Rehabilitation and Preventive Care

Wockhardt Hospitals Rehab and Preventive care facility offers excellent rehabilitative services for inpatients with physical and occupational therapy. Our team of a well-experienced physiotherapist and a highly skilled staff can provide physical, occupational and holistic therapy that can meet a wide array of health care needs of a patient. The centre is geared to provide a Therapeutic Exercise and Wellness Program.

The facility needs the rehabilitation needs of both in-patients and out-patients. Staff members specialize in rehab programs of a varied nature—low back pain, arthritis, breathing techniques, easing delivery, Tai Chi, de-stress and ergonomic counseling. Therapists collaborate in order to ensure that patients receive tailor-made care and service that is the best and the most comprehensive program available.

Therapeutic Exercise and Physiotherapy Program

If you have a medical risk factor that affects your ability to exercise safely, or being physically fit is important to you, worry no more. The answer lies in **Wockhardt** Therapeutic Exercise and Wellness Program. At our facility, a complete health program is the basis for achieving results. Our therapeutic exercise program conforms to well-tested principles of exercise, nutrition and personal wellness. The program is developed keeping each patient's specific needs in mind. It places increasing but controlled demands on the body's regimen for you under close scrutiny. The facility is equipped with the latest technology designed for regular. Neurological, Orthopedic and Cardiac Rehabilitation. This multi-specialty rehab team supplements the state-of-the-art infrastructure offering services such as sports rehabilitation, neurological rehabilitation, cardiac rehabilitation and woman's wellness.

Speciality Wellness Programs

Women's Health

Ante-natal Sessions
Post-natal sessions
Kegels Exercies
Pelvic Floor Toning
Pilates
Yoga and Meditation
Lamaze Exercise
Stress Management

Children's Wellness

Healthy Posture Programs in Schools
Junk Food De-addiction Programs
Yoga in Schools
Musculo-skeletal Assessment
Athletic Potential Evaluation

Senior's Health

Arthritis Management

Frozen Shoulder Management
Posture Control
Breathing Exercises
Joint Range Exercises
Osteoporosis Prevention
Tai Chi

Rehab Services

Stroke
Arthritis
Cerebral Palsy
Parkinsons
Post-Surgical Rehabilitation and Physiotheraphy for all specialists
Weight reduction—Pilates and Core Strengthening

Corporate Wellness

Ergonomics Counselling
Repetitive Strain Injury Prevention
Relaxation Techniques
Breathing Exercises
Posture Correction
De-stress
Fitness Concepts.

Wockhardt hospitals, their doctors, nurses and entire staff and committed to providing you with excellent care both clinical and personal. In addition it is our policy to respect your individuality and dignity. We support your right to know about your health and illness and also the right to participate in the critical/vital decision that affect your well being. It is our sincere intention to deliver your care in a manner that meets your expectations. It is with this intention that we publish your rights as a patient at our hospital.

You have the right to receive the best care (medically) indicated for your problem regardless of race, religion, national origin or the source of (payment) for your care.

You have the right to prompt lifesaving (treatment) in an emergency without discrimination on account of economic status or source of payment unless such discussion can be imposed without risk to your health.

You have the right to be treated respectfully by others and be addressed by your proper name and without undue familiarity.

Your individuality will be respected and (differences) in cultural and educational background taken into account. When you have a question you will be listened to and receive an appropriate and helpful response.

You have the right to privacy.

You may expect to talk with your doctor, nurse or our administration representative in private and know that the information you give will not be overheard or be given to others without your permission. In the hospital when you are in a semi private room you can expect a sincere and reasonable attempt to keep all (conversation) confidential. When you are examined, you are entitled to privacy. If you are hospitalized, no outsiders may see you without your permission. Your hospital records are private as well and no persons or agency beyond those caring for you may be permitted to see those records expect the authorized statutory bodies.

You have the right to seek and receive all the (information) necessary for you to understand your medical condition.

You have the right to know the name of the doctor who is responsible for your care and to talk with that doctor and any other who give you care. You are entitled to know the planned course of diagnosis and treatment and the prognosis for the future. You have the right to ask you doctor or nurse any question that concerns you about your health.

You have the right to select your doctor and your treatment.

You have the right to say "Yes" to the (recommended treatment). You also have the rights to say "No" to treatment at your own medical risk. You have the right to request and receive (additional) medical consultation or a second opinion on you medical condition, if you desire.

You have the right to leave the hospital even if your doctor advises aginst it unless you have an infectious disease that may influence the health of the other patients.

If you decide to leave before the doctors advise, the hospital will not be responsible for any harm that this may cause you and you will be asked to sign a "Discharge Against advice" form.

You have the right to understand and receive information on the payment of hospital bills on a day-to-day basis in accordance with the (policies) of the hospital.

You, your family or your guardian has the right to tell us when something is wrong in the delivery of your care.

If you do complain, your care will not be (affected) in any way. Your feedback is welcome at all times.

You also have some responsibilities—

- Be honest with us, tell us all you know about your present illness, your previous hospitalizations if any and any other matter relating to your health which will help us to treat you better.
- Help us maintain the truth about your medical history for all documentation.
- Please tell us if you donot understand anything concerning your care or if you feel, you are unable to follow the instructions.
- Respect the right of the other patients to receive medical care without being disturbed. Please ensure that your visitors are

considerate of other patients particularly with regards to noise that they observe the "Visiting Hours" schedule of the hospital.

- Observe the "No smoking" and other rules of the hospital.
- Your have the responsibility to be prompt about the paynment of your hospital bills and where necessary to provide information essential for processing your bills always.
- Wockhardt health check up programmes are specifically designed to diagnose, monitor and prevent potential health problems and help you lead healthier lives.

WOCKHARDT HEALTH CHECKUP PROGRAMMES

HEALTH CHECKUP PROGRAMMES

At Wockhardt, we care for your well-being. We strongly recommend practicing prevention and securing health. In a world where lifestyle evolves by the day, it is essential to stay in the pink of health. Wishing you and your family good health and happiness always.

Wockhardt health check-up programmes are specifically designed to diagnose, monitor and prevent potential health problems and help you lead healthier lives.

(A) Basic Health Screening Rs. 950

A basic health check-up to help you assess your health:

Haematology with ESR
Blood Gr and Rh
RBS
Serum Cholesterol
Chest X-ray
VDRL
Urine Routine
ECG
Consultation with Physician

(B) Basic Hearth Check Rs. 1500

Initial stress-related damage to the heart, the most crucial organ in the body, can start early and have little or no symptoms. This programme is invaluable for early detection of heart diseases.

Haematology profile with ESR
FBS
PPBS
Lipid Profile
Sr. Cholesterol
Sr. HDL Cholesterol
Sr. LDL Cholestrol
Sr. Triglycerides
Sr. VLDL Cholesterol
ECG
Chest X-ray
Consultant with Cardiologist
Consultation with Dietician

(C) Diabetic Health Check Rs. 950

Diabetes is a silent yet devastating diseases that has implication on every organ in the body. Early onset of non insulin dependent or Type 2 diabetes is rising very rapidly in India. While there is no cure for diabetes, early detection can keep it under excellent control with diet, exercise and professional supervision.

HB, TC, DC	Urine-Protein
FBS	ECG
PPBS	Consultation with Diabetologist/ Dietician
Fasting Lipid Profile	
Serum Creatinine/Potassium	.

(D) Comprehensive Diabetic Health Check Rs. 2100

HB, TC, DC, ESR	Urine-Microalbunimuria
FBS, PPBS	ECG
Fasting Lipid Profile	Chest X-Ray
Serum Electrolytes	Fundoscopy
Serum Calcium, P, Alkaline Phosphatase	Consultation with Diabetologist/ Dietician
Blood Urea, Serum Creatinine	
HbA1c	

(E) Exclusive Diabetic Health Check Rs. 3650

Fasting Lipid Profile	ECG
Sr. Electrolytes	Chest X-Ray
HB, TC, DC, ESR	Fundoscopy
FBS	TMT
PPBS	Echo
Blood Urea ·	Consultation with Diabetologist, Cardiologist and Dietician
Sr. Creatinine	Consultation with Physiotherapist
Serum Calcium, P, Alkaline Phosphatase	
HbA1c	
Urine—Microalbunimuria	

(F) Senior Citizen's Profile Rs. 1800

A very thoughtful and caring present to ageing parents on all occasions. Ageing brings its own health problems and some of them can certainly be prevented or kept under control

Haematology profile with ESR	Chest X-Ray
FBS	ECG
Liver function Tests	Urine Analysis
Total Protein A/g Ratio	TSH

SGPT, SGOT
Sr. Alkaline Phosphate
Lipid Profile
Sr. Cholesterol
Sr. Triglycerides
Sr. Inorganic Phosphorous
Sr. Calcium
PSA
Consultation with Dietician
Consultation with Geriatrician
Consultation with Opthalmologist

(G) Executive Health Check Rs. 2400

On the move, always under pressure, forced into an irregular lifestyle, executives often neglect their health and ignore the early warning signs. This programme checks all the vital functions of the body.

Haematology with ESR
Fasting Blood Sugar (FBS)
Blood Gr and Rh
PPBS
Kidney Profile
Blood Urea Nitrogen
Serum Creatinine
Uric Acid
Lipid Profile
Sr. Cholesterol
Sr. Triglycerides
Ultra Sound (Abdomen and Pelvis)
Chest X-Ray
ECG
Urine Routine
Stool Routine
VDRL
Liver Function Tests
Total Bilirubin
Total Prorein
A/g Ratio
GGT/SGOT/SGPT
Sr. Alkaline Phosphate
Consultation with Physician and Dietician

(H) Master Health Check Rs. 3500

This is a comprehensive programme which includes investigation of all body organs designed to certify good health as well as detect early symptoms of developing illness.

Haematology with ESR
Blood Gr and Rh
FBS, PPBS
Lipid Profile
Sr. Cholesterol
Sr. Triglycerides
Sr. HDL Cholesterol
Sr. LDL Cholesterol
Sr. VLDL Cholesterol
Kidney Profile
Blood Urea Nitrogen
Sr. Creatinine
Uric Acid
Liver Function Tests
Total Bilirubin
Thyroid Test
TSH
VDRL (Basic STD Screening)
Urine Routine
Stool Routine
Chest X-ray
ECG
Spirometry (Lung Function Study)
Computerised Stress Test
Ultra Sound
(Abdomen and Pelvis)
Consultation with Dietician
Consultation with Physician
Consultation with Physiotherapist

Total Protein Alg Ratio
GGT, SCOT, SGPT
Sr. Alkaline phosphate

(I) Comprehensive Heart Check Rs. 3400

This programme runs through a comprehensive list of investigations for all symptoms related to heart disease.

Haematology profile with ESR
FBS, PPBS
ECG
Lipid Profile
Sr. Cholesterol
Sr. HDL Cholesterol
Sr. LDL Cholesterol
Sr. Triglycerides
Sr. VlDL Cholesterol
Chest X-Ray
Ultra Sound
Computerized Stress Test
Echocardiography with
Color Doppler
Consultation with Cardiologist
Consultation with Dietician
Consultation with Physiotherapist

(J) Wockhardt Health Management Programme Rs. 4800

This is a comprehensive check-up of body and mind, it includes consultation with several specialists, to give a complete health status.

Haematology with ESR
FBS, PPBS
Blood Gr. And Rh
Stool Routine
Urine Analysis
Lipid Profile
Sr. Cholesterol
Sr. Triglycerides
HDL Cholesterol
LDL Cholesterol
VLDL Cholesterol
Kidney Profile
Blood Urea Nitrogen
Sr. Creatinine
Uric Acid
Liver Function Tests
Total Bilirubin
Total Protein A/g ratio
GGT, SCOT, SGPT
Sr. Alkaline Phosphate
Thyroid Test
TSH
Chest X-Ray
Ultrasound Scan—Abdomen
Echocardiography with Col. Doppler
Computerised Stress Test
Spirometry
ECG
PSA (men)
Consultation with Dietician
Consultation with Dentist
Consultation with Opthalmologist
Stress Screening by Psychologist
Consultation with Physician
Consultation with Cardiologist*
Consultation with Physiotherapist

(K) Well Women Profile Rs. 2550

On the top of the routine stresses of modern life, women carry with extra burden of a complex reproductive system. Routine health check—ups help keep a woman in optimum health.

Haematology with ESR	Urine Routine
Blood Gr. And Rh	Ultra Sound—Abdomen and Pelvis
T3, T4, TSH	Mammography
Pap Smear	Consultation with Gynecologist
FBS	Consultation with Physiotherapist
VDRL	

(L) Special Package Women Rs. 800

Mammography and Papsmear

PRACTICE PREVENTION

Balance your diet

Take a reduced calorie diet which is rich in vegetables and whole grams. Substitute whole milk products with skimmed milk and cook with unsaturated vegetable oil.

Give your heart a Workout

Regular program of aerobic exercise like walking, jogging, running or swimming. Schedule at least three sessions a week of at least 30 minutes. Reduce obesity.

Says Yes to

Vegetables and Fruits, lean cuts of meat, chicken without skin, Fish and brown bread.

Cut Cholesterol

Elevated lipids namely cholesterol and triglycerides are best controlled through a.regiment of strict diet which is low on saturated fats such as organ meats, fatty meats and egg yolk. Avoid butter and cheese.

Quit Smoking

Smoking triple chances of a heart attack. Quit today and reduce your risk to half in 2 years.

Control BP

Hypertension makes the hearth work harder to move blood through the body. If you get short of breath when you exert don't ignore it, consult your doctor today. Address hypertension with proper diet, exercise and medication.

Control Diabetes

Check for diabetes today particularly if there is family history. If you have diabetes keep it under check, remember diabetes multiples your risk of heart disease.

Reduce Stress

Chronic stress can increase the risk of heart disease, spend time with yourself and choose to do things that make you happy. Sleep well.

INSTRUCTION

1. Programmes other than A require 12-hour fasting. Please do not have milk/tea/coffee in the morning before the tests. However, you may drink water.
2. For people undergoing other than programmes A and C breakfast will be provided at the hospital as a part of this health check up programmes.
3. Men should shave their chest for Stress Test.
4. You should carry your stool sample with you for health check up programmes GH and J. If required, you may collect your containers from the Pathology Department.
5. Patients needing dilatation during ophthalmology consultation, will not be able to drive or read for 4-6 hours after the procedure.
6. Three-days prior appointment is required for all Wockhardt health check-up programmes.

Please report for your health check up programmes at 8.00 a.m.

Appendix 4

MANIPAL HOSPITAL, BANGALORE

Manipal Hospital, situated on Airport Road, Bangalore is a landmark destination for quality and affordable health care. The 600 bed centrally air-conditioned hospital is the first tertiary care multi superspeciality referral centre in Karnataka.

It is India's first hospital to be ISO 9001:2000 certified for Clinical, Nursing, Diagnostics and Allied Areas. The hospital has been declared winner of the prestigious Golden Peacock National Quality Award 2005 in the service category.

With a team of some of the best doctors in the world, an attentive staff, state-of-the-art equipment, the hospital provides specialized medical services at affordable costs in over 40 specialties.

The world over, this hospital is recognized for its ability to provide the most comprehensive health care.

Manipal Heart Institute

Manipal Heart Institute is one of Asia's largest and most modern Heart care centres dedicated to the prevention and cure of Heart related ailments. A vastly experienced, highly motivated team of expert doctors and support staff with the help of latest treatment facilities work towards the objective of "Healing Hearts Saving lives."

Interventional Cardiology

The Department is equipped with state-of-the-art equipment to handle all kinds of cardiac cases.

Major Treatments Offered

- Coronary Angioplasty and Stenting
- Multi-vessel Coronary Stenting, Left Main Stenting, Chronic Total Occlusion Stenting
- Temporary and Permanent Pacing
- Balloon Valvuloplasty
- *AICD* and Pacemaker implantation
- Electrophysiological Studies and Ablation
- Device closure of ASD, VSD, PDA
- Interventions for various Congenital and Valvular Heart Diseases

Cardiovascular and Thoracic Surgery

The Department is well recognized for its advancements in Cardiology. Apart from routine By-pass Surgeries, Beating Heart Surgeries and Valve Replacements, Manipal Heart Institute has rich experience in conducting rare Congenital and Redo Surgeries.

The Department specializes in Neonatal Cardiac Surgeries and Surgeries under Total Circulatory Arrests (TCAs). In adults it handles rare cases like Triple Valve Replacements, Left Ventricular Aneurysm Reconstruction, Bentall Procedure, Ross Procedure and Surgery for Aortic Dissection.

Facilities

- Two state-of-the-art digital Cath Labs
- Four full-fledged Cardiac Operation Theatres
- Nuclear Cardiology Lab
- Electro-Physiology Lab
- Advanced Intensive Therapy Unit
- Coronary Care Unit (CCU)
- 24 hour Laboratory and Blood Bank
- Mobile Cardiac Care Ambulance

Manipal Institute for Neurological Disorders (MIND)

MIND is one of the premier departments at Manipal Hospital for diagnosis and treatment of Neurological Disorders. Its divisions of Neurology and Neurosurgery with dedicated Neuro Rehabilitation facilities, diagnoses and treats various diseases affecting the Brain, Spinal Cord, Muscles and Nerves. This Department has a reputed and dynamic team of Neurologists and Neurosurgeons.

MIND caters to all subspecialties in Neurosciences. The Department runs special clinics on Parkinson's Disease and Movement Disorders, Peripheral Nerve Disorders, Craniofacial Deformities and Epilepsy. It is linked with the imaging services (CT and MRI) and has modern Neuro. Diagnostic facilities like EEG, ENMG, Evoked Potentials and Telemetric EEG in addition to a dedicated Neuro Trauma and Stroke Unit.

MIND has Reputation for its Services in:

- Brain Tumour Surgery
- Pituitary Surgery
- Neurovascular Surgery
- Deep Brain Stimulation for Parkinson's Disease
- Neuroendoscopic Surgery
- Skull Base Surgery
- Paediatric Neuro Surgery
- Complex Spine Surgery
- Craniofacial Surgery

- Intrathecal Baclofen Pump for Spasticity
- Programmable shunts for Complex and Complicated Hydrocephalus
- Neurorehabilitation and Computer Assisted Cognitive Retraining
- Total Reconstruction of Brachial Plexus Injuries

Manipal Institute of Nephrology and Urology (MINU)

MINU has been in the fore front for the care of patients with kidney diseases in this part of the world. MINU has the largest Dialysis Centre in the country performing over 24,000 Dialysis each year. It has vast experience in Kidney Transplantation and was the first Centre in Karnataka to perform Cadaver Renal Transplantation. The Department has a rich experience in Chronic Ambulatory Peritoneal Dialysis and is the first Centre in Karnataka to use Automated Peritoneal Dialysis using Home Care Machine.

Dialysis on Wheels, which is a unique programme introduced for the first time in the country is a state-of-the-art Dialysis Unit, launched to facilitate Haemodialysis at home. The Department has full-fledged Paediatric Nephrology Unit, including Haemodialysis, CRRT, Peritoneal Dialysis and Transplantation even for infants and children.

MINU was the first Lithotripsy Centre in Karnataka with a programme for the non-invasive management of the stone disease. The Department specializes in Endo-Urology and Laparoscopic Urological Procedures. It has treated a large number of patients with urinary stones and has one of the best equipped Urodynamic unit in the state. MINU was the first Centre in Karnataka to be recognized for training in Nephrology by the National Boards.

Comprehensive Cancer Centre

The Manipal Comprehensive Cancer Centre with its full-fledged sub-divisions of Surgical, Radiation and Medical Oncology takes a multidisciplinary approach to provide Comprehensive Cancer care.

Surgical Oncology

Surgical Oncology constitutes the oldest and the least expensive modality of Cancer treatment. Team of Onco-surgeons in the Department believe in optimum tumour control with maximum preservation of function thereby improving the quality of life. Thoracic, Breast, Abdominal, Head and Neck, Gynaecological Onco Surgeries are routinely performed at the Centre.

The Manipal Comprehensive Cancer Centre is equipped with hand held Gamma Probe, which allows the surgeons to perform Targeted Sentinel Lymph Node Biopsy, mainly in Breast Cancers and Gynaec Cancers, thereby avoiding blind and at times unnecessary surgery. It also facilitates ROLL (Radioisotope Guided Occult Lesion Localisation) wherein very small

Breast Tumours are biopsied using minimally invasive techniques and Radioguided Parathyroid and Endocrine Surgeries.

Radiation Oncology

The Manipal Comprehensive Cancer Centre's Radiation wing consists of a highly qualified and experienced team of Radiation Oncologists, Physicists and Technologists, backed by new generation, state-of-the-art equipments capable of delivering precise doses of radiation accurately to the tumour with minimum damage to normal structures

Some of the hi-tech equipments at the Centre include:

- Precise Digital Linear Accelerator
- ADAC Pinnacle IMRT Planning System
- Simulator (Mevasim), helps to localise the tumour precisely, facilitating accurate radiation therapy
- Eclipse 3 Dimensional Treatment Planning System
- Modern Cobalt 60 machine Theratrone—780°C
- Brachytherapy Gammamed Plus, Remote Controlled HDR System
- SPECTCT
- Dual Headed Gamma Camera with latest processing software
- Gamma Probe (EUROPROBE)

Medical Oncology and Haematology

Chemotherapy for different solid tumours with the most up-to-date drugs and drug combination is routinely performed at the Centre. The Centre has been recognized by the University of Minnesota for Bone Marrow Transplant Programme.

Haematology and Haemato Oncology services are offered by qualified Clinical Haematologists for all Benign and Malignant Haematological Disorders.

International Institute of Dental Sciences

The Department offers the most comprehensive range of Dental services. It is equipped with 16 Ultra Modern Chairs fitted with monitors and Digital X-rays, unique centralized sterilization and a highly sophisticated Full Mouth Digital X-Ray Unit. The Department offers sub-speciality services in the areas of:

- Orthodontics—Correction of Irregular Teeth
- Oral and Maxillo-Facial Surgery, Surgical Dentistry; Injuries to Jaws and Oral Cavity and Infections
- Aesthetic and Cosmetic Dentistry
- Conservative Dentistry and Endodontics
- Root Canal Treatment
- Prosthodontics—Replacing Missing Teeth

- Periodontics—Treatment for Gum Diseases
- Oral Medicine and Maxillofacial Radiology—Diagnosis and Management of Diseases of Oral Cavity and Face

Implantology

The Department facilitates Implants—Fixed type of teeth replacement from single to full mouth. Implanted teeth are just like natural teeth, universally accepted and highly successful. Implants have changed the quality of life in toothless individuals.

Institute of Liver and Digestive Diseases

Manipal Hospital in an effort to provide comprehensive treatment of digestive diseases under one roof has taken the initiative to establish a dedicated Digestive Disease Centre Manipal Institute of Liver and Digestive Diseases (MILDD). MILDD has state-of-the-art diagnostic and therapeutic endoscopic unit equipped with videoscopes. The Centre brings together a team of skilled Gastroenterologists, Endoscopists, Gastrointestinal Surgeons and Interventional Radiologists with special interest in liver and digestive diseases. The major thrust areas for the center are Liver transplantation and Bariatric (morbid obesity) surgery program.

Services

- MILDD offers treatment for a wide spectrum of gastrointestinal diseases which include.
- Hepato-biliary diseases:
  Chronic liver disease and its complications, Surgery for portal hypertension, Liver abscess and tumors, Biliary stone disease gallstones and bile duct stones, Cancers of the biliary tract cholangiocarcinoma and gallbladder cancer, Biliary tract injury.
- Pancreatic diseases:
  Acute pancreatitis and its complications, Chronic pancreatitis, Pancreatic cancer.
- Gastrointestinal disorders:
  Esophageal disorders cancer and benign, Gastric disorders like peptic ulcer and cancer, Colorectal diseases and cancer, Enterocutaneous fistulae, Inflammatory bowel disease, Ulcerative colitis, Crohn's disease, Abdominal tuberculosis.
- Surgery for morbid obesity.

Manipal Andrology and Reproductive Services (MARS)

MARS provides treatment and care for couples seeking help in starting a family.

MARS has a Comprehensive Andrological Laboratory to diagnose male fertility problems. The Department is equipped to do several advanced test for Sperm Egg Interaction to predict fertility. Treatments are offered for severe Sperm Count Problems such as poor or absent Sperm Counts including Surgical Sperm Retrieval and Microsurgery.

Reproductive Medicine caters to both evaluation of female infertility problems like Anovulation and Tubal Problems and Management of Female Fertility Problems by Laparoscopy as well as IVF and ICS. The other facilities are Sperm, Embryo Freezing, Donor Sperm Bank, Testicular and Ovarian Tissue Cryopreservation, all of which ensures management of difficult or complex fertility problems, offering the best of solutions for the couple.

Accident and Emergency

A well established Department for Accident and Emergency provides the much needed care in an emergency. The Department is well equipped with most modern life saving equipment and well-trained staff to provide round-the-clock emergency care services.

Anaesthesiology

Ever since the inception of the hospital, the Department of Anaesthesiology has provided the highest quality of resuscitative care. It has set very high standards in the management of the patient in the Pre-operative Period, Trauma Care, Life Support, Obstetric Analgesia, Post-operative Pain Management, Anaesthesia Care in Critical Diagnostic areas like Cardiac Catheterization, ERCP, CT and MRI, Brachytherapy and so on.

Critical Care Medicine

The Department of Critical Care Medicine at Manipal Hospital recognizes the unique needs of critically ill patients of any age and strives to secure the highest quality care for them. The Department is backed by quality infrastructure, a team of critical care professionals, specialists, trained nurses and support staff.

Service Highlights

- One of the largest multi-disciplinary critical care units in Bangalore
- 3 full time Critical Care Consultants
- 24 hour cover by a team of experienced Registrars (post-MD/ Diploma)
- 1:1 nursing care for all ventilated patients
- 1000 medical/surgical patients treated every year
- Able to provide ventilatory/advanced cardiovascular support
- Facilities for continuous/intermittent renal replacement therapy
- Advanced monitoring available on all beds
- Recognised by the National Board for training towards Fellowship in Critical Care Medicine
- Recognised by the Indian Society of Critical Care Medicine for the Certificate Course and Fellowship in Critical Care Medicine

Dermatology

The Department equipped with state-of the art US FDA approved technologies applies the latest technologies to treat diseases and disorders of the skin, hair and nails. The Department was the first in the state to introduce Laser Surgery, Photo Therapy, Cryotherapy and Allery Testing.

Major Services Include

- Deromato Surgery—Laser Surgery, Electoautery, Electrolysis, Acne Scar Reivions, Hair Transplantation, Crysosurgery, Dermabrasion and Skin Resurfacing, Nail Surgery.
- Vitiligo Surgery—Full Body, Hand and Foot Phototherapy Unit, Micropunch, Grafting and Tatooing, Blister Grafting.
- Paediatric Dermatology
- Cosmetic Dermatology—Chemical Peels, Fillers, Laser, Microdermabrasion, Botox Injection

Dietetics

A good diet helps to maintain a good health. For a patient who is hospitalized, a customized diet aids in faster recovery and shortens the duration of hospitalization. The Department of Dietetics at Manipal Hospital works towards this objective by offering the following services:

- Customized diet is served in the most hygienic manner to all patients based on their medical requirements
- Customized diet counseling for inpatients and outpatients
- Diet counseling for all patients on dialysis and Post Transplant patients in the Department of Nephrology
- Anti-natal nutritional counseling for pregnant women
- Paediatric nutritional counseling
- Community nutrition programme, talks on food and health, awareness session on nutrition
- Nutrition support services for corporates and industrial houses

Diabetes and Endocrinology

The Department is committed to early diagnosis, evidence based management of Type 1 and Type 2 Diabetes and Gestational (Pregnancy related) Diabetes. The Department is on par with ADA, IDF, ACE guidelines in meeting the needs of Diabetes population in order to take care of short and long-term complications. The Department functions with an aim to provide care, concern and commitment to all patients and actively participates in international clinical research/trials and is also accredited to provide following Endocrine treatments:

- Thyroid and Obesity
- Parathyroid (Ca metabolism)

- Growth and Puberty Disorders
- Secondary Hypertension
- Adrenal Disorders

ENT

With the availability of dynamic ENT Surgeons, Audiologists and Auditory Verbal Therapists, the Department provides advanced care in ENT Head and Neck Surgery and Audiological Science. Equipped with all latest equipments and diagnostic methods, like Operating Microscopes, Audiology Lab, Diagnostic Video Endoscopes the Department has served as a bench mark facility in the region.

The Department introduced Radio Frequency Surgery for the first time in South India for Somnoplasty (Snoring) and Turbinoplasty (For Nasal Obstruction). Expertise exists to do Cochlear Impantation, Endoscopic CSF Leak Closure, Trans-nasal Paraseptal Endoscopic Pituitary Surgery, Endoscopic Darocystorhinostomy (OCR), Phono Surgery (Voice Surgery), Laser Surgery and Paediatric Airway Surgery. Otoneurological and Skull Base Surgery is undertaken with the Neuro Surgical team. Neonatal Hearing Screening to detect hearing loss in newborns has been recently introduced.

Fetal Medicine

The Fetal Medicine Department performing about 50-60 Obstetric and Gynaecological scans per day is a tertiary referral unit for complicated Gynaecology and Fetal Scans. Chorionic Villous Sampling, Amniocentesis, Fetal Blood Sampling and Invasive Gynaecological procedures are routinely performed in the unit. Fetal Blood Transfusions have been performed with good results. The Department successfully performed the first EXIT (Ex-utero Intrapartium Treatment) procedure in India, with excellent support from Anaesthetists, Paediatricians, Paediatric Surgeons and Obstetricians.

Services Offered

- 20/30/40 Obstetric and Gynaecology Scanning providing excellent real life image quality
- Invasive Obstetric and Gynaecological procedures for diagnosis and treatment
- Prenatal and antenatal counseling for pregnancy complications
- Observership for short and long-term basis can be provided in agreement with individual consultants

Gastroenterology Medical

The Department deals with patients having Castro-intestinal, Liver and Pancreato Biliary disorders. The Department is well equipped with a diagnostic and therapeutic endoscopy Unit. The routinely performed therapeutic endoscopic procedures include:

- Endoscopic Control of Castro-intestinal Bleed
- Endoscopic Dilatation of Strictures and Placement of Stents in Oesophagus and Castro Intestinal tract
- Percutaneous Endoscopic Gastrostomy
- Removal of Foreign Bodies
- Endoscopic Polypectomy in Castro-intestinal Tract
- Endoscopic Drainage of Cyst in the Pancreas
- ERCP Removal of Stones from Bile Duct, Pancreatic Duct and Stenting
- Endoscopic Ultrasound (EUS) for Castro-intestinal, Hepato Pancreato Biliary Disorders

Surgical

The Department of Surgical Gastroenterology provides diagnosis and surgical treatment for patients with common and complex Abdominal, Castro-intestinal, Morbid Obesity (Bariatric), Hepatobiliary and Pancreatic Surgical Problems. The department also plans to embark on Liver Transplantation Programme.

Major Services Offered

Basic and advanced Laparoscopic Procedures:

- Cholecystectomy
- Fundoplication (Nissen's)
- Cardiomyotomy for Achalasia
- Vagotomy and Castro Jejunostomy (Ulcer Disease)
- Small Bowel Resections
- Colorectal Resections (Benign and malignant)
- Thoracoscopic Esophagectomy (Esophageal Cancer)
- Splenectomy
- Gastric Bypass/Lap Band (Morbid Obesity Surgery)

Other Complex Abdominal Procedures such as:

- Surgery for Corrosive Stricture
- Surgery for Bile Duct Strictures and Choledochal Cyst
- Whipple's Pancreatico Duodenectomy
- Pancreatic Necrosectomy
- Major Liver Resections (Benign and Malignant)
- Surgery for Portal Hypertension
- Restorative Proctocolectomy for Ulcerative Colitis and FAP
- Sphincter Preserving Procedures for Rectal Cancer

Re-operative Abdominal Surgery
Management of Enterocutaneous Fistulae

General Medicine

The Department of Medicine has a dedicated team of well trained and experienced Physicians. All kinds of medical problems, both acute and chronic diseases are seen and if required patients are referred to the respective super speciality clinics available at the hospital.

International Patient Care Centre

Over the years Manipal Hospital has treated international patients from more than 55 countries including the USA, UK, Malaysia, Oman, the U AE, Tanzania, Srilanka and Mauritius. Our dedicated International Patient Care staff have decades of experience in handling all the requirements and special needs of our international patients. This ensures that our international patients' visits are smooth and hassle-free.

Services Offered Include:

Travel, transport and accommodation arrangements, scheduling appointments with consultants, money exchange, insurance liaison and legal assistance, visa registration and extension formalities, sight-seeing and shopping arrangements, language interpretation assistance, provision of cuisine options.

Health Check

At Manipal Hospital, we continue to emphasis the age old adage that 'Prevention is better than cure". The Department offers a set of comprehensive and reliable Preventive Health Check Packages, designed keeping in mind the varied requirements of all members of a family. Regular health checks ensure that you enjoy uninterrupted good health over a long period of time.

Manipal Health Check Offers

- Diabetic Check
- Comprehensive Check
- Check Plus
- Routine Plus Check
- Routine Check
- Manipal Health Check Offers
- Corporate Annual Health Checks

Regular health checks ensure that you enjoy uninterrupted good health over a long period of time.

Medical Genetics

In its commitment to give patients a comprehensive and upto date medical care, Manipal Hospital has started the Clinical and Molecular Cytogenetics Division.

Services Offered Include:

- Clinical Diagnosis and Genetic Counselling
- Peripheral Blood Karyotyping
- Prenatal Diagnosis
- Bone Marrow studies in Haemato Oncological Disorders
- FISH Studies in instances of Complex Chromosomal re-arrangements and Micro Deletion Syndromes such as Congenital Heart Defects
- Molecular Studies

Obstetrics and Gynaecology

The Department offers comprehensive Gynaecology services to address the health care needs of women from their adolescence, through pregnancy to menopause and beyond. Apart from efficient management of routine Gynaecological services, the Department has established various sub-specialities namely Fetal Medicine, Gynaec Endoscopic Surgery and Gynaec Oncology services. Well monitored state-of-the-art labour wards with Birthing Suites, 24 hour Epidural and Anaesthetic services on par with western standards are available in the Department.

Ophthalmology

The Department of Ophthalmology houses a well-equipped facility for the complete examination, diagnosis, and treatment of various Ocular Diseases in both adult and paediatric patients. Most eye disorders can be diagnosed and treated at the hospital, including Refractive Disorders, Cornea and External Diseases, Uveal Diseases, Cataract, Glaucoma, Strabismus and Amblyopia, Orbital and Lid Orders Retinal Disorders, complex Vitreo Retinal Surgeries in addition to vast array of other ocular surgeries/procedures. The Department has introduced various sub-speciality clinics like Diabetic Retinopathy, Retinopathy of Prematurity and Glauçoma care.

Facilities Include:

- Argon Laser
- Ophthalmic Ultrasound
- YAG Laser
- Phaco Emulsification Unit for Cataract Surgery
- LASIK Laser Refractive Surgery
- PIT for Macular Degeneration

Orthopaedics

Paediatrics

The Paediatric Department is highly reputed and caters to all health care needs of children, from birth to adolescence. From specialized care for sick and premature babies to routine checkups, our Paediatricians have the expertise and experience to help parents give their children the right start to a healthy life. The Department highlights include:

Service Highlights:

- Well equipped 35 bed Neonatal ICU with New Generation Ventilators and High Frequency Oscillators and advanced technology to markedly reduce the mortality and morbidity rates of new borns and children with complex illnesses.
- Kangaroo Mother care Programme adopted in the NICU for pre-term and low birth weight babies helping babies to maintain warmth, have breast feeds, have better nutrition, growth and development.
- Neonatal Transport Team with advanced life support equipment transports sick babies from other hospitals by road as well as air.
- Fully equipped 8 bed Paediatric ICU provides care for sick children with various illnesses including trauma, poisoning, drowning, etc.
- Pulmonary Function Lab provides care for children with lung illnesses.
- Sleep lab is on the anvil of being acquired.
- Active Paediatric Pulomonology Wing catering to children with complex lung disorders.
- Only Centre in the state offering Paediatric Flexible Bronchoscopies and Paediatric Sleep studies.
- Paediatric Emergency room to provide emergency care for the sick neonates and children.
- The Emergency room has 6 beds in addition to a rapid assessment and treatment care area. Sick neonates and children including trauma patients are taken care by trained personnel round the clock.
- The Department runs speciality clinics in high-risk newborns, Paediatric Endocrinology, Paediatric Hematology, Paediatric Pulmonology, Paediatric ENT, Paediatric Neurology and Development Disability Clinic under renowned specialists in their respective fields.

Manipal Hospital is one of the few hospitals in the country and the first in the state to offer Paediatric Endocrinology service. Some of the disorders diagnosed and treated by our Paediatric Endocrinologist include:

- Growth Disorders including short stature and tall stature
- Obesity
- Pituitary dysfunction which the child could be born with or develop during the course of radiation therapy to brain, or due to brain tumors and their treatment
- Diabetes
- *Thyroid Disorders*: overactive and underactive thyroid gland, thyroid nodules, goiter
- *Pubertal Disorders*: early or delayed pubertal development, irregular; irregular, heavy or absent menstrual periods in an adolescent; polycystic ovarian syndrome
- Intersex Disorders which could manifest as abnormality in genital appearance or as a lack of pubertal development
- Disorders of water balance which manifests as either a low or high sodium level
- *Bone and Calcium Disorders*: Low and high Blood Calcium Levels, Rickets, Osteoporosis, Osteogenesis Imperfecta
- Adrenal Disorders
- Genetic Disorders like Down Syndrome, Klinefelters and Turner Syndrome that are associated with hormonal abnormalities
- Bone and Calcium Disorders Low and high Blood Calcium Levels, Rickets, Osteoporosis, Osteogenesis Imperfecta
- Adrenal Disorders
- Genetic Disorders like Down Syndrome, Klinefelters and Turner Syndrome that are associated with hormonal abnormalities

Paediatric Surgery

The Department functions in conjunction with department of Paediatrics and Neonatology to provide comprehensive care to the neonate, infant and child. All surgical conditions in children right from birth are managed in this Department.

This includes Congenital Disorders (Birth Disorders), Infective, Traumatic and Neoplastic conditions, which need surgery such as Cleft Lip and Palate, Anomalies of the Ano-rectum, Kidney, Ureter and Bladder, Hypospadias, Anomalies of the Gastro-Intestinal System, etc. These surgeries include both the conventional open surgery as well as endoscopic (keyhole) surgeries of the Chest and Abdomen. The services offered include Neonatal Surgery, Paediatric Urology, Paediatric Oncology and Paediatric Laparoscopic Surgery

Physical Medicine and Rehabilitation

The Department offers complete range of rehabilitation services and is specifically devoted to the evaluation, management and prevention of disability and disabling conditions. It aims at restoring lost abilities of a person who has been disabled as a result of disease, disorder or injury.

The Department has a team of well qualified, dedicated, skilled and experienced Rehabilitation Professionals like Physiatrist, Physiotherapists, Occupational Therapists, Speech and Language Therapists, Neuro Developmental Therapists and Cognitive Therapist, Orthotists and Prosthetists, Social Worker and Psychologists. Each patient is evaluated by Rehabilitation Specialist and discussed with the rehabilitation team for comprehensive rehabilitation programme.

Along with Physiotherapy section, Occupational Therapy section and Speech Therapy section, the Department also has exclusive Rehabilitation Ward, Neurodevelopment Therapy Unit, Neuro-rehabilitation Unit, Sports Medicine Unit and Fitness Centre.

Experts from the Department run Speciality Clinics

- Cerebral Palsy Clinic
- Geriatric Clinic
- Work and Ergonomics Clinic
- Hand Rehabilitation Clinic
- Antenatal and Postnatal Clinic
- Home Care Management

Plastic Surgery

Department of Plastic Surgery is manned by highly qualified and skilled doctors in cosmetic and reconstructive surgery. Their skills are sought by other Departments like Neurosurgery, Oncology and Orthopaedics at one time or other.

- The Department renders services in the following specializations
- General Plastic and Cosmetic surgery
- Reconstructive Micro-Neuro-Vascular surgery
- Cleft lip/Palate deformities
- Cranio-Maxilo-Facial surgery
- Hand Surgery
- Cancer Reconstruction and Free Vascularized Tissue Transfer
- Trauma Care

Psychiatry

The Psychiatrists at Manipal Hospital are friendly and have at their command a variety of the latest test and equipment to assess mental functioning. Special emphasis is laid on detailed medical, emotional and psychological evaluation before treatment.

Areas addressed include:

- Child and adolescent problems
- Anxiety and Depression
- Suicidal ideas or attempt
- Alcohol and other substance dependence
- Marital counseling including sex education and sex counseling
- Problems of the elderly
- Help patients with chronic physical illnesses cope with their illness better

Respiratory Medicine

The Department of Respiratory Medicine is committed to provide a high quality service, working in partnership with patients, to improve the quality of life of people who have respiratory problems. Patients with respiratory problems such as Asthma, Pneumonia, Lung Cancer, TB, Fibrotic Lung Diseases and Sleep Apnoea Syndromes (Snoring with disturbed sleep) are dealt with and treated by reputed respiratory consultants in the Department. There are comprehensive and sophisticated facilities like Spirometry, Fibre Optic Bronchoscopy, Bronchoscopic Biopsy and Lavage, Non-invasive Ventilation and Sleep Lab for the diagnosis and treatment. Facilities for Open Lung Biospy are also available.

Rheumatology

Rheumatology Department at the hospital is a pioneering Department in the field of Rheumatology in the country and provides comprehensive care for patients with Rheumatological and many Autoimmune Diseases. The diseases managed by the Department include:

- Arthritis of many kinds (Rheumatoid Arthritis, Osteoarthritis, Gout etc.)
- Musculoskeletal disorders like Low Back Ache and Tennis Elbow
- Metabolic Bone Disorders like Osteoporosis
- Autoimmune Connective Tissue Diseases like Lupus (SLE)
- Paediatric Rheumatology

The Department provides support to many other Departments in providing Immunosuppressive Therapy. The Department also provides expertise in chronic pain management and has the support of Pain Psychologist and Rehabilitation Specialist.

Stem Cell

The Centre has most accomplished team of stem cell research leaders who experimentally apply new techniques to a wide range of human disorders, including many types of Cancer, Neurological Diseases and Spinal Cord Injuries.

The Centre is providing a comprehensive and coordinated "bench to bedside" approach to cell therapy, including basic and clinical research programs, and the development and administration of new therapies to patients. The Centre is building on existing excellence at the affiliated institutions in Heart Disease, Bone Marrow Transplantation, Vascular Disease, Neuro Degenerative Diseases such as Parkinson's Disease and Spinal Cord Injury.

Social Work

Manipal Hospital Bangalore does yeoman services in providing free and concessional health care to the deserving and needy. Organizations that have benefited by the free and concessional health policy of the hospital include:

- Orphanages
- Institution for physical and other handicaps
- Institutions working with street/working children
- Leprosy rehabilitation clinics
- Homes for children/people affected by HIV
- Shelter for destitute women

Sports and Exercise Medicine

The Department of Sports and Exercise Medicine at Manipal Hospital address the growing societal concerns about fitness, wellness, sport, injury prevention, and rehabilitation. The services provided at the Department are comprehensive and tailored to the individual's needs after careful assessment and evaluation. This is accomplished by providing services in:

- Evaluating specific components of fitness
- Providing advice on training methods
- Prescribing specific exercises
- Identifying factors that might lead to injury
- Planning rehabilitation
- Providing access to advice about diet and psychological aspects of exercise Clinics and Treatment Methods Offered
- Sports Injury Clinic : Acute and Chronic
- Focused Treatment for Focused Individuals
- Musculo-Skeletal Medicine (MSMed)
- Osteopathic Medicine
- Medical Strengthening Therapy
- Medical Acupuncture/Dry Needling
- Mesotherapy
- Treadmill Gait Analvsis

Surgery

General Surgery

A variety of surgical procedures are carried out at the Department by highly experienced and talented specialists. These include operations on Breast, Thyroid, Hernia, Salivary Glands, Gastrointestinal Tract, Liver, Pancreas and Spleen apart from all surgical emergencies and abdominal trauma. The Department has an active academic programme with Post-Graduate training recognized by National Board and Royal College of Surgeons of UK.

The Operation Theatres are well equipped with most modern instruments like Harmonic Scalpel, Laser, etc. Other departments like Anesthesia, Intensive Care Unit, Radiology and Clinical laboratory offer excellent support services.

Minimally Invasive Surgery

Manipal Hospital is the first to introduce Minimally Invasive/ Laparoscopic/Keyhole Surgery in the state. This surgical procedure has revolutionized the surgical management of many diseases with minimal discomfort to the patients and faster recovery. A number of operative procedures are done Laparoscopically which include:

- Cholecystectomy
- Appendicectomy and Hernia Repair
- Splenectomy and Colectomy
- Pancreatic Pseudocyst Drainage
- Surgery for Morbid Obesity
- Hepatobiliray and Pancreatic Disease
- Endocrine and Colorectal Surgery

Telemedicine

The Manipal Hospital Telemedicine Network enables patients in remote locations in the country and abroad to see and interact with the specialists at Manipal Hospital, Bangalore. Using this facility all the patient's medical information including investigations like ECG, X Ray, Cr, MRI, and real time images like Angiogram can be transmitted live, which the specialists at Manipal Hospital can view along with the patient and decide the course of treatment. The facility helps to avoid the patient's inconvenience in coming all the way to Bangalore for getting expert opinion from specialists at Manipal Hospital.

Vascular Sciences

The Department of Vascular Sciences along with Radiology and Cardiology Units offer a wide range of services like Duplex Scan, Angiogram, Angioplasty and Stenting for Carotid and Peripheral Arteries, Venacaval Filter Insertion. It has also introduced Endolaser treatment for

Varicose Veins (ELVeS), a new minimally invasive method with faster recovery. In addition, Sub Facial Endoscopic Perforator Surgery (SEPS) another technical innovation in the management of patients with Venous Ulcers has also been introduced. Recently the Vascular Surgery Department has started Stem Cell Therapy for End Stage Peripheral Vascular Diseases. The commonly performed procedures includes:

- Infra Inguinal Bypass and Aortic Aneurysm Repair
- Carotid Endarterectomy
- Aorta Bifemoral Bypass and Upper Limb Bypass
- AV Malformations
- Vascular access for Haemodialysis
- Venous Procedures like Varicose Vein Surgery, Venous Bypass and Valve Repair for Chronic Venous Insufficiency
- Podiatric foot care for Diabetic patients

Diagnostic Services

The Diagnostic Laboratory in the hospital fulfils a longstanding need for a well equipped laboratory capable of providing a complete range of investigations in the areas of Haematology, Clinical Pathology, Biochemistry, Histopathology, Cytopathology, Microbiology and Immunology. The laboratory is the first hospital-based laboratory in India to get the prestigious accreditation by the NABL. The Department functions 24 hours a day, with emphasis on accuracy, precision, reproducibility and prompt reporting. The Molecular Pathology Unit is equipped with a variety of molecular assays that helps in better, faster and precise diagnosis.

Transfusion Services (Blood Bank)

Manipal Hospital houses one of the largest blood banks in the state and is recognized as the Regional Blood Transfusion Centre. Keeping in tune with the hospital policy of harnessing latest technology, the Blood Bank uses modern equipments and new technologies.

Recent Developments Include:

- The only Blood Bank in South India with ISO Certification
- Nucleic Acid Testing of blood bags for HIV/HBV/HCV for the first time in the country
- Thalassemia Transfusion Centre
- Blood Component Therapy with Automated Component Extractor (T-ACE)
- Apheresis Unit including Stern Cell Unit

Nuclear Medicine

- The Department of Nuclear Medicine performs both diagnostic as well as therapeutic procedures.

- State-of-the-art SPECT CT dual headed GE Infinia Hawkeye Gamma Camera with latest processing software
- Discovery STE 16-Slice Pet-CT Scanner.

Radiology

Manipal Hospital houses one of the latest technology in the Department of Radiology. The Department of Radiology is well equipped for diagnostic work as well as therapeutic procedures. It has a light speed 64 slice high resolution CT Scanner, PET with 16 Slice CT Scanner, 1.5 T twin speed MR scanner with complete cardiac capability, Perfusion Studies, Spectroscopy, and Whole Body MR Angiography, Modern Ultrasound, Colour Doppler, 2D Doppler, Bone Densitometry and Mammography. The Department is in the process of implementing PACS and Digital Radiography.

Manipal Speciality Hospital

363, Halagevaderahalli, Rajarajeshwari Nagar, Bangalore 560098. Phone: + 91 80 2860 8888, 2699 9850 Fax: + 91 80 2699 9870 Email: msh@manipalhospital.org www.manipalhospital.com

Manipal Speciality Hospital in Rajarajeshwarinagar, Bangalore is a recent health care venture by Manipal Health Systems. This 120 bed multi speciality secondary care hospital, further strengthens the availability of quality health care by offering state-of-the-art diagnostics and consultancy services in all major clinical specialities, in an upcoming satellite town, on the outskirts of Bangalore.

The hospital endeavors to provide total health care solutions at an affordable cost to patients across every strata of the society with its eminent doctors, well trained nursing team and para medical support staff.

Manipal Northside Hospital

71, 11th Main, Malleswaram, Opp. Malleswaram Railway Station, Bangalore 560003. Ph: 2346 0468/2346 0469

mnsh.admin@manipalhospital.org www.manipalhospital.com

Manipal North Side Hospital is a friendly neighborhood hospital situated at Malleswaram, Bangalore. This 70 bed facility is renowned for its medical expertise in the areas of General Medicine, Orthopaedics and Gynaecological services. The secondary care hospital supported by a team of dedicated doctors, nurses and well trained support staff extends quality health care at highly affordable costs. Manipal Clinic, located at Jayanagar is a unit of Manipal Health Systems. Its broad range of services include consultations, diagnostic services, preventive health check packages and a 24-hour pharmacy, all under one roof. The multi-speciality clinic endeavors to provide one stop solution to the primary health care needs of the whole family at an affordable cost.

Manipal Clinic JP Nagar

Kothanur Main Road, JP Nagar 7th Phase, Bangalore-78 Phone: 4166 3616

Manipal Clinic, JP Nagar provides specialist consultation with leading doctors and facilitates comprehensive range of diagnostic services. The Clinic houses the latest, world-class medical equipment, thus ensuring correct diagnosis and treatment. Manipal Clinic JP Nagar also facilitates exclusive health packages designed for various age groups. One of the unique features of the Clinic is its "Mobile Blood Test" facility where in blood samples for laboratory investigations is collected right at the door steps. The other one being the 24-hour Pharmacy which stocks a wide range of 100% genuine medicines that also offers free home delivery within a certain radius in the city to increase customer

Index

Deep 8 Deep 27/9/10
5465 5×5